Leadership and Medicine is far more than the title suggests. This book is a compelling mix of wisdom and practical advice from one of medicine's most thoughtful and experienced leaders. Dr. Loop provides insightful analysis of the keys to leadership as he explains how our healthcare organizations actually work. Every aspiring healthcare leader should read—and heed—his words.

— Jack Rowe, M.D.
    Professor, Department of Health Policy and Management, Columbia University Mailman School of Public Health
    Former Chairman and CEO of Aetna, Inc.

Having served as his trustee chairman, I can say without reservation that Dr. Loop is to academic medicine what Abraham Lincoln was to American presidents. He is a great recruiter, a rare visionary, highly respected by his team, yet in Sam Walton's words, a "great servant leader." I once asked him how he so effectively led 1,200 physicians and scientists. He replied, "Mal, sometimes you just drink a little muddy water." Dr. Loop demanded excellence from himself and the enterprise. The results speak for themselves. *Leadership and Medicine* will become the bible for physicians who aspire to positions of leadership in medicine.

— Mal Mixon
 Chairman and Chief Executive Officer, Invacare Corporation
 Chairman of the Board of Trustees, Cleveland Clinic

Leadership and Medicine

by Floyd D. Loop, M.D.

Published by:
Fire Starter Publishing
913 Gulf Breeze Parkway, Suite 6
Gulf Breeze, FL 32561
Phone: 850-934-1099
Fax: 850-934-1384
www.firestarterpublishing.com

ISBN: 978-0-9749986-8-8

Library of Congress Control Number: 2009926378

Printed in the United States of America

To Bernadine

…for what she means to me.

TABLE OF CONTENTS

FOREWORD

Leadership and Medicine takes a thorough, introspective look at one of the world's most renowned academic medical centers, the Cleveland Clinic, through the eyes of former chief executive officer Floyd D. Loop, M.D. The book sheds light on how Dr. Loop led the transformation of this respected but financially struggling monolithic medical enterprise into one of the most successful, comprehensive and integrated health systems in the world.

The book is a virtual road map outlining the journey of Dr. Loop, a distinguished cardiac surgeon who assumed the leadership post at the highly acclaimed medical institution in 1989. After almost 70 years of existence, the Cleveland Clinic was facing daunting problems. But over the span of the next decade, under Dr. Loop's stewardship, the Clinic developed into a large, premier medical delivery system. The unique character and values of the enterprise were never compromised in the process. Devoted to patient care, education and research, the Clinic is now viewed as an industry model of quality, efficiency, growth and innovation.

Dr. Loop is critically honest in assessing and analyzing both his triumphs and travails along the way, allowing the reader to "ride along" with him as he dissects the many challenges and opportunities that he faced during his tenure as chief executive. As he looks ahead to the future of medicine and healthcare in general, his advice and admonitions must not be ignored. He lays out a compelling case for fundamental change and offers a clear and concise blueprint for advancing the development of leading-edge medical care while taming the rapid rise in costs.

The book is a true masterpiece on a subject that is in short supply these days, both in and out of healthcare. *Leadership and Medicine* is written by a real doctor who is intimately familiar with what it takes to be a leader. It is filled with practical, down-to-earth, common-sense gems of wisdom not only from Dr. Loop but from many other great leaders and writers and philosophers he has studied, all showing how to bring out the very best in those who lead others. The result is a veritable treasure trove of wisdom, sagacity and practical knowledge.

In the very first chapter, Dr. Loop shares with us a remark attributed to Abraham Lincoln: "Nearly all men can stand adversity, but if you want to test a man's character, give him power." That statement actually sets the tone for the rest of the book, which I consider one of the best works I have read during my 50 years in healthcare. Once you start reading *Leadership and Medicine*, I guarantee you will have a tough time putting it down.

— Charles Lauer
Former Publisher and Editorial Director of *Modern Healthcare*

INTRODUCTION

I am going to return my borrowed life today with [a] little interest.

— Colonel Masajiro Furimiya
Commander, 29th Infantry, Guadalcanal
Cited in Frank RB. *Guadalcanal.*
The Definitive Account of the Landmark
Battle. Penguin, NY, 1990, p. 366.

Former executives consider writing about their careers as they leave the "great theatre of action." [±] Although one cannot teach experience, 15 years as chief executive of a large academic medical center may provide a perspective about patients and personnel, the business of medicine, changes in healthcare, and the staff model of medicine. Personal history is based on recollections. If you don't write it, you will forget it.

Leadership in healthcare is critical today. First, we are beginning an era of increased consumer knowledge and responsibility for personal health. Second, we are in the business of superior results, which demands leadership for quality assurance, automated business transactions, and translation of science into clinical application. Third, leadership is important to assure that healthcare does not devolve into a commodity that stifles innovation. Healthcare is now subject to the economic risks of commercial business. Yet, we are a unique service industry. Our product is a changed human being.[1]

± George Washington, Address to Congress resigning his commission, 23 December 1783.

This book is not written solely for physician executives in academics. The commentary applies to anyone in a healthcare leadership role. All administrators or physicians who have an interest in executive positions may appreciate a treatise on medical leadership that gives them a new perspective about interaction and values. Leaders as physicians, nurses and medical administrators, individually and collectively, have an extraordinary impact on the mission of their organizations. The provision of value will depend on the caliber of all the staff, their experience and dedication. Staff input, teamwork, and helping people realize their potential are vital for progress. In the 21st century, the great medical organizations will lead an accelerating pace of change. Their aligned interests strengthen the academic mission and result in greater healthcare value for the communities that they serve.

Although not-for-profit, many academic medical centers and community hospitals have become large enterprises. Their fiduciary duty is a dual responsibility that rests ultimately with trusteeship. Hospital trustees generally come from other businesses and at the outset believe that not-for-profit healthcare should be run more "like a real business." New trustees readily see the apparent inefficiencies in healthcare, specifically administrative expense, constant litigation, supply chain wastage, reimbursement complexities, incomplete information, and service complaints, to name a few. Invariably, their opinion early on is that these problems should be managed to the irreducible minimum by no-nonsense leadership and more attention to detail. After a few meetings, the same majority tends to be more tolerant as they learn about excessive regulations and the challenges of running a large service organization with the daily variables of complex patients, physician interactions, inexplicable payment and compliance.

The lessons that I write about are from my own observations without rationalization or a precise formula for medical leadership. Instead, the purpose is to acquaint the interested reader with personal experiences in leading a large healthcare system. The word *leading* must be qualified, because a leader presides over good governance, and if he or she succeeds and grows in the position, wise counsel is sought from an unintimidated executive team and trustees from other professions. In addition to understanding as much as possible about the healthcare field, a successful leader must hold everyone accountable, top to bottom. Advancing the mission, personal accountability and sense of responsibility are incentives, not threats. The convergence of innovation, clinical value, effective communication and follow-up comprise real leadership.

The background material and lessons herein will serve as a foundation for new healthcare leaders and a perspective for those more experienced. These and other reflections are basically common sense that improves with experience. No one in this field can write a "how-to" book because of healthcare trends, market differences, contractual issues, differing hospital sizes, academic responsibilities and scope of practice. If there is one notable axiom, it is that great physicians and great scientists make great academic medical centers. Effective leadership must understand the local and regional market demands, guide the response to changes in science and technology, emphasize the importance of growing the academic enterprise and, above all, figure out how to get everyone to "act as a unit."[±]

It was a privilege to lead the Cleveland Clinic in a time of significant achievement. Our reputation, known around the world, has grown through the actions of each successive administration. Today, the Cleveland Clinic inspires respect and admiration and signifies great advances in science and medicine. It has been a great voyage and before I reach the last harbor, I have organized my thoughts and personal lessons. When one looks back on a career, all the memories of intensity and stress and responsibilities tend to fade, but the memories of successes shared with patients and colleagues remain forever. It has been argued that we all know more than we can express verbally.[2] One of the reasons for writing is to see how much of one's experience can be expressed clearly and for effect.

[±] George Crile. Entry on August 27, 1918. Diary, May to November 1918.

LEADERSHIP

Nearly all men can stand adversity, but if you want to test a man's character, give him power.

— Abraham Lincoln, 1809-1865
Attributed

The word *leader* first appears in English in about 1300 as *ledere,* and it is anciently derived from the words for path, or road, or the course of a ship at sea. Sir Gordon Brunton defined leadership as the intelligent and sensitive use of power.[1] Leaders are able to set compelling goals and get others to share and pursue those goals. The bond between leader and follower is one of trust, flowing in both directions. John Gardner calls it "the capacity to move people to action, to communicate persuasively, to strengthen the confidence of followers."[2] In every organization, good leadership is essential for sustained success. As the Asian proverb reminds us: No leader; no land.

We all have our heroes – business legends, revered presidents, great scientists, influential educators, mentors, and so on. They all have characteristics that command our respect. However, leadership comes with no set formula. Baxter Black, the columnist and veterinarian, observes that, "The world is made up of the tough and the strong, the quick and the fast, the intelligent and the smart. Not to mention the idealistic and the pragmatic, the overconfident and the cautious, the ready and the hesitant, the blinded and the blind, the patsy and the hard-sell, the forgiving and the grudge holders, the bashful and the watchful, and of course the wordy and the taciturn. We are all in there somewhere...."[3]

A whole lot of time is spent distinguishing leadership from management. I have never understood why the line has to be so sharp. Leadership is direct, organizational, and strategic. Therefore, leaders have to understand a wider range of issues compared with managers; however, managers, no matter how big or small their responsibility, must be leaders. One cannot successfully supervise a group of people and be effective without having leadership qualities. Both leaders and managers provide direction, insist on accountability, and oversee an environment that strives for exceptional performance. Managers tend to "adopt impersonal if not passive attitudes towards goals. The goals arrive out of necessities rather than desires. Managers see work as an enabling process. Leaders work to develop fresh approaches and have more active attitudes towards goals." [4] They are more cognizant of risk and reward. They interact face-to-face with executives and key personnel, articulate priorities, influence decisions, oversee implementation, and communicate the reasons for the intended direction. Therefore, leaders must also manage. Leaders are much more visible and have larger responsibilities of direction, team building, assessment, and inspiration. They must react quickly and with confidence to an unexpected crisis. Leaders are held to a higher standard. They are expected to be flexible, but not to vacillate. Specifically, leaders are operating on a longer time horizon while managers are generally focused on delivering commitments already in place. [5]

Power and leadership are not synonymous. Power is the capacity to mobilize resources. Leaders who see their role solely in terms of power are usually ineffective. They waste energy and goodwill telling people how powerful they are and running around… "killing the chickens to scare the monkeys." Power involves the ability, based on the personal qualities of the leader, to elicit the followers' voluntary compliance in a broad range of matters. Leadership achieves its goals through influence. Power simply holds its subjects' preferences in abeyance. [6] When George Shultz testified before a Senate Committee during the Iran-Contra hearings, Senator Inouye, the committee chairman, asked him "…we thank you for being here and sharing your views with us. Do you have any advice for the American public?" Shultz said, "Yes. Just remember one thing, Senator: Don't give power to people who can't live without it." [7]

CHARACTERISTICS OF REAL LEADERSHIP

Leadership did not originate in the military. In fact, it is "management" that is a military term. Some may feel it is inappropriate to draw parallels between the military during war and healthcare where the most inviolate precept is "first, do no harm." But the comparison is not as ironic as it may first appear. The principal function of a strong military is to keep the peace. In healthcare, the best use of medical knowledge is to encourage wellness and prevent disease. When peace fails or disease occurs, competent leadership is critical for success. In both fields, a hierarchy is evident and respected. Few other professions demand so much responsibility and often require life-and-death decisions under intense pressure.

The Cleveland Clinic itself was founded by physicians who worked in military hospitals for the American Expeditionary Force in France in World War I. These physicians, who had already enjoyed successful careers before joining the service, were impressed by the multi-specialty collaboration that they saw in the military hospitals of that time. The Cleveland Clinic founders drew from their army experience to recreate a unique staff model in the civilian setting.

As we read about leadership, we search for unique characteristics and the lessons they impart to us. The armed forces take leadership and management very seriously. Training and staff colleges emphasize leadership fundamentals and management theories and practice. Many officers have carried their military experiences into business careers.

Beginning with the essentials of leadership, one historical leader, not well-known here and not even American, is from a military campaign. A long time ago I read a book by George MacDonald Fraser titled *Quartered Safe Out Here* – a minor classic.[8] The book is a recollection of a period in jungle warfare experienced by a handful of ordinary young soldiers[±] who, together, survived – the ending is poignant and I won't spoil it. In that short tale of World War II combat in central Burma, Fraser wrote that the British troops, of which he was one as a young man, felt secure because of their commander, General W. J. Slim. The thought of him "was like home and safety."[9]

A great deal has been written about General Slim, who intrigued me even more as I read about the India-Burma campaign, "the forgotten war." Most of us who were born during World War II know about General MacArthur, the fall of Singapore, the Pacific island campaigns and naval battles, and the Bataan Death March, but most of us didn't realize the extent of the war along the Indo-Burmese border, which was the longest campaign in World War II.

I became interested in this leader who inspired such confidence.[†] He did not court popularity, hated publicity, but inspired great trust. Who was this man who was considered by Lord Mountbatten "the finest general the Second World War produced"? He was, to begin with, a tactical genius who knew what had to be done in a real soldier's war – and did it.[10] It was said that where defeat was predicted, he triumphed. Against the highest odds, his army recaptured Burma, which, in his

---

±   18-19-year-old Cumbrian men (Northern England near the Scottish border) who were in Section 9, Company B, 9th Battalion, Border Regiment in 17th Indian "Black Cat" Division.

†   "Tell me who your admired leaders are, and you have bared your soul." (Wills G. *Certain Trumpets. The Call of Leaders*. Simon & Schuster, New York, 1994.)

words, "could fairly be described as some of the world's worst country, breeding the world's worst diseases, and having for half the year at least the world's worst climate."± Confronted constantly by anxieties over supply, health, and morale, he realized that morale is a state of mind – an intangible force that will move a whole group of men to give their last ounce... without counting the cost to themselves as long as the men feel they are part of something greater than themselves.[11]

Bill Slim believed that the foundation of morale was *spiritual, intellectual,* and *material,* in that order of importance. It was *spiritual* because only spiritual people can stand real strain in pursuit of a vital, active, and noble objective that gives one a sense of purpose; *intellectual,* because man is swayed by reason and confidence as well as feelings (colleagues want to have confidence in leadership, but they want to see progress); and *material,* because people need the best tools for the job and want nothing more than to be treated fairly in the best possible environment conducive to success. Be critical of ideas, not people.[12] You can't lead unless you love those whom you lead.†

"Experience had taught me," Slim wrote, "that before rushing into action, it is advisable to get quite clearly fixed in mind what the object of it all is."[13] There is nothing worse than the "arrogance of ignorance." Leadership is not solely about endless activity. There are times that thinking is more appropriate than doing. Slim had little patience for excuses. The best excuses are of no use for next time; what is wanted are causes and remedies. Leadership of a successful organization is, for the most part, exhilarating. But leading people is invariably problematic. If you are going to command, you have to shake off all regrets because they claw at will and self-confidence. "Forget them and remember only the *lessons* to be learned from defeat – they are more [instructive] than from victory."

> We have found that tremendously so in the Army, because the world in material and scientific matters has advanced so much. As soon as you get into any position of command, you find yourself surrounded by new and changing factors. What it was right to do yesterday may well be wrong today; some scientific invention, some new process or political change may have come along overnight and you have got to adjust yourself and your organization to it.

±   As Atlee said, "Slim... he may do with the scrapings of the barrel."

†   You must love those you lead before you can be an effective leader. You can certainly command without that sense of commitment, but you cannot lead without it. And without leadership, command is a hollow experience, a vacuum often filled with mistrust and arrogance. (Shinseki EK. Retirement Ceremony Speech. June 11, 2003, from http://www.army.mil/features/ShinsekiFarewell/FarewellArticle.htm)

After all, it is the organism which can adjust itself to changed conditions which survives. This quality of flexibility of mind is increasingly vital. Time and again you will see in leaders a conflict between flexibility of mind and strength of will. I have known fellows who were very good commanders in many ways — I have served with them and under them — who had strength of will but who translated it into refusal to change their minds or to receive suggestions from outside, whether from above or below. I have seen commanders who had such flexibility of mind and strength of will, to watch that your strength of will does not become just obstinacy, that your flexibility of mind does not become vacillation. Every man must work this balance out for himself. One word of warning: if you go about reminding yourself that you are a strong man you'd better take a good look at yourself; there's something wrong.[14]

Leadership is an extremely personal thing, and everybody exercises that a bit differently from everybody else... it is the combination of persuasion, compulsion, and determination. Even in the army, much more is done by persuasion, by gaining the confidence of your soldiers, than by barking harsh orders at them... the purest form of leadership and in many ways the most effective... instead of saying "go on" says "come on" and men will always respond to that much better.[15]

General Slim, later Field Marshal and Viscount Slim, led tactically and philosophically against near-impossible odds. He had the head of a general and the heart of a private soldier. He personally took part in battles; he knew the field; he had clear objectives and attained them; he was a keen observer of human nature and a student of leadership itself; finally, he had that which he called "the quality that makes people trust you." If you are to be a leader... then I think you must have one more quality, and that is not so much of a quality as an element in which all the other qualities work and that I would call integrity.[±]

The men of the Fourteenth Army trusted Slim and thought of him as one of themselves; perhaps his real secret was that the feeling was mutual.

±   President Dwight Eisenhower summed up his thoughts on leadership: "The supreme quality for leadership is unquestionably integrity. Without it, no real success is possible." After integrity, Eisenhower listed these timeless characteristics for successful leadership: 1) single-minded and selfless dedication to the task at hand; 2) courage and conviction; 3) fortitude of spirit, the capacity to stand strong under reverses and to rise from defeat; 4) humility (As one of his commanders used to say, "Always take your job seriously, not yourself."); 5) thorough homework; 6) the power of persuasion. Eisenhower believed that a sense of humility was a quality that he observed in every leader whom he had deeply admired. (Eisenhower DD. *What is Leadership?* Reader's Digest: June 1965: 49-54.)

RELEVANCE TO HEALTHCARE

The above attributes are fundamental to leadership in any profession or business. Each of us will have different experiences, but your integrity, courage, wide-ranging knowledge, and the abilities to concentrate and deliver remain essential to your organization. The basic characteristics of leadership have long stood the test of time and won't change, but your philosophy will evolve from your experiences. If you are beginning a new role, the best advice that I can offer is to stick to the basics of the mission and remember that healthcare is a service organization. Avoid mission creep until you have everything in order and even then be very selective.

The role of a leader begins with team building. There's no point in delegating unless you have a great team around you. When your team is in place, it is easy to share power and credit. Development of a good executive team gives you time to think and reflect about the direction of the organization. Insist on proactive management. Don't get into the thick of every issue; that is why you have an organizational chart. Celebrate the big achievements. Otherwise, not too many victory laps.

In healthcare, the first test of leadership relates to the quality of the medical staff, which is emphasized throughout this book. By medical staff, I mean doctors and nurses of all stripes and personnel who don't directly touch the patient. In a large healthcare organization, the challenge is to recruit outstanding leadership in every specialty and in every area of research and educational endeavor. The word outstanding means scientists and physicians recognized in their field, good clinical doctors who have the ability to perform or oversee clinical research and who can recruit and retain the very best talent around them. An enthusiastic staff is the single greatest factor in patient satisfaction.

In healthcare, leaders generally fall into three categories. The first is the *ossified* leader, who is frozen, indecisive: the sort of person who, if you see him on the stairs, you can't tell if he is going up or down. The second is the *confused* leader, who may have big dreams or good intentions, but doesn't know the field or how to establish market priorities. The confused leader is lost in a big house, and like the ossified leader, is an empty suit. What we're talking about in this book is the third category, *performance leadership* – having a plan, achieving goals, consistently advancing the mission, and delivering increasing value to the patients and the community.

The leader has to be an "effective learner."[16] If the leader is progressive and scientific, so will the staff be progressive and scientific. It is the leader who exemplifies, embodies, and personifies the character of the institution. If the physician leader is a scholar, the staff will follow this example. If he (or she) is merely holding his job to earn a salary, then staff will likely assume the same attitude.

As the healthcare leader, you are in the business of managing people, not inanimate production. Talk straight at all times and be sure that the executives and physician managers do the same. Don't dump critical issues on your key executives. Your interactions should be thoughtful, supportive, and measured at all times. Engaging personnel does not mean taking sides and getting into political disputes. If you make promises, keep them. The best way to avoid breaking promises is to make them only rarely, and then only in alliances or to recruit key staff. The staff expects you as the leader to be presidential.

I learned a lot from people around me, throughout my tenure as chief executive and in a surgical career, from non-profit and corporate boards, the Medicare Payment Commission, and from the literature. Whatever opportunities are present, you have to be an "effective learner." In a world of increasing knowledge, you, as the leader, must know your field, and from that knowledge, set the course, communicate, and make it happen.

Leaders develop their styles as they interact with their constituents. My style was understated, which seemed to work for us but is not necessarily best for every organization. Some leaders need constant attention and adulation, which works only if there is real performance to back it up.

Healthcare is less of a cyclical business today. The hard times that we are experiencing may prevail for a long time, maybe forever. Yet, there are many opportunities. And that's what you are there for – to seize the best opportunities and advance the organization. Throughout this book there are points of view and lessons learned that apply to our environment, and they are not always transferable. The core elements of leadership are transferable, and that's what I am writing about.

PERFORMANCE LEADERSHIP

Although success in a healthcare organization starts at the top, the concept of one leader is flawed. In medical organizations there have to be many leaders. Virtually every institute, department, and section requires authentic leadership. Leadership, especially in medicine, is a function performed by many, not a position held by one. Knowing where the organization is going is the one task the chief executive cannot delegate. Performance is more than trying to compete with everyone in the market. An academic medical center grows through innovation, by acquiring new facilities or building services. And effective competition depends foremost on consistent good service and outcomes. Effective leadership requires a sense of urgency. A lot of ideas coupled with proactive[±] management are the keys to endurance and success.

The responsibility of a leader is to always define reality.[†] The first task for a chief executive is to declare what is core.[17] A leader must enshrine the institutional values; articulate a vision; set the course to that vision; assure performance; empower the people (and get out of their way).[18] As a leader GE's Jack Welch said he had three jobs: 1) selecting the right people;[§] (2) locating the capital resources; 3) spreading ideas quickly (you may find communications easy or difficult; but don't forget, it's not what you say – it's what people hear).[19] In 1943, Eisenhower wrote to his son John, a cadet at West Point, "The only quality that can be developed by studious reflections and practice is deciding what to do, and then getting men to *want* to do it."[20]

It has been said that the rules attributed to Jack Welch are obsolete and that America needs a new play book.[21] Not so fast. The Welch rules may need some tweaking, but they're still sound. Strength and leading market share are always the right goals as long as you achieve results to back them up. Welch's goal was to get his swollen conglomerate lean, agile, and thinking like a small company.[22] Bigger can be better, he said, as long as it runs efficiently. "Admire a little ship, but put your cargo in a big one."[23] The so-called new rules concentrate on agility, innovation, and service. The old and the new rules together are what every organization should strive for.

In addition to knowing the field and setting the course, leadership involves learning from dialogue with other leaders and managers. The best leaders know they have to delegate and are comfortable doing so because they have a good team. Jim Collins calls the best leadership Level V, which is the triumph of humility and fierce resolve, the ability to build enduring greatness through a paradoxical combination of personal humility plus professional will.[24] Powerlessness, in contrast, tends to breed

---

±   Proactive is said to be a "tired" word, overused. In the absence of a good synonym, proactive means get off your position; know what's going on; anticipate change; find opportunities and do something about it; inspire those who report to you and hold them accountable. Proactive carries a sense of urgency, the need to demonstrate progress. Be active, not reactive or inactive.

†   De Pree wrote that the first responsibility is to define reality. The last is to say thank you. In between the two, the leader must become a servant and a debtor. (De Pree M. Leadership is an Art. Chapter 4. Collaborative Leadership. Cited in; Marshall EM: *Transforming the Way We Work: The Power of the Collaborative Workplace.* New York, American Management Association, 1995, p. 68).

§   Eisenhower writing to General Keyes. "Every commander is made, in the long run, by his subordinates" in Atkinson R. *The Day of Battle: The War in Sicily and Italy, 1943-1944.* New York: Henry Holt and Company, 2007, p. 334.

bossiness rather than true leadership. In large organizations, it is powerlessness that often creates ineffective, desultory management and petty, dictatorial, rules-minded managerial styles.[25] The leader should make every effort to tone down the politics – especially the corrosive kind. Conflict within a large institution can't always be prevented. Formal authority does not guarantee influence. Conflict usually occurs, however, at the department level, and it can generally be managed by intercession and communication. If everyone understands the goals and direction, conflict should be infrequent. If conflict is rampant, something is wrong with leadership. Find out the issues and fix the problem right away.

As former Indiana University basketball coach Bob Knight observed, "Popular people don't make particularly good leaders; decisive people with judgment who aren't afraid to tell other people who don't have such good judgment that their judgment isn't very good, make good leaders."[26] And when you have to intervene, that sometimes takes courage. "'Tisn't life that matters," one of Hugh Walpole's characters said, "but the courage yer bring to it."[27] In courage, our assets are discipline and tenacity – in short, ourselves. Try to be better than your previous performance. It's a lot more stimulating and rewarding than competing with colleagues. President Ronald Reagan often said, "Courage is contagious."[28] Keep your fears to yourself, but share your courage with others. Good leadership is a carrier of courage.

All good surgeons know that 99 percent of postoperative morbidity emanates from events in the operating room. Morbidity is infrequent and mortality rare from events outside the operating room, such as errors in management, procedures, or prescriptions. In other words, your strategy and decisions are predictive of the end result. If one can't shoulder the responsibility for patient care, the team, or the performance of the healthcare system, don't lead; follow instead. The insecure always blame others. Japanese managers have a saying, "When you point a finger at someone, always remember that three fingers are pointing back at you."[29] Criticism is part of human nature, and some revel in others' misfortune, either for personal career gain or jealousy.

Some leaders expect undying loyalty. Instead, emphasize loyalty to the institution and its mission. If you are constantly worried about praise and devotion, you are in the wrong job. There is an old saying that if you want loyalty, buy a dog. Frankly, I say *Pro me; si merear, in me*: Employ this sword for me, but if I deserve it, turn it against me.[30] In other words, as we succeed, thank you for your support; no strategic success, no support.

Leaders are better able to shape people's perceptions of their interest and alternatives when they are respected, considered trustworthy, and perceived to possess the experience to make good judgments. They are also more persuasive when their approval is highly valued. Leaders who demand and reward excellence and who spotlight and condemn inadequate performance are likely to find their approval a rare and sought-after commodity. A leader who takes this too far might earn a reputation for never being satisfied, but a reputation for not being fair or strong enough is probably more damaging. Make your approval as sought-after and valued as gold. Dispense it rarely, but fairly. A reputation for being hard to satisfy is better than a reputation for being indecisive and insincere.

Adair[31] offers a short course on leadership starting with the six most important words: I'll admit I made a mistake. Next, the five most important words: I am proud of you. The four most important words: What is your opinion? The three most important words: If you please. The two most important words: Thank you. The one most important word: We – and the least most important word: I. An added admonition: You should not miss an opportunity to keep your mouth shut.

VISION

Leadership in medicine today has greatly changed from earlier times, especially so in the past 10 years. Responsibilities have multiplied. Charisma alone will not do it. The leader is accountable to everyone across the organization and scrutinized closely by trustees and staff. As a new leader, it's good to challenge the conventional wisdom, but it's also good to define the issues before you do so. Learn the history of your organization. Talk about it. The penalty for historic illiteracy is the repetition of old mistakes. Beyond that, the history of an organization usually contains the seeds of its vision – that mystical blending of inspiration, imagination, and initiative that can energize and direct personal and organizational development.[32]± Vision is knowing and articulating your future priorities. The problem with "vision" is that you have to follow where you want to go.

Every medical organization, profit or not-for-profit, large or small, is in effect a fate-sharing vessel. If there's no sense of teamwork, ownership, commitment, or ethos, it's very difficult to act on a vision. Fuzzy goals are unattainable. Some people laugh at the idea of vision. Years ago, two New York hospitals found their vision of a merger opposed by the faculty in both organizations. The newspapers quoted a dissatisfied psychiatrist who said, "In my line of work, only *schizophrenics* have a vision, and we give them medication."[33] Well, maybe, under those circumstances, the vision was cloudy, but whatever you think of vision, you need to know your

---

± Father Theodore Hesburgh, former president of the University of Notre Dame, said, "The very essence of leadership is [that] you have to have a vision. It's got to be a vision you articulate clearly and forcefully on every occasion. You can't blow an uncertain trumpet." (Bowen E. *His Trumpet Was Never Uncertain.* Time, May 18, 1987.)

priorities, and where you're headed personally and professionally, and to go there hand-in-hand with the institution where you practice. The effective leader knows the field, provides direction, protects the guiding principles, and articulates a vision that is based on integrity and trust.

Leadership is far more than solving problems; it requires finding and acting on great opportunities. There's an Arab proverb that says four things "come not back": the spoken word, the sped arrow, the past life, and the neglected opportunity. My family and I once went to a furniture store to buy a new sofa. My son Frederick accompanied us. The owner, John Sedlak, took a shine to Fred and while we were looking through the store he asked Fred to come to his office. John asked my son if he had a table next to his bed. The answer, "Yes." What's on it? "A telephone." What else? Frederick said, "A clock." John said, "What kind?" Frederick said, "An alarm clock." John Sedlak said, "No, not alarm… it's *opportunity*." Opportunities are everywhere if you know the market and the profession and are actively innovating and constantly looking for the edge. One of the most important lessons in leadership is that results are obtained by exploiting opportunities.

Seizing the opportunities prevents stagnation. If you can't demonstrate real progress, the organization will slip. If the healthcare enterprise is big enough, it will take a lot of unwinding before it unravels; but hospitals without demonstrable and favorable changes in the delivery system, in recruitment, informatics, service, patient communication, and continuous innovation will, I assure you, eventually unravel. Medicine tends to be a cyclical business, some of which is driven by reimbursement and complicated regulations. Sustained progress overcomes the cyclical problems in healthcare management. Left unattended, the dynamic of change is decline.[34]

Vision is formed from many sources. In my experience, many ideas culminate in a unified vision. Also, reading diverse literature gives one a broad perspective and encourages lateral thinking.[±] De Bono coined the term to mean "idea creativity." Reading health policy, management, or medical journals doesn't tell you exactly what to do, but it stimulates thoughts on many other subjects. As Harvey Firestone observed, "I noticed that when all a man's information is confined to the field in which he is working, the work is never as good as it ought to be. A man has to get perspective, and he can get it from books or from people – preferably from both."[35]

Forty years ago, Michael DeBakey gave me some advice I've always followed. He advised me to do my work *before* I went to work. Many years later, during the

---

[±]   Lateral thinking is an operational skill for developing new ideas… based on an understanding of how the brain works as a self-organizing information system. The mind makes asymmetric patterns, and lateral thinking is a way of cutting across patterns laterally, rather than moving along them sequentially. (Watt S. *Questions for Edward de Bono*. Rotman Magazine, Winter 2008, pp. 70-72.)

succession process at our institution, our trustees asked me to describe my schedule as chief executive. They were amazed to hear how much "homework" could be done in the morning – hours of reading before the daily schedule. Steven J. Ross, former chief executive of Time Warner, recalled his father's advice, "There are those who work all day; those who dream all day and those who spend an hour dreaming before setting to work to fulfill those dreams. Go in to the third category because there is virtually no competition."[36] This exercise will stimulate your vision. There are no exceptions – you have to know the field, and without intense devotion to scholarship, a great deal of potential learning is lost. Intuition is based on knowledge. Serendipity is the effect of a chance occurrence on a prepared mind.

PERSONAL GROWTH

"Every leader, early on, is disobedient."[±] Probably so, but real leaders grow wiser as they mature. The wise temper their aggression and become assertive in a thoughtful way. Eisenhower wrote in Omar Bradley's yearbook at West Point: "True merit is like a river. The deeper it is, the less noise it makes."[37] Showing your power through confrontation is rarely necessary and doesn't give you, the chief executive, more stature or even contribute to personal growth. If a good member of the staff argues forcefully, first try to see their side of the story because more often than not, unless they are chronically unmanageable, they may have a good idea. At least they are thinking. Whatever the situation, avoid public quarrels.[†] And be sure that it's over a big issue vetted in a calm environment. Henry Kissinger quotes a Chinese proverb, "When there is turmoil under the heavens, little problems are dealt with as if they were big problems, and big problems are not dealt with at all. When there is order under the heavens, big problems are reduced to small problems and small problems will not obsess us."[38]

A person who is elected or appointed to a position of title and responsibility either grows or swells. Tom Coughlin, a former Wal-Mart executive, used to say, "Don't think you are such hot stuff; a lot happened before you got here."[39] To put it another way, there are two types of people in this world: those who want to be somebody and those who want to do something.[40][§] Ambition is something more than looking at the point you want to reach. Ambition is taking off your coat and pulling and dragging your boat up the stream.[41] To grow, you need to learn the business, anticipate change,

---

±   Asian proverb, anonymous.

†   "Beware of entrance to a quarrel; but, being in, bear't, that the opposed may beware of thee." (Shakespeare W. *Hamlet*, Act I, Scene 3).

§   Told to Jean Monnet by Dwight Morrow, who was Coolidge's ambassador to Mexico and father of Anne Morrow, who married Charles Lindbergh.

expand relationships, enact a good strategy, and develop talent. Swelling is acting mainly on ceremony. If you're going to be arrogant and self-aggrandizing, you'd better be real smart and never make any mistakes. Remember, Narcissus[±] was not in love with himself; he was in love with his reflection. The world of business today doesn't tolerate a ceremonial administration for long. Today we are in the business of results.

Personal growth involves resolve. You know what persistence is: Persistence is the hard work you do after you get tired of doing the hard work you already did. And persistence is genius in disguise as exemplified in this anecdote from the historian Stephen Ambrose. He tells about trying to find a subject for a graduate thesis. Finally he came upon an obscure historical figure, about whom little had been written. His research was tiring, but his work eventually resulted in his first book.

> I sent my MA thesis to LSU Press in Baton Rouge; they sent the script around for expert readers' opinion; it passed, and in 1962 my first real book, not an edited collection, appeared as *Halleck: Lincoln's Chief of Staff.* It got some fair reviews with some faint praise and a bit of criticism. It won no prizes and had a limited, at best, readership. But one of the readers made up for the absence of prizes or a front-page or any page in the *New York Times Book Review.* Two years after publication, [Dwight D. Eisenhower] called me to Gettysburg to ask me to work on his papers, to be published by Johns Hopkins University… I went to meet him and we talked for a few days about what would be involved in editing his papers. At one point, General Eisenhower said, "Son, you must have a lot of questions."
>
> "Yes, Sir, I sure do," I replied. "But first of all, why me?" I was then 28 years old.
>
> He replied, "*I read your book on Halleck.*"[42]

± Narcissism is "a pervasive pattern of grandiosity (in fantasy or behavior), need for admiration and lack of empathy…" The condition is said to exist in a person when five (or more) of the following nine criteria (stated in abridged from) are evident: 1) grandiose sense of self-importance; 2) preoccupation with fantasies of unlimited success, power, brilliance, beauty, or ideal love; 3) billed as being "special" and unique; 4) request for excessive admiration; 5) sense of entitlement to especially favorable treatment; 6) exploitation of others; 7) lack of empathy; 8) belief that others are envious of them; 9) arrogant and haughty behavior and attitude. (Amernic JH, Craig RJ. *Guidelines for CEO-speak: Editing the Language of Corporate Leadership.* Strategy & Leadership 2007: 35 (3); 25-31)

Academic medical activities operate in an increasingly complex and changing environment. Money is tight; the intensity of care increases; the cost structure is difficult to maintain and managing disparate personnel is much like coaching a professional sports team. Continuous personal improvement is the essence of professional growth. What is the prescription for personal growth? The answer to these and many other leadership questions comes with experience. Growth around you is all about acquiring the experience to lead and manage better each year. Ask yourself, are you better after each measurement period? Is the team better coordinated – do you receive knowledgeable input, on-time goals, great ideas, good dialogue, and create mutual respect?

If trends are not favorable, do you take the lead in finding causes and remedies? Are you consistent in your approach to management? Does your staff know what to expect each day? Is the organization tuned for efficiency and exploitation of opportunities? If results are trending favorably, the leader has to stay ahead of the curve in knowledge about the industry, the market, and healthcare innovation. The willingness to learn, to be involved, and to accept risk are the responsibilities of leadership and the price of success. A prominent cardiothoracic surgeon reminded me, "It is not bad to be ignorant, although you may be wrong, but it is disastrous when you know a lot but cannot be taught."[43]

Personal growth also comes from an open environment conducive to challenging ideas. Stories and analogies are useful to emphasize a point as long as you are not wasting too much time. One observer told me that our administrative meetings reminded her of the Knesset – in our case, it seemed to be effective because a lot of good ideas came out and we made progress. Jamie Dimon, who heads JPMorgan Chase, also emphasizes an open environment. "If you sat through one of my management meetings, you wouldn't know who was the boss."[44] In building a team, the leaders must actively resist the tendency to attract and promote like personalities and skills.[45] Find independent thinkers who understand the collective goals and are secure in their profession. Above all, you don't want to be like Samuel Goldwyn, who reportedly said, "I want everybody to tell me the truth – even though it costs him his job."

MENTORING

Mentoring is at the heart of medicine. "When you become a leader, success is all about growing others."[46] Acquiring, developing, and retaining talent is part of leadership. Mentoring builds experience on both the giving and receiving ends, but it takes maturity, self-confidence, and a willingness to commit time and energy beyond that required for teaching.[47] A good mentor needs to be knowledgeable and collegial and have the common sense, competence, good judgment, and a strong enough ego to be able to share credit.[48] You can't teach courage or experience, but you can emphasize the importance of sticking to your principles and being more than "steady under light fire."[49]

Mentoring is crucial for the development of the highest personal standards and ethics. A mentor is someone who may be a teacher and advisor and even a loyal friend and confidant. A real mentor derives satisfaction from the responsibility of mentoring. The most effective mentors share their knowledge and experience, offer new ideas and perspectives, are patient and enthusiastic, and teach values and ethics.[50] Salacuse lists the seven principles that govern all advising: 1) know the person who will use the advice; 2) help or at least do no harm – recognize that advice matters and can have serious consequences; 3) understand your role beforehand; 4) develop a partnership between advisor and client (the word client comes from the Latin *cliens*, a person who has someone to lean on); 5) tailor advice to life, needs, and objectives; 6) keep advice pure of self-interest, prejudices, biases, and personal shortcomings; and, 7) know when to stop.[51]

To be a real mentor is part of being an educator. Early on the young doctor learns to be a good or great physician more so from a wise mentor than from books or journals. When I contemplated a thoracic surgery career, I went to see one of my mentors, Brian Blades, professor of surgery at George Washington University. I had plans of my own about where to go and what to do, and he listened patiently. Then he pointed out another option. He told me that a whole new era of surgical endeavor was beginning, one that related to coronary arteries. He suggested that I go to the Cleveland Clinic to train and then return to the university. To this day, I do not know how he could have anticipated direct coronary artery surgery, because there was only one surgical method of revascularizing the heart at that time (the Vineberg implant), and it was not consistently effective. But, I followed his advice and, looking back, I can see that it was probably the defining moment of my life. Brian Blades' advice to me was mentoring at its best: sharing wisdom and showing personal regard for a young pupil. I am not the only one to have benefited from his wisdom and foresight over the years. As a leader, you have an unusual opportunity to communicate with young people, to help define their careers, and to "bring those who sat in darkness to see a great light."[52]

When Dr. William J. Mayo, on the occasion of his 70th birthday, was feted by associates of the American College of Surgeons, he talked about mentoring: "As I have watched older men come down the ladder, as down they must come, with younger men passing them, as they must pass to go up, it so often has been an unhappy time for both. The older man is not always able to see the necessity or perhaps the justice of his descent and resents his slipping from the position he had held, instead of gently and peacefully helping this passing by assisting the younger man. What pleasure and comfort I have had from my hours with younger men! They still have their imagination, their vision, and the future is bright before them. Each day, as I go through the hospitals surrounded by younger men, they give me of their dreams and I give them of my experience, and I get the better of the exchange."[53]

We can't teach experience, but we can teach perseverance and the importance of scholarship, ingenuity, and enterprise. We *can* teach resolve and conviction. And even if it can't be taught, a mentor must emphasize the importance of character. *The only thing in the world not for sale is character.*[54]

> A story about character was told to a doctor friend of mine, John Costin, who listened to an elderly patient reminiscing about his brother Jack who had recently died. There were a number of strong memories about Jack from WW II. The brothers were on Guadalcanal. The patient, recalling the story, had been assigned to Air Force support. On Thanksgiving Day, the air group was treated to a large turkey dinner. The brother asked his commanding officer if he could take some of the Thanksgiving meal to his brother Jack who was in the field. He loaded up a jeep, drove into the jungle and found his brother, who was sitting in front of a muddy pup tent, boiling water in his helmet to make coffee. After a heartfelt greeting one brother told the other that he had brought him a Thanksgiving dinner of turkey, mashed potatoes, gravy and pumpkin pie. His brother's face lit up and then he asked, "Did you bring enough for the other men in my squad?" The first brother indicated that he did not because he wasn't given permission to do so. The marine brother said, "Bill, thanks for thinking of me, but you better take it back." The message was clear; if he didn't have enough to share with the other marines in his squad, he wasn't going to have any Thanksgiving celebration. This left a very strong impression on the brother who, 60 years later, could not forget this act of selfless leadership.[55]

General Schwarzkopf said that "leadership is a potent combination of strategy and character. But if you must be without one, be without the strategy."[56]

DECISIONS

Leadership is largely about decisions that first require discussion with a great team. The chief executive should facilitate the discussion and help it to reach a timely conclusion. There is nothing more boring than waiting for orders from the top.[57] Many rely on intuition or "gut feel" to make a decision. But intuition can't gather information by way of evidence, and may be influenced by fatigue, boredom, and distractions. The only advantage is: It's fast. It takes less time.[58]

Some leaders believe that all decisions must be grand in scope. The facts are that most decision making involves small details that add up to a larger goal. Nicolas Sarkozy, the French President, said, "I have always favored modest effectiveness over sterile grandiloquence."[59] The decision makers, the principal executives, physician leadership, and managers, must thoroughly understand the issue and the options. A leader who is risk-averse sows inertia that can be hard to eradicate. I used to keep a file labeled "great ideas." Looking back, I can see that most of them came from team discussions. We used to teach "*no one is as smart as everyone.*" Ideas are part of the return on management, but then comes the hard part – implementation. Well done is always better than well said.

Decisions and their implementation don't travel in a straight line. Execution often calls for tacking maneuvers, and your list of options should include a return to port to await more favorable winds. Mistakes are inevitable; analyze them, don't forget, and move on. A smart organization makes relatively few errors in its decisions, but when they happen – learn from them. Discipline is the art of ignoring distractions from the business at hand.

Historically, victors don't learn nearly as much or as well as those who have lost. Mistakes are lessons, and an analysis of errors is more important than any victory laps. Figuring out what went wrong – really understanding it – is part of gaining experience. Learn from coaches – study the films, analyze what went wrong, understand your mistakes, and sharpen your judgment before the next game. Every leader would do well to memorize John Gardner's definition of judgment as the ability to combine hard data, questionable data, and intuitive guesses to arrive at a conclusion that events prove to be correct. Most important, perhaps, it includes the capacity to appraise the potentialities of coworkers and opponents.[60] Are judgment and experience the same thing? Not necessarily. Experience is an accumulation of lessons learned, good and bad. Judgment may be formed by experience, but it is acquired more quickly. In my experience, people generally have consistently good judgment or consistently bad judgment – rarely a mix.

A flawed and floundering leader who makes poor decisions gives off distinct distress signals. Leaders who are inflexible, overconfident, intolerant of dissent, focused on image, and married to their past successes have difficulty making the course changes necessary for progress. By these signs, you will know the end is near: Trustees and loyalists will protect and coach; critics will magnify the leader's deficiencies, hoping to provoke a quick resignation; the leader him or herself will hide and wait for others to act. Finally, talented staff will leave – a really bad sign.[61]

Author Sydney Finkelstein has analyzed executive decision failures and takes a contrarian view of most explanations. He dismisses what he calls the "usual theories" that the executives were stupid, didn't know what was coming, didn't execute, weren't trying hard enough, lacked leadership ability, were starved of resources, or were simply a bunch of crooks. Instead, he attributes failure to: 1) flawed executive mind-sets that throw off a company's perception of reality; 2) delusional attitudes that keep this inaccurate reality in place; 3) breakdowns in communications developed to handle potentially urgent information; 4) leadership qualities that prevent executives from correcting their course.[62]

The majority of problems that arise in any business, including healthcare, are much deeper than just bad decisions. They relate to teamwork and trust, just as they do in the physician-patient relationship. As a leader, you must remember that "a leader doesn't build a business – a leader builds an *organization* that builds a business."[63] In healthcare, we are part of a process, a community, a movement, and a historical continuum that exists by the mutuality and trust of all involved. Without trust, a leader cannot practice or lead in medicine. With trust, you can energize staff and employees to reach heights they may never have imagined possible. You might not be able to always inspire the team, but you can stretch their performance. Measure your success the way Hall of Fame basketball player Bill Russell did: "I'll judge the game on how I made my teammates good enough to win."[64]

CHAPTER 2

THE PHYSICIAN CHIEF EXECUTIVE

Henry in disguise speaks with soldiers before the Battle at Agincourt:

For, though I speak it to you, I think the king is but the man, as I am; the violet smells to him as it doth to me; the element shows to him as it doth to me; all his senses have but human condition; his ceremonies laid by, in his nakedness he appears but a man; and though his affections are higher mounted than ours, yet, when they stoop, they stoop with the like wing. Therefore when he sees reason of fears, as we do, his fears, out of doubt, be of the same relish as ours are; yet in reason, no man should possess him with any appearance of fear, lest he, by showing it, should dishearten his army.

— William Shakespeare
King Henry V
Act IV, Scene 1

The great majority of hospitals are ably run by laity, not physician executives. Notable exceptions are the larger teaching hospitals that are often led by a physician or scientist. The single greatest lesson I have learned throughout my career is that larger medical centers should be led by physicians. The rationale is that a physician may better understand the challenges of academic medicine and the needs of the patient. In theory, colleagues want to believe that the physician chief executive may interpret their interests and fairly integrate the three pursuits of academic healthcare: patient care, teaching, and research. It is easier for a physician to learn the fundamentals of business than for a businessman to learn medicine.[±] Leadership draws on the same qualities whether it is directing an academic medical center or heading a department or a group of physicians or even running a commercial business: knowledge, good decisions, and vision based on integrity and trust... and in our case upholding the academic principle.[1]

In succession planning and during an active search for a new chief executive, one of the first questions is whether the academic organization should have a physician in the leadership role. Can a doctor of medicine truly communicate more effectively about academic principles, quality and innovation, as well as drive financial performance for reinvestment in science, education and clinical medicine? The answer, of course, depends on the candidate. Physicians could be ideal leaders if they 1) have demonstrated recognized leadership in medicine or research; 2) have achieved success clinically and academically; 3) understand medical operations and basic finance; 4) possess a high level of organization; and 5) are prepared to master the changing elements in healthcare management. While not a prerequisite, a master's degree in business is increasingly preparatory for the leadership of a medical center.

SELECTION OF THE MEDICAL CHIEF EXECUTIVE

Whoever is chosen should have the characteristics of personal (mental) security, credibility, fairness, good judgment and a reputation for accomplishment. It is very hard for any committee to hold a candidate "up to the light" and see what's really inside. Selecting a leader is a singular event in history that will determine the intermediate-term fate of the organization. The ideal source of candidates is generally inside a large organization. Start this process *before* the current CEO's expected departure.

The search committee should review the leading candidates carefully to assure no evidence of dissemblance. The candidates must understand the reality of the chief executive position. This is not a ceremonial role. Academic medicine is far more than

---

[±] "Physician leadership does not necessarily mean physician management of everything, but physician leadership is an essential element in the direction of everything... that makes the physician accountable for what happens throughout the institution. If the institution fails, the physicians have only themselves to blame." (Herrell, JH. *The Physician-Administrator Partnership at Mayo Clinic.* Mayo Clinic Proceedings, January 2001, p. 108.)

a coalition of group practices. It is truly a scientific cooperative for the welfare of the sick, which integrates medical education and all forms of research into the practice of medicine. There are no hard and fast psychological traits to look for except honesty. Their past must not be checkered in regard to trust. An organized mind is essential – inherent credibility is not worth anything if you forget your priorities. Ask the candidates about their plans, management styles, and perceived challenges. Look for individuals who *listen* rather than those who reply before others have even finished talking. Get a sense of their ethics, their stability (evidenced by family and other non-work activities), and their tolerance for pressure.[2]

Look for the qualities that, as Bertrand Russell says, "confer authority, self-confidence, quick decision making and skill in deciding upon the right measures."[3] As physician chief executive, he or she will be company president, coach, executive recruiter, and in charge not only of strategy, but follow-through and measurement. Nobody controls an academic enterprise or even manages it. However, from time to time, the chief executive must direct and influence it. When the game is over, they can't complain that the offensive line didn't protect him. Responsibility for success or failure, deserved or undeserved, will come to rest in his office. They must recognize that much of top management in medicine is on the shop floor,[4] the nurses and support personnel, the physicians and the scientists, and the dedicated educators. Those are the skilled professionals who advance a great medical center. In summary, the best candidate has to "shine in every direction."[5]

Search committees should be ready with a core set of questions. Do you believe that you can advance this organization? If so, how? Do you have a history of plans and implementation? Do you have the necessary capacity for organization? Are learning and scholarship part of your makeup? Do you have the skills to build consensus? Are you tough enough to withstand challenges? Are you worried about a career risk? Can you get things done, make it happen? Give us your priorities – what is your agenda, early on? In summary, does the candidate have the abilities, intellect and conviction to lead a large academic enterprise? Courage is fundamental: courage of convictions and courage to implement convictions. As Teddy Roosevelt said after nearly eight years as president, "While President, I have been President—*emphatically*."[6]

Can the appointed physician executive communicate the principles of the organization better than a lay administrator? That's what the organization is banking on. The physician, having been in practice or functioning as a physician scientist, should understand compassionate care and the foibles and frustrations involved in medical practice, scientific investigation and medical education. This is a people-intensive enterprise. The first order of importance is always the patient, followed by the welfare of the institution and, finally, the personnel, including the medical staff. In other words, it's not about you, the individual; it's about working together to make the environment successful. Value to the patient and personal success for all the staff depend on "acting as a unit."[±]

CHARACTERISTICS OF THE HEALTHCARE CHIEF EXECUTIVE

In no particular order, I offer twelve qualities that ideally enable a physician to lead and manage a large medical center:

1) A past record of outstanding leadership with proven success – i.e., the ability to take charge, execute, motivate, and hold everyone accountable, including himself.[†]
2) Ability to articulate and implement a clear vision. A leading-edge thinker who provides ideas and serves as a catalyst for moving the organization forward.
3) The capacity to absorb and integrate information from many sources.
4) Evidence of intellectual depth, intuition and decisiveness.
5) Confidence as chief strategist who enjoys developing plans, methods and resources for achieving goals and objectives.
6) Fundamental knowledge of business principles.
7) Willingness to challenge the status quo.[§]
8) Courage to take measured risks. The new chief executive's job is not just to solve problems – look for potential and implement it.
9) Devotion to academic superiority and the need for clinical excellence.
10) Ability to write, speak and communicate… possesses excellent interpersonal

---

[±] When Marshall selected Eisenhower… he did so on the basis of qualities that had little or nothing to do with leading men in battle. Eisenhower's orderly mind, his intelligence, his experience in administration, his ability to get along with others, and his penchant for making others get along with each other – these were some of the traits that impressed Marshall. The Chief knew that if unity of command were to work in an Allied theater, the commander-in-chief had to be a man who could force a mixed staff to work together. (Ambrose SE. *The Supreme Commander. The War Years of Dwight D. Eisenhower.* Jackson, MS: University Press of Mississippi, 1999.)

[†] Mandela's eight lessons of leadership were revisited on the occasion of his 90th birthday: 1) courage is not the absence of fear – it's inspiring others to move beyond it; 2) lead from the front but don't leave your base behind; 3) lead from the back and let others believe they are in front; 4) know your enemy – and learn about his favorite sport (Mandela learned Afrikaans and learned about the Afrikaners' sport of rugby); 5) keep your friends close – and your rivals even closer; 6) appearances matter – and remember to smile; 7) nothing is black or white; 8) quitting is leading too (face reality). (Stengel R. *Mandela: His Eight Lessons of Leadership.* Time, July 2008)

[§] "It is not within the power of the properly constructed human mind to be satisfied. Progress would cease if this were the case. The greatest joy in life is to accomplish. It is the guessing, not the having. It is the giving, not the keeping." (Frederick Banting, discoverer of insulin)

skills, exhibiting tact and diplomacy. The objective here is to persuade people to work together, to show them the advantages of doing so, and to show them that beyond differences of opinion, they have a common interest.

11) Constancy of purpose and great persistence... demonstrates executive presence in guiding the organization toward fulfillment of its mission.

12) A proven record of good recruitment.

The search group and the candidates should understand that the chief executive has to create a winning strategy, recruit the best talent, execute alliances, raise capital, interact appropriately during bond rating and contracting, keep multiple projects in play and bring them to successful closure, and advance the academic mission. Trust and absolute integrity in all matters are the indispensable characteristics.[±]

INFLUENCE

Now you are in a real leadership position. You are the chief executive. You have influence and responsibility. You are ready for the job. However, you have not yet cast a shadow. Just remember the observation by Sarkozy: "Look. I have everything to be happy. I dreamed of having a political party. I have one. I wanted top ministerial posts. I've had them. I've dreamed of being where I am now. I'm here. But I am not excited. It's hard. I'm already president. I'm no longer in the *before*."[7][†]

When I began my career as a physician chief executive, the key issues that were facing American medicine included a growing sensitivity to cost, erosion of professional autonomy, and unresolved access problems. Added to this were the destabilizing effects of cost shifting, the entry of for-profit hospital systems into local markets, rapid technological and scientific advances, and the growth of uncompensated care. Staff felt insecure. Rumor and speculation were rife. Under these conditions, a new physician chief executive should host a question and answer session in selected departments, periodically. Looking back it might have been better

---

[±]   Whoever is careless with the truth in small matters cannot be trusted with the important matters. (Albert Einstein)

[†]   If you have a desire to officiate, know what the office holds. Opportunities are in abundance for the man who volunteers to give of himself, but nothing calls for greater care in choice. Some offices demand courage, and others shrewdness. It is easy to manage in those establishments which call merely for honesty, but most difficult in those which call for skill. It is a wearying business to govern men, who often include the neurotic and fool; and double brains are needed to deal with those who have none. (Fuller, T. *Leading and Leadership*. Notre Dame, IN: University of Notre Dame Press. 2000 p. 55)

to call it a worry session or rumor day. I'd listen to audience concerns, quash or confirm rumors, and comment until all questions were answered. As a new leader, one of the first things I noticed is that pessimism seems to carry a certain prestige. It is somehow regarded as being more scholarly than optimism.[8] In the interchange, it's okay to say "I don't know." Straight talk eventually leads to mutual respect.

Blogging is part of the "groundswell" of interconnectivity. However, a blog is only a small part of management. If leaders or managers rely on e-mail as a primary management tool, they will be ineffective. Incessant e-mails will overwhelm your constituents to the point of numbness. In healthcare, physicians and scientists are absorbed in their work and not terribly interested in administrative details. As Gardner notes humorously, "Apathy is rampant, but who cares!"[9] It is best to get off your position and talk face-to-face whenever issues are important. Bennis and Nanus write that a major task of leadership is the management of attention.[10] E-mails are often written from emotion or to fortify a position rather than directive. A memorandum is written not to inform the reader but to protect the writer.[11] John Adair, who has studied and written extensively about leadership, describes what is called "walking around" management: The president of Toyota, who, when asked why he spent so much time out of the office, replied, "It's very simple. We do not make Toyota cars in my office."[12]

As you make your rounds, gauge the attitude of staff (all personnel) throughout the ranks. Morale is a critical sign and symptom of institutional health. If morale is down, the message should be: When we are really successful, morale will improve. Psychiatrist W. Walter Menninger[13] has listed the signs of low institutional morale:

- increased absenteeism
- diminished time on the job
- reduced production
- increased staff turnover
- an increase in the frequency of mistakes and poor quality
- an increase in accidents
- a decrease in maintaining and repairing equipment
- a tendency for employee communications to become more constricted particularly with reduced communication to supervisors
- an increase in scapegoating

Contention among the staff does not necessarily mean low morale, and high morale does not necessarily mean that people get along together. As Drucker put it, the test is performance, not conformance.[14] When you want to persuade people about a course of action, give them a clear overview of the issues, a list of options with assumptions and, if possible, a list of unintended consequences. As Benjamin Franklin said, "Would you persuade, speak of Interest, not of Reason."[15]

Influence means that you, the leader, are responsible for development of your key executives, the physician leaders, and especially *yourself.*

RECRUITMENT

A medical institution is first and foremost its talent base. Recruitment is one important area where physician chief executives must excel. Great physician leaders in clinical medicine and science are able to recruit on the basis of the academic environment, a large and varied clinical practice, respected colleagues, and the reputation of the academic medical center. Occasionally, department heads or search committees need help in finalizing a search for new staff. The physician chief executive must tell the story of the organization and show the candidate why this great medical enterprise would be his or her best career choice.

The physician chief executive depends first on outstanding department heads for clinical performance and for recruitment. The chief executive may be called on to "close the deal." We had excellent department leadership and our successful healthcare organization was a magnet for clinicians and scientists. Reputation, department leadership, organizational success and relative autonomy in clinical practice and scientific investigation are elements that attract new staff. Recruitment, however, is an art.[±]

If you are intent on attracting a particular talented individual, go the extra mile. Jack Shewmaker, a multi-talented former Wal-Mart executive, tells a story about his first encounter with Sam Walton. As a young man, Shewmaker had quit his job and was in the process of interviewing with several large retailers around the country, including Wal-Mart, which at that time had only a few stores in Arkansas. Because Sam Walton wasn't there at the time, Shewmaker saw only some of the managers. After the interview, he thought that he might have a better offer elsewhere so he drove back to a relative's home in Missouri. That night, Sam Walton called Shewmaker to tell him that the interviewers were impressed and that he would like him to come back for more discussion. Jack Shewmaker replied that a trip back took too long and he really didn't see any point because he was going to look elsewhere. Sam Walton said, "*I'll meet you halfway.*"

±   Warren Buffett wrote, "In looking for people to hire, you look for three qualities: integrity, intelligence and energy. And if they don't have the first, the other two will kill you." (Reynolds S. *Thoughts of Chairman Buffett: Thirty Years of Unconventional Wisdom From the Sage of Omaha.* New York, NY: HarperCollins Publications 1998).

The first task in recruitment is to showcase an environment where medical and scientific candidates believe they can achieve success. There's no point in parading a candidate through a disgruntled department. That is a prescription for unsuccessful recruitment. The interview process does not need a fixed protocol. It depends on the candidate. High-profile recruits may need to see the chief executive first. Many times I have walked leading clinicians or scientists around the campus talking about the history or department excellence and how the organization is governed. The topic of money gets addressed at some point. Personally, I tended to overpay star talent, and on that subject, I can't remember making a mistake by doing so. The return was tenfold, or more. An environment to achieve success is more important than money, but a good salary goes a long way.

NEGOTIATIONS

You don't get what you deserve in life; you get what you negotiate. There are times when the chief executive needs to be present in the negotiation process, whether it be payer contracts, labor, compensation, acquisition, or fundraising. Your being there makes a statement. Most contract negotiations are performed by procurement officers, managed care executives and lawyers. In the medical "business," it is good to know the basic issues that your delegates face. When supply chain or payer contracts are renegotiated, physicians and nurses are consulted infrequently. Their input can be valuable. Healthcare insurance contracting is the most problematic – worse in some markets than others.

Successful negotiations depend on "the art of letting them have your way."[16] An associate of communication magnate Rupert Murdoch, who observed his negotiating style for many years, remarked that as a buyer Murdoch "understands the seller – and, whatever the guy's trying to do, he crafts his offer that way. He is able to see what the person most wants out of the deal."[17]

One of the most fundamental and recurring problems that we faced was that the contracting teams turned the negotiations into something akin to unions vs. management. The people on the other side of the table can be like some parties in the Northern Ireland struggle, who would reportedly "drive 100 miles out of their way to receive an insult." These were people whose attitude was said to be: "Forget the future; let's get on with the past."[18] My point is that a leader occasionally has to intercede but before doing so must understand all issues. If the chief executive has to break too many log jams, something is wrong with the negotiating team.

Charm is often easy to see through, but presence shows sincerity and interest and indicates that the chief executive understands why the deal is important and how it can be mutually beneficial. There's nothing like the personal touch. Berkshire

Hathaway had wanted to purchase Business Wire for years. But Cathy Baron Tamraz, Business Wire's chief executive, feared her company would be cost-cut and sold. After reading a journalist's profile of Berkshire Hathaway's Warren Buffett, Tamraz wrote him a letter explaining her problems with the deal. Buffett read the letter, picked up the phone and called Tamraz directly. "He makes you feel like you're the greatest manager in the world," said Tamraz, who went on to take what was Berkshire's original offer.[19]

PHYSICIAN COUNSEL

Part of leadership is to work with all kinds of people, those with exaggerated self-importance and those who are unsure. Many good doctors have massive egos. Architect Frank Lloyd Wright said he made the choice at an early age between "hypocritical humility and honest arrogance."[20] The facts are that talented physicians frequently have "an immature, unbridled desire for unmanaged freedom."[21] "The smaller the field, the greater the megalocephaly. Imagine if Dr. Osler could view the medical world today!"[22] Personally, I don't have any problem with large egos unless their need for the tumult of applause doesn't match performance expectations. "Why are you dressed like that?" asks the Jewish mother of her son when he visits her wearing the uniform of a naval officer. "Because, Mama," he explains, "I just bought a boat and I'm the captain," to which she replies, smiling fondly, "Well, by you, you're a captain. And, by me, you're a captain. But by a captain, are you a captain?"[23]

The problematic doctor is often one who is the greatest contributor. However, faculty members have to be worth the trouble they cause.[24] Therefore, an equal and important aspect of leadership is to offer guidance to the physician who is too far out of step with the organization. If this behavior is repulsive, it may affect colleagues, patients and donors. You may be famous, but you have to have character. The doctor may have 100 patients, but the patient doesn't have 100 doctors. Jim Willerson, former editor of the journal *Circulation*, pointed out that "while we are observing and trying to understand the patient, we must remember that they are observing and evaluating us."[25] This thought goes back many centuries. John Donne remarked in *Devotions*, "I observed the physician with the same diligence as he the disease."[26] Patients who make an appointment with a doctor and encounter a jerk may shrug their shoulders and simply go elsewhere. But you can be sure they'll tell their friends. Many good doctors don't realize their faults. Anyone can have an off day, but if complaints become a chorus, counsel is in order.[±]

±   "Say you're educated and you can't throw strikes; then they don't leave you in too long."
    (Casey Stengel)

Generally department leaders remain motivated, but occasionally good doctors burn out or become bored or somehow lose their way. Why do medical personnel leave the organization? 1) They dislike the working environment or the department head; 2) They're offered more money elsewhere; 3) They find an attractive relocation; 4) They'd like to spend more time with the family; 5) They don't like their colleagues; 6) They're not interested in academics. Star performers sometimes have "fatal personality flaws."[27] You have seen them all: the hero (egomaniac), the dictator, the bulldozer, the pessimist, the rebel, and the home run hitter who tries to do too much too soon. All of these can be managed to varying degrees of success. Some need a bridle and a few others need a spur.[28] And the *opera buffo* is a waste of everyone's time. An organization gets the behavior it tolerates.

The biggest executive management problem that I've seen personally concerns those who are enormously talented but when left totally to themselves are "wackers," meaning that they are too tough for the wrong reasons and inspire fear, not confidence. At the other end are the pretty good doctors who show up every day and do good work but have no academic interest. That's okay. As they say out west, "If a man can't skin, he must hold a leg while somebody else does."[29] The point is to get the best out of everyone and also acknowledge your own mistakes. You as the leader have to engage and advise, proactively. Good leadership understands that the organization has to motivate the motivators. Remember, you, the leader, have to get better every year, too. "Guys that improve every year are always adding something to their game."[30]

It goes without saying that you can't keep everyone happy and sometimes you have to let people with a bad attitude simply go and find another job or another line of work. Mark Twain wrote: "If you pick up a starving dog and make him prosperous, he will not bite you. This is the principal difference between a dog and a man."[31] But they are the exceptions. For me, the medical profession has always commanded, and continues to command, my greatest respect. "Now, I've known my share of arrogant doctors," columnist Charles Krauthammer wrote, "and a few given to opulence, but I have found them as a class to be admirable, unusually hard working, and dedicated… in fact, if all American industry operated at the level of the medical profession, we would not be talking endlessly about the failure of American competitiveness."[32]

Medicine tends to attract real individualists. They want freedom without too much interference. Don't be too directive; cut them some slack. As Ronald Reagan said to his chief of staff, "I'll take 80 percent of what I want, rather than to go over the cliff with the flag flying."[±] They desire relatively autonomous practices and some want time for academic pursuits. Physicians have a strong tendency to view the organization as an institutional support service, which otherwise interferes with

---

±   Cited in Baker III JA. *The Big Ten: The Case for Pragmatic Idealism*. The National Interest *online*, August 29, 2007. http://www.nationalinterest.org/PrinterFriendly.aspx?id=15370

what is good for their specialty or practice.[33] In their department rounds, one of the principles that physician executives have to prove is that the administration is not the enemy.

What is important to staff physicians in an academic medical center? In no special order, I'd say it is the expertise of their colleagues, a departmental environment that fosters creativity, empowerment at some level, good management and governance, and professional security. Academic physicians, and probably physicians in general, are focused on personal and group endeavors with little regard, if not disdain, for the administrative dynamic, unless bad performance affects their needs or otherwise restrains their pursuit of the ideal practice. Some really great physicians and scientists don't have, and possibly won't ever have, interest in the infrastructure of the institution or even their own department. It makes sense to tolerate a certain amount of unawareness among good staff. Not everyone will walk in lockstep and you should not insist on it. Gene Blackstone[34] reminded me about his father's lesson to his children:

> Some know and know they know
> Others know but don't know they know
> Some don't know and know they don't know
> Yet others don't know but they don't know they don't know.

In this regard, don't look to physicians for administrative change. In a study of ten well-managed hospitals, physicians were found to be reactors rather than initiators of change.[35] They are generally imperturbable and prefer to be left alone, but they also want to be proud of the institution in which they work. Inherently they have faith in talented leadership. At the same time, they want someone to listen to their complaints and ideas. They want to be heard but not necessarily to respond to initiatives from above. Like all personnel, doctors want to be recognized for outstanding performance. Empower the doctors who can influence their colleagues positively.

There comes a time for many physicians when they question their role in life and wonder "what is expected of me." I would suggest that anyone having doubts read *Language of God*,[36] by Francis S. Collins, best known as the director of the Human Genome Project. As a young doctor, Collins did missionary work in Nigeria:

> One afternoon in the clinic a young farmer was brought in by his
> family with progressive weakness and massive swelling of his
> legs. Taking his pulse, I was startled to note that it essentially
> disappeared every time he took in a breath. Though I had never seen

this classic physical sign (referred to as a "paradoxical pulse") so dramatically demonstrated, I was pretty sure this must mean that this young farmer had accumulated a large amount of fluid in the pericardial sac around his heart. This fluid was threatening to choke off his circulation and take his life....

No ultrasound was available. No other physician present in this small Nigerian hospital had ever undertaken this procedure. The choice was for me to attempt a highly risky and invasive needle aspiration or watch the farmer die. I explained the situation to the young man, who was now fully aware of his own precarious state. He calmly urged me to proceed. With my heart in my mouth and a prayer on my lips, I inserted a large needle just under his sternum and aimed for his left shoulder, all the while fearing that I might have made the wrong diagnosis, in which case I was almost certainly going to kill him.

I didn't have to wait long. The rush of dark red fluid in my syringe initially made me panic that I might have entered the heart chamber, but it soon became apparent that this was not normal heart's blood. It was a massive amount of bloody tuberculous effusion from the pericardial sac around the heart.

Nearly a quart of fluid was drawn off. The young man's response was dramatic. His paradoxical pulse disappeared almost at once, and within the next twenty-four hours the swelling of his legs rapidly improved.

For a few hours after this experience I felt a great sense of relief, even elation, at what had happened. But by the next morning, the same familiar gloom began to settle over me.... Even if he survived the disease, some other preventable disorder, born of dirty water, inadequate nutrition, and a dangerous environment, probably lay not too far in his future. The chances for long life in a Nigerian farmer are poor.

With those discouraging thoughts in my head, I approached his bedside the next morning, to find him reading his Bible. He looked at me quizzically, and asked whether I had worked at the hospital for a long time. I admitted that I was new, feeling somewhat irritated and embarrassed that it had been so easy for him to figure that out. But then this young Nigerian farmer, just about as different from me in culture, experience, and ancestry as any two humans could be, spoke the words that will forever be emblazoned in my mind: "I get the sense you are wondering why you came here," he said. "I have an answer for you. *You came here for one reason. You came here for me.*"

INTERACTION WITH THE BOARD OF TRUSTEES

Approximately 85 percent of hospitals are nonprofit state-chartered institutions that derive their status from the work they do in education, research, and charitable care. A board of trustees holds the fiduciary responsibility to see that those criteria are honored. In today's world in which good governance has become a compelling issue for public corporate boards, it has also become of vital importance to nonprofit hospitals and medical centers. Invariably, successful medical organizations have a strong board of trustees. Apart from fiduciary responsibility, a knowledgeable and dynamic board provides an independent perspective on finance and operations and, if composed of the right people, the trustees are an excellent sounding board for strategies, fundraising, and insight into community involvement. A board has to have clarity about the mission of the organization and understand its vision.

What is a dynamic board? In smaller institutions internal resources are more limited and the need for board contributions to operating issues is greater; while in larger organizations, the typical focus is on oversight of operating performance, business strategy, enterprise risk management and succession. In the assembling of a board, look for these characteristics: 1) *business experience*; 2) *available time*; 3) *attitude*; 4) *organizational ability*; 5) *public board experience*; 6) *diversity*; 7) *collegiality*. The five Ws of work, will, wisdom, wit and wealth are good places to start. If you are the chief executive, you have to judge whether the new board candidate is someone who can add value to the board composition and whose interests coincide with the goals of the organization. Is this a person who can be a trusted advisor?

In large medical centers, a rigorous nominating process for trusteeship is preferred over the good old boy network. Too often the chair or a senior trustee intends to install a friend or business associate on the board without review, or worse, has already made a promise to that person that he or she will become a member of the board. The chief executive, the board chairman, or a nominating group should interview each candidate and start with the question, what do you want to contribute?

Not money, at least initially. Instead, where and how can you help our organization? What knowledge, skills and perspective do you offer? The right board should be a team of mentors with experience, intellect, and business acumen.[37] Ideally, all advice should be accompanied by a check (from the trustee who gives the advice).

New board members should be oriented in a concise manner. Don't overwhelm them. Begin by acquainting them with the guiding principles of the institution, their responsibilities, the need for independence, and the mission and administrative structure of the institution. Encourage them to read up on the theory and history of trusteeship. There are some good board books such as the *Governing Board Orientation Manual* published by the Washington State Hospital Association[38] and other books about directorship.[39, 40] When orientation is complete, the new trustee should be conversant with the medical center and its delivery system and be aware of key medical and operational indicators and financial trends. He or she should understand the academic enterprise, how it differs from a conventional hospital, and how the academic medical center helps to support the community.

In 2005, there were 369 nonprofit health *systems* comprising 56 percent of U.S. hospitals. A recent survey about nonprofit board governance conducted by the University of Iowa[41] analyzes newer trends in governance and regulation. It finds increasing involvement of physicians and nurses on boards of community health systems. This report contains extensive references related to board governance. Since the enactment of Public Law 107-204 (Sarbanes-Oxley Act) and revisions to the Federal Sentencing Guidelines in 2004, attention has also been focused on nonprofit organizations including hospitals and health systems. The boards of these organizations must now "manage the additional responsibility of overseeing the organization's regulatory compliance mechanisms and tax-exempt status."[42]

Most boards, more so in the not-for-profit sector, look at performance based on finances only. Of all the other clinical, operational and academic factors that make up a leading health center, I believe that patient and personnel satisfaction top the list. Those are the surrogates for quality and operational effectiveness. Attrition rates in every category of employment are an important metric and with other metrics should be viewed as trends. As will be mentioned later on, the number of new patients enrolled in the system is a crucial sign of progress or lack thereof. Trustees must look at outpatient metrics as well as hospital indicators. A quarterly report on strategy is an area where leadership can benefit from trustee oversight. The point is that trusteeship extends beyond celebrations and other social interactions. Healthcare is increasingly businesslike, and there are parameters for measurement today that were not attended to in the past.

One of the fundamental benchmarks of good governance involves fair, objective, and regular leadership evaluation. Boards should hold leadership accountable for finance, quality, safety, team building and community benefit. As part of the discussion of charity care and community benefits for tax-exempt organizations, the IRS has modified Form 990 (Schedule H), which requires not-for-profit hospitals to report charity care, community benefits, executive and board compensation, and organizational governance. In the Iowa survey, only 36 percent of the health systems had a formal community benefit plan with measurable objectives.

The relationship between the chief executive and the board chair must be complementary. There is a separation of these roles in nonprofit healthcare (for true independence). The board chair and chief executive appoint the best and most qualified members for key committee chairmanship. In addition to the nominating committee, the key committees include medical staff relations (compensation), finance (which may or may not include investments), audit, marketing, buildings and grounds, and community relations. Each medical center has its own committee structure depending upon the market, the extent of research and education, and current health policy. The relationship between a chairman and chief executive should be close, synergistic and above politics. "I knew," wrote General William Sherman to General Ulysses Grant, "wherever I was you thought of me, and if I got into a tight place you would help me out of it alive."[43]

BOARDS THAT DELIVER

A weak board generally indicates weak management. In Ram Charan's book *Boards That Deliver*,[44] he poses ten questions that every director should ask periodically. Since the fiduciary responsibility of a board includes operating effectiveness, the following questions are especially pertinent for an academic medical center.

1) Do you have the right chief executive?
2) How well are reports linked to actual performance?
3) Do you have a precise understanding of the long-term strategy?
4) Is the management team looking at external trends and diagnosing the opportunities and threats that they present?
5) What are the sources of organic growth?
6) How rigorous is the process for developing the leadership gene pool?
7) Do you have the right approach for diagnosing financial health?
8) Are you examining measures that capture the root causes of performance?
9) Do you hear bad news from management in time and unvarnished?
10) How productive are the executive sessions?

The warning signs of a flawed chief executive have to be recognized before disaster hits (also see chapter 1). This is one of the jobs of governance, including trusteeship. Look for these signals: an overt zeal for prestige, power and wealth; shameless self-promotion; a proclivity for developing grandiose strategies with little thought toward implementation; lack of consensus building; impulsive style; a penchant for inconsiderate acts; poor listening skills; contempt for the ideas of others; energy without objective; a career marked by numerous misunderstandings; and chronic rationalization of misdeeds.[45] Of all these signs, the most important, in my estimation, would be the lack of strategic thinking and inability to execute. The first decision a board must make during a crisis is to decide whether the chief executive should lead the organization through the crisis.

The board is not there to set strategy. It is there to approve strategy, or disapprove it as necessary. Further, it is there to see that approved strategy is implemented.[46] As chief executive, you need to make the case for your strategy in a fair but effective way to the board. You need to inform them of short-term risks, even as you prove that the long-term strategy is viable and will contribute to growth in performance and reputation. Trustees, for their part, are responsible for understanding the direction the organization is moving, and assuring that the ship is not dismasted. The board has to be absolutely sure that reports are not sugarcoated and are 100 percent accurate. It is a good idea for a hospital board to meet once a year for a strategy discussion. Concentrate on long-term value. Above all, encourage open discussion on all pertinent matters.

A dysfunctional board will spend too much time on trivial matters, focus on short-term interests, and will prefer to react to events rather than make things happen. It will review, rehash, redo, diffuse authority, and look for ways to "get around" the chief executive.[47] Vigilant input and an appreciation of economic trends are the essentials of trusteeship. However, trustees are not line managers. The chair should remind board members that if they don't have a proposed solution to a problem, then they are part of the problem. The business experience of most trustees gives them an appreciation of the fact that when things are going well, that is often the time of greatest danger.

Risk assessment is one of the most important activities that a board can engage in. Just as the role of directors is changing in the corporate world, trustees of nonprofit organizations should be increasingly focused on compliance. This is the responsibility of your key board appointments, or your chairs of audit, investments, and buildings and grounds. The board needs to educate administration on the points of risk: investments, quality, privacy, medical liability, and legal compliance. It should not neglect material risk, including environment, finances, operations, litigation, terrorism, and strategy. Does the organization have an enterprise risk strategy to identify and react to potential risks (and opportunities) in a timely way?

Wars of succession have been known to tear organizations apart. A well-developed succession plan is essential to assure the orderly transfer of power. But according to a 2004 American College of Healthcare Executives study, only 21 percent of 722 hospitals engaged in succession planning.[48] A strong "bench" of potential successors should be developed across the organization. I don't believe that it is in the purview of the executive committee to review the profile of potential successors for each department; however, the chief executive should be encouraged to nominate a pool of qualified individuals who have been groomed for leadership.

Trustees can be of enormous value to physician chief executives who lack experience with public companies, or with the kind of scrutiny that comes from government regulators and the investment community. They are called "trustees" because their legal obligation is fiduciary, that is to say, exercised on behalf of others. Through the Volunteer Protection Act, federal law provides that volunteers in nonprofit organizations who are paid less than $500 per year are immune to personal liability for actions taken in good faith. Most states have similar laws for trustees of nonprofit organizations.[49] Although the Sarbanes-Oxley Act does not yet apply to nonprofit organizations, it is mandatory to be compliant, especially in regard to certification of financial statements, audit committee expertise, and strict adherence to laws such as IRC-4958, IRC-501(c)3, the Stark Law, and the Medicare Anti-Kickback Law.

A summary of directors' obligations, including oversight, fiduciary liability exposure, and compliance plan effectiveness, is summarized in a publication from the American Health Lawyers Association.[50] Chief among these issues is the subject of conflict of interest. Trustees are comprised of community leaders, and virtually every one of them has some conflict of interest if you look hard enough into their professions or businesses. At the outset, trustees should be aware that solicitation is forbidden and there will always be scrutiny regarding conflict of interest. Strict confidentiality is also a given.

The healthcare industry operates in a heavily regulated environment with a variety of identifiable risk areas.[±] The organization must provide an appropriate level

---

± A good nonprofit board self-evaluation form may be found in the previously referenced appendix from the Bulletin of the National Center for Healthcare Leadership (Nonprofit Board Self-Evaluation of Effectiveness). In addition, the Office of the Inspector General of the U. S. Department of Health and Human Services and the American Health Lawyers Association published a resource for healthcare boards of directors titled *Corporate Responsibility and Corporate Compliance* (http://oig.hhs.gov/fraud/docs/complianceguidance/040203CorpRespRsce Guide.pdf.) In this context, the terms directors and trustees are used interchangeably and the term corporate applies to the healthcare organization.

of due diligence to allow directors to make informed decisions. Directors need to be able to "ask knowledgeable and appropriate questions related to healthcare corporate compliance." Boards have the legal obligation known as "duty of care." Duty of care demands that directors act in good faith, be prudent in avoiding or preventing harm to others, and to act in a manner that can be recognized as being in the best interests of the organization. Duty of care includes a board's oversight as well as decision making functions. Compliance is more than a reactive activity; it requires proactive thinking about compliance legal standards.[51] While the compliance officer needs to address significant risks, the organization must also provide adequate resources to implement and sustain a compliance program.

In healthcare, active compliance programs have increased from a prevalence of 55 percent in 1999 to 87 percent in 2002. Every large hospital should designate a compliance officer to serve as the focal point for compliance activities. Trustees are urged to inquire how compliance programs are structured, to review and receive reports on compliance issues, and to understand the goals of the compliance program. The main question is whether the compliance officer addresses the significant risks to the organization and has substantial resources dedicated to implementing and sustaining a compliance program.

The Office of Inspector General believes that it is prudent to separate the compliance function from key management. More specifically, it should not be in the office of the general counsel. For independence, the auditor and the compliance officer should report directly to the trustees of the organization. The oversight function is enhanced if the board understands the complementary roles of the general counsel and the chief compliance officer in their support of the board's oversight responsibilities.[52] When the general counsel or internal auditor serves as a chief compliance officer, boards are encouraged to adopt a recusal process in which either the officer or auditor may be recused from a compliance investigation. If the organization currently has the chief compliance officer report to the general counsel, consider moving that report to the board. This doesn't mean that the two offices and their functions should be totally severed. There is great value in having the general counsel periodically involved in risk assessment. It can also help review proposed policies and reports on compliance processes, conduct investigations, and address legal violations.

Although I was in the minority, I believe term limits are essential for a healthy board of trustees. Unfortunately, it's hard to remove hospital trustees except by term limits. Case Western Reserve University (CWRU) limits the terms of its board by what I consider a model of term-limit regulations.[53] The term of CWRU trustees commences the day after their election. Trustees who were in office at the initiation of term limits were allowed to serve three more years. New trustees serve a four-year term and are permitted to serve no more than two consecutive terms (could be modified to three terms). Trustees' terms expire as they reach age 72, and they may not be reelected (this age limit should be modified upward). The number of trustees may be increased or decreased by affirmative vote of a majority of trustees present, provided that the vote does not shorten the term of any incumbent trustee. Boards, like executives, need renewal.

CRISIS MANAGEMENT

Asked what worried him most during his time of leadership, Harold Macmillan is said to have replied, "Events, dear boy, events."[54]

"Events," in the form of crises, come to all large operations at one point or another. How you as a leader handle them can be the difference between a passing storm and Hurricane Katrina. Remember that your stakeholders include your staff and the media. Brief the staff personally. Answer their questions in a straightforward manner. Don't fix blame. Apologize only when necessary and then mean it. Remember, it's not what you say to the public; it's what they hear. Be absolutely sure that you have the facts and then make the facts available in a forthright and absolutely honest way. The leader has to accept responsibility. Don't blame, disavow, or overstate the problem. If you can be very brief, do so. Ideally, your response will be some variation on, "It happened; it shouldn't have happened; it won't happen again."[55]

Be alert to the signals of a brewing crisis: complaints, suspicions, rumors, and warnings. If your standards are lax, crises are more likely to occur. Sometimes the signals don't reach your office. This is the sort of thing you learn from a post-crisis review, where performance is analyzed and lessons are drawn to prevent recurrences. You'll find that every crisis has its enablers. Sometimes they're your own lax standards.[56] How you handle a crisis is important, but your leverage and status upon entering the crisis is the biggest determinant of outcome.[±]

In a high-grade crisis, it's best to call in the trauma surgeons of public relations, the crisis consultants. Your executive team would do well to read about damage control and the variables that spell doom or survival.[57] Most of the literature on crises will advise the organization to take the initiative, avoid casting blame, and communicate effectively. Anyone who communicates with personnel or the media should have authority. There's a difference between crisis management and crisis leadership. Crisis management is primarily reactive. Crisis leadership is proactive, which means identify, prepare, and communicate effectively. In serious matters, the chief executive meets with the media to control the message and accept responsibility.

±   In conversation with Richard Landgarten, Managing Director, Global Healthcare Group. Global Investment Banking. Citigroup Global Markets, Inc.

When the communication director takes over, make sure that you are all speaking in the same voice and delivering the same message. The public will not be conned. If you're avoiding the issues, they'll see right through you. "No comment" is not an acceptable response. Avoid denial and the appearance of weakness.

ADVICE TO NEW PHYSICIAN LEADERS

When I started in the executive role, things didn't look too good. So I pointed out to the staff that the largest ship in the Navy at that time was the aircraft carrier *Enterprise*. It is comprised of an air group and the ship's company. The air group often works night and day and is concerned only about the number of strikes, but the ship's company enjoys the status quo of the maintenance of the vessel. To keep that ship functioning, these units are mutually dependent on each other. The process is rather slow and it requires great momentum to turn the *Enterprise* around. In fact, it takes about five miles for a turning radius. However, once it has been turned around and is headed in the right direction, it's capable of incredible speed and power. We were turning our ship around immediately.

It's hard to estimate how many new chief executives are appointed because of a need for improvement. My guess is that about half the time there is a normal succession process, and the other half the hospital organization is in some sort of trouble and the previous administration has been removed because of perceived deficiencies. Change happens when: 1) people are dissatisfied with the status quo; 2) the new direction is obvious; 3) there is confidence that it will succeed; 4) they accept that change can be messy, marked by episodes of confusion and anxiety that must be endured.[58] Trustees must be committed to the need for transformation.

The new chief executive, if he or she is a change agent, will encounter a mixed attitude in personnel. Remember, "When a leader arrives, people are full of panic, uncertain what to do and defeatist about the future. When the authentic leader has spoken, they have been given back their courage."[59] Forget the naysayers. Search for the energized personnel for whom the status quo is unacceptable. Communication begins with a rational plan including strict timelines and a relatively short horizon to accomplish prioritized change – and should not include railing against the previous administration. Initially the focus is concentrated on turnaround, but that is not a long-term strategic plan. The proper role of the chief executive is to make sure the ship gets out of the harbor but not beyond the horizon where it can no longer be seen. In the late 18th century, when the British navy experienced a series of mutinies, the admiralty learned a twofold lesson from those events – namely that legitimate grievances from the lower deck should be promptly redressed and that impossible demands were best resisted without compromise.[60]

The transformational leader[61] may sweep the executive offices clean. When transformation is urgent, that may be a necessity. As Rupert Murdoch said, "…when you take over a company and you want to make changes, it is good to do everything you can to change the culture. And a physical move is a big and useful thing to do."[62] Murray Weidenbaum, who chaired Reagan's Council of Economic Advisers, caught the prevailing mood: "Don't just stand there; undo something."[63] Michael Feuer, founder of OfficeMax, advises the new chief executive: "First, do no harm." [64] However you effect change, retain great talent. Don't identify with Henry Ford, who accomplished a great deal, but managing talent was not his strong suit. He said, "I let him go not because he wasn't good, but because he was too good – for me." In effect, Ford removed all the people who had a talent equal to his or the temerity to argue with him….[65] The key lesson is that turnaround succeeds only by affirmative change. Remember the Basuto proverb "If a man does away with his traditional way of living and throws away his good customs, he had better first make certain that he has something of value to replace them."[66]

In my experience, the leverage to progress further each year depends on: 1) taking advantage of the tools and technologies that are available to help you manage a very complex business; 2) developing a better workflow design that improves efficiency; 3) paying attention to human resources (The level of talent and experience required of employees is greater now than ever before); 4) building an effective partnership with all your colleagues; 5) staying focused on the mission, which is primarily to take care of patients – all this other stuff, complicated and beneficial as it is, is really a means to an end; and, 6) attending social functions is part of the job. If you show up, act like you want to be there.

Choose your ground carefully. As former University of California President Clark Kerr noted, "You must [sometimes] find satisfaction in being equally distasteful to each of the constituencies; you must reconcile yourself to the harsh reality that successes are shrouded in silence while failures are spotlighted in notoriety."[67] You can't keep everybody happy. If you just set out to be liked, you would be prepared to compromise on anything at any time, and you would achieve nothing.[68] *There are no 100 percent heroes.*[69] Your responsibility as the leader is to invest in the strong, rehabilitate the weak, and eliminate the unnecessary.

Some healthcare chief executives are travelers, spending a great deal of time at national meetings pertaining to hospital issues, health policy, quality, etc. In order to accomplish their outside committee work, one of their administrative team members assumes control and directs the day-to-day operations. This style may work for some executives, but I've found a fairly low yield on the road and preferred to stay at home and be there for most of the key executive meetings. My role was to set the agenda, approve the goals, listen to the periodic reports, educate and mentor, follow up on tactics, analyze mistakes and celebrate success. Incidentally, "If you're not in control of your calendar, you're not in control."[70]

PERSONAL LESSONS

Prior to retirement, I passed on these ten lessons to my successor.

1) This is not still life; progress requires calculated risk taking.
2) Be courageous – weakness will kill you.
3) Don't expect loyalty, but always give it, unconditionally.
4) The single greatest competitive advantage is speed of sound action.
5) Power should be invisible.
6) Give all credit to others.
7) No one is as smart as everyone.
8) Your conscience is your religion.[±]
9) Don't fret about competition; we compete with ourselves (to get better each year).
10) Set the course; be credible; communicate; make it happen.

Each successive administration governs during different times and circumstances. We are only temporary stewards in the life history of our respective medical organizations, and our mission is to have our organizations thrive much longer than the biological lives of their current members. This can be done only by hard work, fresh ideas and persistence.

One admonition that cannot safely be ignored is to pace yourself. Reeling from one meeting to another every day all week long will grind you down quickly. Determine relatively soon what is unnecessary and can be eliminated or delegated. I don't understand why delegation is ever controversial. Of course you should delegate. Those to whom you delegate should do their jobs and communicate with you. The chief executive shouldn't meddle unless there are major problems. The inability to delegate is widely recognized as a counter-indicator of success in leadership. If you can't delegate, there's something wrong with you, your organization, or the people who work for you. Delegate, that is, but don't abdicate.

Frequently ask yourself and your team: Are you just going through the motions, or is the organization making measurable progress? Whatever your style, do not tolerate inertia. Don't measure yourself by what you accomplished, but rather by what you should have accomplished with your ability.[71] Effective, intelligent plans

---

±   Taught to me by Dick Jacobs.

are made to move the organization ahead, and those plans have to be acted on with deliberation and speed, and when implemented, add value to all intents and purposes. Don't spend an inordinate amount of time on distant projects. Avoid politics, cronyisms, empty gestures and promises. You cannot just go along to get along.

Bad days? You bet. In the great parabola of life, there are days and sometimes a string of them that will make you wish you were never born. The only people who don't have problems are the people who don't do anything. Or maybe the results are not that bad, but you are plowing mud and not making progress. In that case, take out a legal pad and list your concerns. When you write down your frustrations, you might be able to reprioritize your goals or even find a solution for immediate problems. Remedies often take time. At the outset of World War II, Churchill wrote to the King, "Better days will come – though not yet." [72]

Cleveland Clinic Founder George Crile suffered his greatest setback in the 1929 Clinic x-ray fire that killed 123 people. Boston's Dr. Ernest A. Codman wrote to him:[73]

> I am writing to ask a question.
>
> I always think of you as an eagle able to look directly into the sun, looking down, perhaps, on the rest of us common birds, who are controlled by our sympathies, petty desires, and emotions.
>
> You have climbed the ladder of surgical ambition high into the skies of Fame. You have done more good by your introduction of blood pressure measurements, of transfusion… and gas-oxygen anesthesia than could be counteracted by (the bad events). In the haste of your upward progress you have known that some wings would break and lives be lost. Now comes this accident which is not the least your fault, and which will do untold good, as every x-ray laboratory in the world will be safer for it.
>
> And now, my question: Since you have known both "Triumph and Disaster" – did you "treat those two Imposters just the same"?[±]

George Crile and his successors were able to answer that question and it contributed to their successful leadership. In each successive administration, medical activities operate in an increasingly complex environment. Money is tight, the intensity

---

[±]   From Kipling's *If*.

of care increases, the cost structure is difficult to improve upon, and managing disparate personnel is much like coaching a sports team. As everyone knows, sports metaphors are overdone in business writing. But my example comes from personal observation. Some years ago, I had the privilege of visiting the New England Patriots' training camp. Watching the team work out, practice and interact, I was impressed by what I can only call an intangible impression of complete competence. One needed only to spend the briefest time with these players, their coaches, and their managers to know that they would win – methodically, consistently and overwhelmingly. I attribute the New England Patriots' air of competence, and consistent success in the regular and post-season, to the leadership of their coach, Bill Belichick.[±]

The National Football League is somewhat like the business of medicine in that each level of success puts you in an environment of greater complexity. Winning teams face a more challenging schedule the following season. They draft lower, their schedules are tougher, they are hit by free agency and salary caps: In short, everything is arranged to make it harder for them to win again next year. Under these circumstances, you'd think it would be impossible to create a dynasty that can rise to the top of the league year after year. Yet Belichick has done it. He seems to excel in proportion to the intensity of the competition. You as a healthcare leader can and should aspire to similar consistency. If you can pull it off, the fans will love you.

[±]   See Halberstam D. *The Education of a Coach*. New York, Hyperion, 2005.

THE ACADEMIC MEDICAL CENTER

Geronte: It was very clearly explained, but there was just one thing, which surprised me – that was the positions of the liver and the heart. It seemed to me that you got them the wrong way about, that the heart should be on the left side, and the liver on the right.

Sganarelle: Yes, it used to be so but we have changed all that. Everything's quite different in medicine nowadays.

— Molière
Cited in *Le Médecin Malgré Lui*

Great scientists and great physicians make great medical centers. All hospitals strive for a healing environment conducive to success for the patient and the staff, and the term *staff* should mean all personnel. The word "academic" signifies the scholarly activity of teaching, research and learning. It is more than intellectual inquiry; it is the creation of medical progress through discovery and innovation. These are the building blocks. In the arts it is the artist, and in the sciences it is discovery.[1] Academic healthcare generates new knowledge for clinical application. This "academification"[±] touches all medical specialties. The purpose of academic endeavors is to add greater value to patient care, and as such is no longer an ivory tower exercise.

[±]   *Academification*: a term used by Dr. Eric Topol, who was formerly the Chief Academic Officer of the Cleveland Clinic

In 1921, at the dedication of the clinic and hospital he founded, George Crile said it this way, "… that throughout the Cleveland Clinic Foundation, we will have a continual policy of active investigation of disease and this policy will be assured. That is to say, we are considering not only our duty to the patient of today, but no less our duty to the patient of tomorrow."[2] These are timeless words… as medical research adapts to better fit the patient's needs, basic research has become more directed to clinical problems. The resulting translational research aims for practical clinical significance. Louis Pasteur wrote: "To him who devotes his life to science, nothing can give more happiness than increasing the number of discoveries, but his cup of joy is full when the results of his studies immediately find practical application."[3]

Although a great deal of the activity in academic medical centers relates to research and education, the "product" of an academic health center is medicine, or as it is more blandly referred to today, healthcare. Sometimes highly motivated people in academic endeavors don't understand the importance of patient care. Dr. Jerome Groopman criticizes academic medicine for arrogance because he believes it applauds research, takes teaching for granted, gives writing precedence over clinical medicine, and makes taking care of patients a low priority.[4] The academic medical center staff is often, and sometimes rightly so, accused of arrogance where research, often not contributory, is given precedence ahead of patient care. Patient care is why we are here. Patient care helps fund the academic activities. Patient care is what we return to the community. The joy of healthcare is the privilege of taking care of the patient. The importance of clinical activity is memorialized by another founder of the Cleveland Clinic, William E. Lower, whose words are as true today as they were 70 years ago:

> A patient is the most important person; the patient is not someone to argue or match wits with; a patient is not dependent on us; we are dependent on them; a patient is not an interruption of our work – it is the purpose of it; the patient is not outside our business – they are our business; the patient is a person, not a statistic.[±5]

SCIENCE AND EDUCATION

Darwin wrote that "Great scientific discoveries are like sunrises. They illuminate first the steeples of the unknown, then its dark hollows."[6] The best academic centers

---

±   This quote was adapted by Dr. Lower from a very old "commercial creed," which is widely repeated in business, and which for many decades has appeared on a large sign over the counter at the L.L. Bean store in Maine – with the word "customer" where Dr. Lower uses the word "patient."

have a research system of discovery. We believe that research begets research as discoveries yield more material for investigation, more grants, more citations, and more discoveries. Clinical medicine is "an art which utilizes the sciences."[7] Essentially all new treatments emerge from the discoveries in clinical research or basic science. As these activities are integrated, we build the intellectual endowment. In a progressive academic medical center, the bonds between research and clinical medicine are powerful and indissoluble. An integrated academic and patient care environment attracts the best talent.

In a landmark report on science, Vannevar Bush advised President Franklin Roosevelt, "In the last analysis, the future of science in this country will be determined by our basic educational policy."[8] The aura of good science and education that surrounds clinical medicine defines the academic organization's culture. The unification of basic (translational)[±] and clinical sciences with medical and postgraduate education can only strengthen patient care. In his introduction to *The Origin of the Species*, Darwin wrote:

> Therefore my success as a man of science, whatever this may have amounted to, has been determined, as far as I can judge, by complex and diversified mental qualities and conditions. Of these, the most important have been – the love of science – unbounded patience in long reflecting over any subject – industry in observing and collecting facts – and a fair share of invention as well as of common sense. [9]

From the beginning of our medical training, doctors are involved in scholarship. Whether it's termed education or learning, knowledge is a fundamental requisite of our being and we pursue it all throughout our lives. What makes lifelong learning difficult is not so much the forgetting of what we have learned, but the struggle to acquire new knowledge. New knowledge is the real wealth today, far more than material assets. The information revolution is actually a knowledge revolution.[10]

± "...effective translation of the new knowledge, mechanisms, and techniques generated by advances in basic science research into new approaches for prevention, diagnosis, and treatment of disease" (Fontanarosa PB, DeAngelis CD. *Basic Science and Translational Research*, JAMA. 2002: 287 (13); 1728). The second area of translational research seeks to close the gap and improve quality by improving access, reorganizing and coordinating systems of care, helping clinicians and patients to change behaviors and make more informed choices, providing reminders and point-of-care decision support tools, and strengthening the patient-clinician relationship. (Sung NS, Crowley Jr. WF, Genel M, et al. *Central Challenges Facing the National Clinical Research Enterprise*. JAMA. 2003: 289 (10);1278-87)

As John Locke observed, the purpose of education is not to learn facts but to acquire a relish for knowledge.[11] Knowledge spans many activities, all of which potentially improve patient care. There are many incentives for scholarship – for vigilance, humanism, and personal renewal. We may be dissatisfied with current medical results or we may try to stay abreast of technical advances – both necessary to prevent the isolation of a practice, which may happen with a physician's advancing age. Thus, the academic medical center has a broad mantle of educational responsibilities. Academics include continuing medical education and other health schools such as nursing, dentistry, pharmacy, public health, and the allied health professions. Yet, as physicians, we tend to overlook what may be the greatest educational responsibility of all: educating the patient. All good doctors are both students and teachers. Charles H. Mayo wrote that the patient is safest in the hands of a person engaged in teaching medicine. In order to teach, the doctor must always be a student.[12] Being a teacher offers a second opportunity to improve on our initial education. "To teach is to learn twice."[13]

Medical education in America is still the envy of the world and a precious resource that benefits the public and the profession enormously. It is driven by science but is still a humanitarian art. What motivates anyone to undertake the rigors of a medical career? Why suffer grueling hours, life-and-death responsibilities, and the obligation to study? Money alone cannot account for it. What motivates physicians, and especially academics, is the love of scholarship, a sense of accomplishment and a deep desire to help the sick and afflicted. Of all professions, medicine is one of the most knowledge-intensive, intellectually stimulating and emotionally satisfying pursuits. As the physician and poet John Bland-Sutton wrote:[±]

> I divided my life into three parts:
> In the first I learned my profession;
> In the second I taught it;
> In the third I enjoyed it.

The real-world challenges of a medical education cannot be ignored, however. The monetary rewards of medicine are declining relative to the expense of training. The great majority of students borrow to pay for college and medical school and acquire substantial debt. In 2004 the median educational debt for those graduating from private medical schools was more than $130,000; debt for those graduating from state schools was approximately $100,000.[14, 15] The length of medical education and the debt incurred by students can discourage careers in basic or clinical research.

±   Quoted in: Etziony MB. *The Physician's Creed.* Springfield, IL: Charles C. Thomas Publisher. 1973.

Until now, medical education had enjoyed the same broad support of other public initiatives, but perceptions are changing. Medical education has been criticized for concentrating on disease management while ignoring prevention, access, practical research, and cost management. Most of these issues are not emphasized in medical school. Exaggerated reports of physician surpluses and too many specialists, along with reports of medical errors and physician greed, have eroded the practicing doctor's reputation. The problem is less an over- or under-supply of physicians, but more the crisis is the current and projected shortage of nurses, allied health professionals and other skilled personnel.

In the recent report on American medical education, a century after the Flexner report, the authors denounced the commercial atmosphere that has permeated many academic centers.[16] Students hear educators speaking more about productivity or market share or relative value units and the financial bottom line rather than about prevention and relief of suffering. Students learn from this culture that healthcare as a business may threaten medicine as a calling and turn it into a commodity rather than a profession.

Some dissatisfied physicians join the critics of medicine to denigrate their own profession. And this is not new. Osler[17] reminded them a century ago:

> Some will tell you that the profession is underrated, unhonored, underpaid, its members social drudges – the very last profession they would recommend a young man take up. Listen not to these croakers; there are such in every calling, and the secret of their discontent is not hard to discover. The evils which they deprecate… in themselves lie… [and] in failure to grasp those principles of their science without which the practice of medicine does indeed become a drudgery, for it degenerates into a business.

All too often, the practicing physician is not trained to understand "health policy," leaving the resolution of these issues to economists, statisticians, and politicians. The academic medical center has a responsibility to meet this educational challenge, which will enable students to navigate and even participate in policies that influence their practice. To begin with, seniors in medical school and residents-in-training should have some knowledge of both health policy± and how to build a practice: 1) how to organize your office for operations and service; 2) how to communicate with patients and with referring physicians; 3) how to provide responsible patient

± Barr DA. *Introduction to U.S. Health Policy: The Organization, Financing, and Delivery of Healthcare in America.* Baltimore, MD: The Johns Hopkins University Press, 2nd ed., 2007, should be required reading for medical students.

follow-up; and 4) how to pace yourself. This is not commercialization; this is common sense. We may be in an academic environment, but the product is clinical medicine – the patient's welfare above all else.

"The real work of a doctor... is not an affair of health centers, or public clinics, or operating theaters, or laboratories, or hospital beds. These techniques have their place in medicine, but they are not medicine. The essential unit of medical practice is the occasion when, in the intimacy of the consulting... or sick room, a person who is ill or believes himself to be ill, seeks the advice of a doctor whom he trusts."[18]

THE CLEVELAND CLINIC MODEL

The Cleveland Clinic was founded in 1921 by four physicians who were viewed as rebels, if not Bolsheviks, for promoting this radical innovation – called group practice.[19] ± The Mayo Clinic, which became not-for-profit in 1919, was founded on the same principles. Dr. William Mayo was the keynote speaker at the dedication of the Cleveland Clinic. He used that opportunity to explain the reason and purpose of the new organization.

> The medical profession can be the greatest factor for the good in America. The greatest asset of a nation is the health of its people.... The real job of the medical profession is the extension of knowledge of what the medicine of today is doing and can do in the future, and this must be done by collective effort.... One of the signs of the times is the development of such institutions as the Cleveland Clinic.... It recognizes that the cause of the sick man in this and in future generations depends on education and research.... Properly considered, medicine (is)... a scientific cooperation for the welfare of the sick. Medicine's place is fixed by its services to mankind; if we fail to measure up to our opportunity, it means state medicine, political control, mediocrity, and loss of professional ideals. The members of the medical fraternity must cooperate in this work and they can do so without interfering with private professional practice.... Union of all these forces will lengthen by many years the span of human life and as a by-product will do much to improve professional ethics by overcoming some of the evils of competitive medicine.[20]

± Today in the U.S. there are 600 multispecialty group practices with more than 50 physicians. (AMA Data)

Throughout its nearly 90-year history, the Cleveland Clinic has integrated the medical staff into the life and mission of the organization. Physicians are employed and completely aligned with the hospital and clinic and with education and research; this staff model encourages loyalty to the system rather than to factions. Physicians, along with other executive leaders, are in charge of the multidivisional organizational design. This unique hierarchy has the rare ability to act quickly and in unison. The integrated model enhances recruitment and retention. All staff members are reviewed annually by their peers and by the Board of Governors. The value to the public is assured by these reviews. The Cleveland Clinic is more than a business. It is, in effect, a public trust.

Having spent my career at the Cleveland Clinic, beginning as a fellow in Thoracic and Cardiac Surgery, becoming chairman of that department in 1975 and chief executive in 1989, I share Dr. Mayo's thoughts and passion. Many of my impressions are drawn from my academic life. I would like to emphasize that the lessons, observations and conclusions from my experience are not *ex cathedra*. However, I must also declare that I am distinctly partial to the Cleveland Clinic model of medicine – a not-for-profit group practice, where salaried specialists collaborate on patient care, enhanced by research and education. The founders of the Cleveland Clinic believed that the staff model would underscore cooperation rather than competition, and guarantee an altruistic practice of medicine.

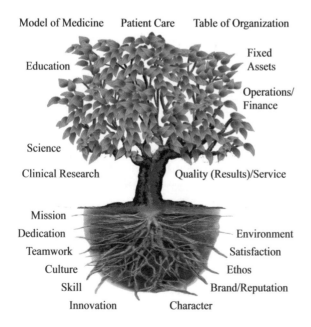

I would compare the Cleveland Clinic to a large tree with a wide canopy and many branches; the tree needs maximum light and nourishment to grow and to bear fruit – some years more than others. Above the ground are the measurable essentials of the organization: patient care; our staff model; the table of organization; our academic performance, in the form of education, grants, publications, discoveries; fixed assets; operations and finance; outcomes and other quality indicators.

Below the surface are the roots, the characteristics that are less measurable. These are the intangibles: mission; dedication; teamwork; culture; skill; innovation; character; brand and reputation; ethos; satisfaction; environment. *Ethos* means honesty, integrity, morality and reliability. Ethos is responsible for many of the academic center's intangible assets: reputation, brand equity, capacity for innovation, advancing the mission – none of these appear on the balance sheet, but are intangible assets that distinguish one institution from another. These values, norms and beliefs reflect the organization's culture. These are the roots from which we derive our reputation.± Our intellectual capital is the main source of academic performance and is our principal source of future revenue. Somehow profit in medicine became a dirty word. As anyone who has ever managed a business will tell you, if an enterprise is not profitable, it can't deliver good service. The purposes of profitability are to 1) keep the mission intact; 2) provide workforce security; 3) invest in research and education; and 4) pay off the debt.

In the event that anyone had the idea to later convert the medical organization into a for-profit venture, the Cleveland Clinic founders took precautions in the charter. Dr. Crile described the incorporation… "Should the successors seek to convert it into an institution solely for profit or personal exploitations, or otherwise materially alter the purpose for which it was organized, the whole property shall be turned over to one of the institutions of learning or science of this city."[21]†

A strong academic enterprise requires that the key executives, all staff and trustees value science and education as complementary and as important as clinical medicine is to the enterprise. The interlocking groups at the Cleveland Clinic during my experience there included a Board of Governors, the majority of whom were elected physicians and scientists who set policy; a division (now institutes) executive committee, also composed largely of physicians, which implemented plans; and

---

±   Brand is a "customer-centric" concept that focuses on what we have promised to our customers (patients) and what the commitment means to them. Reputation is a "company-centric" concept that indicates credibility and respect that an organization has among a broad set of constituencies including personnel, regulators, media, community, and patients. Brand is about relevancy and differentiation (with respect to the customer), and reputation is about legitimacy of the organization with respect to a wide range of stakeholder groups. (Ettenson R, Knowles J. *Don't Confuse Reputation with Brand.* MIT Sloan Mgmt Rev: Winter 2008: 49 (2); 19-21)

†   The Cleveland Clinic is a not-for-profit, tax-exempt Ohio corporation. No part of the net income or assets of the Cleveland Clinic are distributed to its members, trustees, officers or other persons as there are no shareholder or partnership interests in the Cleveland Clinic. Therefore, no one "owns" the Cleveland Clinic. Excess revenues over expenses are reinvested to carry out its corporate purposes, which include the treatment of the sick, the operation of a hospital and related research and education activities. If the Cleveland Clinic were to liquidate, its net assets would be distributed to other tax-exempt organizations as determined by the Board of Trustees or the Cuyahoga County Court of Common Pleas.

an administrative group, which dealt with operational management and included the chiefs of staff, regional practice, medical operations, finance, health affairs, insurance contracting and human resources – some of whom were physicians. There were also physicians on the Board of Trustees, which had the fiduciary responsibility and oversight described earlier. All of these committees and boards were interactive in planning and guidance, and were ultimately responsible for the results of the health system. In succession planning, the governors and trustees participated in the selection of a new chief executive. All of these committees and boards were involved in strategic planning and were responsible for the results of the health system. Selected governors and trustees participated in the appointment of a new chief executive.

It is expected that each governance member must represent the mission of the organization: "To the better care of the sick, investigation of their problems, and to further education of those who serve."[22] Boards must exemplify what is good and right about the organization. Its members cannot misrepresent any facts at the meetings or discuss any confidential material because it could jeopardize the entire organization. Integrity, collegiality, objectivity, ability to listen, intellect, management experience, and loyalty are said to be the characteristics of good board members. To me, all of these are given. What every integrated system needs are ideas, participation, and understanding of the changes in medicine, research, and the market. Trustees add pragmatism and focus. Trustees should be people who are committed to healthcare and its success, men and women with experience in business, education, research, and management. Debate is healthy. Progress has to be measured and excellence is sustained by unity of purpose. These meetings are not séances; this is a business, although it is a unique kind of business.

There can be problems in any hospital governance: 1) not understanding or having objectives; 2) exclusion from decision making; 3) not knowing strategy, and therefore not having the ability to implement strategy; 4) conflict within the board because of weak or indecisive leadership.[23]

Carl Wasmuth, M.D., Chairman, Board of Governors (Jan. 1969-Sept. 1976), summed it up: "The evolution of our present system was not along an easy path. A method had to be found whereby freedom of professional activity could be guaranteed within the rigid fiscal controls dictated by good administration. …Today, the Board of Governors decides all professional policy of the entire complex, and directs the implementation by the administrative officers, subject to review and ratification by the Board of Trustees. The advice and counsel of all echelons are welded into the decisions of the Board of Governors. Thus we, in fact, follow the admonition of the founders '…to act as a unit.'"[24]

ACADEMIC PARTNERSHIPS

There has been a slowly declining interest in biomedical research among residents, fellows and young faculty across the United States, ceding more research to full-time Ph.D. scientists.[25-27] While the absolute number of physician-scientists has held steady, they are an aging cohort welcoming fewer and fewer new members over the past two decades.[28] The percentage of physicians actually engaged in research has fallen from a peak of 4.6 percent in 1985 to 1.8 percent in 2003. Although there seems to be a renewed interest in research careers by medical students, the national population of M.D.-Ph.D. matriculates was still fewer than 600 in 2005, or 4 percent of the total medical student population.

This finding is attributed to personal debt and possibly to the composition of the admission committee. Since there are declining numbers of physician-scientists among medical school faculties, committees often lack the same phenotype as potential physician-scientists. On interview day, every admissions committee should tell its applicants: We want to teach you to be great doctors. But this is a minimal expectation. We also want you to think about what else you might do for the profession and for human health beyond the individual patient; some of you should consider medical science as a career.[29]

Academicians at Case Western Reserve University (CWRU) saw the advantages of a medical school partnership with the Cleveland Clinic. In 2002, the Cleveland Clinic opened a new medical school in partnership with the University, dedicated to the training and mentoring of physician-investigators. During my time in office, CWRU provided the structure and the partnership for this new medical school. Reality was made possible by a $100 million gift by the great humanitarian Al Lerner and his family, who had previously endowed the Lerner Research Institute. Mr. Lerner understood the approaching crisis in biomedical science. He saw it as an opportunity to create a unique legacy and to perform a signal service to science and medicine. The Cleveland Clinic Lerner College of Medicine of Case Western Reserve University is a landmark in the history of medical education, only one of two U.S. medical schools that opened in the past quarter century and the only one solely devoted to the education of physician-scientists. Al Lerner knew the value of an investment and he knew that contribution to science and education was the best investment in the world. Henry Ward Beecher said that, "In this world, it is not what we take up, but what we give up that makes us rich."

The Cleveland Clinic Lerner College of Medicine combined the legacies of two major research institutions, each with its own history of innovation. The five-year program replaces lectures with a unique problem-based curriculum devised by Cleveland Clinic staff physicians and scientists. Its objective is to nurture its students' passion for scientific inquiry and to give them the skills and lifelong learning habits that will lead to successful careers as physician-investigators.

The unique elements of the new College are: 1) each of the 32 students in every class has a physician mentor and a research mentor; 2) each student prepares a thesis based on independent research; 3) all students are exposed to a curriculum including epidemiology, statistics and a broad range of research seminars; 4) a clinical skills center uses videotaping and simulators for primary care training; 5) a double helix curriculum includes nutrition, prevention, ethics and law, diversity, healthcare financing and organization – these components are integrated into problem-based learning coupled with interdisciplinary basic science and research courses; and 6) in addition, there is minimal debt burden for all students in order for them to pursue academic career paths.

In 2008, the Cleveland Clinic announced that the Lerner College of Medicine of Case Western Reserve University will provide all incoming students with full-tuition scholarships in an effort to reduce post-graduate debt and attract more students to the field of academic medicine.[30±] It thus became the first U.S. medical school to forego tuition for all students. The students have to pay for living expenses, equipment, and books. Other medical schools offer tuition subsidy or partial scholarships.

TRADITION

Tradition has received a bad name because it is confused with conventionality. Tradition is not the opposite of innovation. Tradition is in the roots of innovation when it provides stability, a good working environment, and inspiration. We honor tradition so that the staff can know the history of the organization, appreciate the founders' premise, understand the culture and visualize how the medical center evolved. Traditions are passed down from person to person and generation to generation. Our traditions help define the culture of the medical organization. In our case, the core of our tradition was physician leadership and teamwork.

The history of the organization includes the important milestones in medical and scientific advancement. How did the institution grow and what were the key elements in the formation of the academic enterprise? The great doctors, present and former residents, major clinical accomplishments, investigators who made significant contributions to science – all these people and events depict traditions in the evolving health system.

±   In round numbers, by the time they graduate, including premedical debts, students owe on average $150,000, but it varies widely up to $300,000. The question is: What is the effect of educational debt on the choice of careers? And how does the debt burden relate to a return on investment? (Steinbrook R. *Medical Student Debt – Is There A Limit?* N Engl J Med 2008: 359; (25): 2629-32).

Traditions can be illustrated in various ways throughout the organization, including permanent displays at a selected site on the campus. We were fortunately able to renovate a lovely old mansion on our campus, and use it to display some artifacts of our history. The purpose is to honor the great physicians, scientists, nurses and notable leaders who were responsible for the achievements in their respective eras. One may show examples of hallmark scientific papers and pictorial essays that demonstrate the regional and national growth. Many of the intangibles of our legacy are reflected by these exhibits, which are featured during social occasions and often open to the public. Donors especially appreciate the story of the organization where many of them have received care and compassion.

A great medical organization is more than just a place to work. It is a place to be inspired. Knowing what your organization has contributed to the community in the past can motivate achievement in the present and indicate the course for the future.

THE ANNUAL PROFESSIONAL REVIEW

Medicine can never be better than the quality of its physicians. The Cleveland Clinic has conducted annual professional reviews of each individual staff member for more than 40 years. These reviews are more than a ritual and are modified periodically. If an annual review is a tool for institutional renewal, it can't be static. The reviewer is invited to ask the reviewee, "What can I do to help you be more successful?"[31] It is an opportunity for each member of the staff to formally express themselves and to balance the expectations of the Cleveland Clinic against their personal performance. It is a way for staff to measure the administration and vice versa. Performance appraisals serve as the basis for determining salary adjustments.

Before annual reviews were taken seriously, the old era of medicine just involved good doctors showing up. You saw your patients, worked hard, put in some long hours and found the time to study, write, teach and lecture. Most of the time, individuals were oblivious to the support necessary behind that professional lifestyle. Physician complaints arose only if that support failed or interfered with space or efficiency. The new era of medicine is relentless in its pressure to deliver ever-higher quality coordinated care, including doing more with less. We want the staff to have an uncompromising and unwavering commitment to quality. Today, each physician and department is expected to exceed past clinical performance and still find time for academic pursuits. Each staff physician should understand that he or she, individually and collectively, is in charge of cost, quality and service.

In the past, the annual reviews concentrated on eight areas: patient care, education, research, administration, national and other external activities, patient satisfaction, an evaluation of leadership and collegiality. More recently, reviews evolved from a subjective conversation to objective evaluation. In addition to the above, department leadership is also judged by the performance of a particular residency program on the basis of USMLE 1 and 2 scores, peer-reviewed scientific publications by residents and staff, specialty board pass rates, department-sponsored CME courses, teaching scores compiled by residents, and program accreditation status. For patient care, we were interested in how well the department progressed in scorecard metrics and continuous quality improvement. The interactions between leadership and the support staff were evaluated. Access, patient satisfaction, and new patients became increasingly important. What process innovations were enacted in the department during the past year? How was clinical capacity managed? There are many questions to be asked and all are modified over time.

As our medical center staff grew in size, and more recently the department/ division structure has reorganized into institutes, the conduct of the annual review will doubtless be modified. However, the department chair's interview and report is the key to a valuable interchange. This can't be an entirely freewheeling process. A format should be provided to cover more than a ventilation of grievances. It's more than a discussion of productivity; it's about overall performance, including the solicitation of ideas.

A key management principle is that all components of income, such as clinical quality, productivity, academic achievements, and where applicable, leadership performance, are evaluated. A high-performance physician who publishes high-impact papers may reach a high income. Award-winning teachers, outstanding physicians, clinical investigators, and laboratory-based scientists can all earn very competitive salaries. The busy practitioners with modest academic achievements should also be rewarded financially for their revenue generation and quality medicine.

There is a tendency for executives who are responsible for physician compensation to give fixed-percentage raises to individual doctors in a department. I fought that, often unsuccessfully. The great doctors should make more than their average colleagues. Treat everyone fairly, but don't treat everyone the same in regard to compensation. Motivate the motivators. The same advice applies to budgets and salaries in bad times. The worst action is to cut all departments by the same percent. This indiscriminate practice will destroy morale and may compromise strategic initiatives.

The annual professional review is an important index of performance. All of the objective measurements are part of a formula to reward success. Those whose reviews fall short must be given explicit suggestions for improvement. The department chair should provide counsel and follow-up. Mentoring at the department level is part of leadership.

Firing a staff physician should be a highly unusual occurrence. In our staff model, each clinical doctor, scientist, and executive, top to bottom, was given an annual appointment letter to be signed by the individual. If the staff person did not meet the criteria for continued privileges (reappointment), he was told so and necessary arrangements were made for his departure. These events were rare but were handled professionally and, depending on the circumstances, job counseling and support were provided. We did not numerically rank the professional staff except to justify salary adjustment. Our standards were high – everyone was expected to be above the nationwide average and quite a few were exceptional performers.

What do we expect of you, the doctor? We expect each of you to be more than just a good doctor. We expect you to be an outstanding physician, to strive consistently for excellence and to build your practice. We want you to be thoughtful and understand that results are important and that satisfied patients are the best advertisement. More than prescriptions, medicine involves communication, tolerance, flexibility, listening, hard work and a passion for the practice. Maimonides defined the great doctor as... "very accomplished, whose knowledge has been verified, and whose experience has been attested."[32] The knowledge, skill and judgment of the physician are still the greatest determinants of the quality of healthcare.

NOT-FOR-PROFIT STATUS

Academic medical centers have grown into major economic players. They are likely to be the largest employer in the region, a major tax-exempt business and a landowner. Thus medical organizations, like other large businesses, have to follow a bewildering set of rules for environmental protection, occupational safety, hiring and firing practices, wages, overtime and fringe benefits, workers' compensation, and affirmative action—not to mention sensitive and time-consuming negotiations with community planning boards and local citizen groups. This complexity is a "large order for a collection of doctor scholars."[33]

Recently, not-for-profit medical centers have come under attack by opportunistic politicians looking for something new to tax. State law establishes real estate tax exemption for a 501(c)3 charitable institution because such institutions provide a well-defined community benefit.[±] This benefit includes participation in Medicare and Medicaid, the provision of graduate and postgraduate education, research, community education, public health, 24-hour emergency departments, and charity care (in addition to absorbing a great deal of bad debt). It may also include the

±   Approximately 1.5 million organizations are certified by the Internal Revenue Service as satisfying requirements for tax exemption under sections 501(c)3 and 501(c)4 of the Federal Tax Code, which defines charitable and mutual-benefit organizations.

development of a communitywide healthcare system and overall positive economic impact (jobs, local purchasing, payroll taxes, etc.). Not only does a medical center add to the quality of life in a city, but when the academic medical center collaborates with a local university on clinical care and research, it can boost regional economic development.

Tax-exempt hospitals are under more scrutiny today because many believe that this exemption provides a screen for "for-profit" activities, including those outside healthcare.[34] The Internal Revenue Service is investigating how much hospitals measure, bill and report uncompensated care, how they report community benefit programs and how much they pay for executive compensation. In addition to accurately defining and recording charity care, hospitals need to review their billing practices for low income and self-pay patients, audit physician arrangements (payments to doctors), and account for research payments. Princeton economist Uwe Reinhardt has argued for eliminating hospital tax exemptions while allowing hospitals to credit back the real cost of community benefits that they provide against their tax liability.[35] If that happens, some medical centers would get a check from the government.

In a very real sense, the academic medical enterprise is "owned" by the community it serves. It is a valuable asset because it elevates the standards of medical care and attracts highly educated, talented people to work and live in the region – reversing brain drain in some cities. Although the medical center doesn't pay property taxes, it generates substantial payroll taxes. Staff and employees are often enthusiastic community volunteers. All of this is in addition to the institution's basic function of providing healthcare to all who go there. Today, academic medical centers have the additional benefit of serving as generators of innovation, incubators of new companies, and magnets for established biomedical enterprises. Throughout America, the research and technology sectors have grown at twice the rate of the economy. Biotechnology is one of the best wealth generators and provides the greatest prospects for new jobs. Academic medical center governance may wish to quantify their community benefits by conducting an economic impact study and sharing it with the community.[±] This type of study documents the reservoir of good work.

PHILANTHROPY

An academic medical center's success in attracting charitable dollars is a measure of what it has contributed to the community. But more so, such income is critical to renewing and creating infrastructure and supporting efforts in research and

---

±   Our 2003 economic impact study was conducted by Angelou Economics, 2801 Via Fortuna, Suite 430, Austin, TX 78746. (www.angeloueconomics.com)

education. With a shrinking reimbursement dollar, such philanthropic investment becomes even more vital to institutional growth and development.

To give you facts about philanthropy in America, here are some significant figures. In 2005, nationwide voluntary contributions to all causes totaled approximately $260 *billion*. Of this amount, 83.2 percent was given by individuals, 11.5 percent by foundations and, 5.3 percent by corporations. In 2005, there were 68,000 foundations of all kinds controlling about a half-trillion dollars and making grants totaling nearly $34 billion. Approximately 70 percent of all foundation assets are controlled by 2 percent of foundations, with 46 foundations having assets over $1 billion and another 64 with assets between $500 million and $1 billion.[36]

An excellent development officer taught us that professional fundraisers are not there primarily to raise money by themselves. Their most important role is to teach *us* how to raise money. This is something to keep in mind when organizing institutional advancement. Although the person in charge of philanthropy helps to identify potential donors, it is up to the chief executive, the executive team, physicians, educators, and scientists to participate and collaborate in fundraising. Although many universities have fund development activities reporting to the chief financial officer, healthcare philanthropic activities are better organized through the chief executive. There is a lot of competition out there. Most not-for-profit hospitals now understand the importance of philanthropy. At one time, a third of our construction financing came from philanthropy. In years ahead, income in the academic medical sector will rely even more heavily on donors.

A lot of people, especially grateful patients, want to give money. They are searching for a way to give something back. But why give specifically to a medical organization? Why not do as Bill Gates did and target your donation for global poverty or to eradicate specific diseases in undeveloped areas? The answer is that a strong medical organization makes for a strong community. In addition to healthcare, medical education and scientific investigation, academic medical centers figure prominently in public education. Some donors want to fund a new idea or to honor someone in the family or a friend. Others will respond with matching gifts for a specific cause, and many donate to find a cure for a specific disease.[±] Eli Broad, a billionaire businessman who has given more than $650 million dollars for medical research, art museums and urban education, said, "I think there is a

---

±   On a visit to Israel as mayor of West Berlin, Willy Brandt (1913-1992) was invited to view the great new Mann auditorium in Tel Aviv. Having expressed his appreciation of Israel naming the concert hall for Thomas Mann, the German writer, Brandt was politely corrected by his host. The hall was actually named for a certain Frederic Mann of Philadelphia. "What did he ever write?" exclaimed Brandt. "A check," came the reply. (Fadiman C, Bernard A. *Bartlett's Book of Anecdotes*, Boston, MA: Little, Brown & Co., 2000, pp. 75-6)

multiplier effect. What smart entrepreneurial philanthropists and their foundations do is get greater value for how they invest their money than if the government were doing it. I believe the public benefit is significantly greater than the tax benefit an individual receives."[37]

In his essay on wealth, J.P. Morgan argued that it was morally acceptable to become rich; what was reprehensible was to hang onto it – "The man who dies thus rich dies disgraced."[38] There are as many motives for philanthropy as there are donors. Some, of course, want their name on a building or a department or a named professorship, while others donate without expecting recognition. What amazes me is that so many people give money but never know what happens to it. They don't manage their gift or request follow-up on how the money is being used. Accountability is necessary to assure a return on philanthropic investment. Grant money that is part of a multiyear gift should be terminated unless its use meets the expectations of the donor. As leader of a recipient institution, one thing you don't want to hear is, "If the original donors were still alive, they would be turning over in their graves."[39] What is even more astonishing is that some people have no charitable gifts in their estate planning. They must prefer to contribute more to the government. It must be easier to make money than it is to give it away.

John D. Rockefeller said, "Giving is investing."[40] Prospective donors must understand that science and education is the single greatest investment opportunity in America. All progress in our quality of life depends on scientific research in one form or another. So far, medicine has fallen behind other not-for-profit sectors in cultivating philanthropy. According to a 2004 study by the Center on Philanthropy at Indiana University, 18.5 percent of all revenue for higher education comes from philanthropy compared with only 1.5 percent in hospitals.[41] It is said that physicians are not very good fundraisers.[42] But fundraising requires patience and practice. Incredibly, some doctors are reluctant to ask for money because they believe it will impair the physician-patient relationship. Clinical or scientific staff may not be able to see beyond their own interests and resist participation in general fundraising. Intervention by the chief executive and the development officer can help physicians and scientists solicit contributions on behalf of the organization as a whole, or for that staff member's own specialty or department. Part of that process is to make sure that the staff understands the importance of solvency, whether it's building or preserving. Progress always involves new programs, new construction, technological advances and supporting research and education. Everybody can be a good fundraiser. Publicly recognize the donor… and the solicitor.

A decade ago, I had the privilege of being involved in what promised to be a uniquely interesting philanthropic project with Al Lerner, who was the president of our Board of Trustees. The founder of credit card giant MBNA, Mr. Lerner was a genius beyond finance and was greatly admired by all of us. We called our plan the Archimedes project, because we believed it could lever our clinical and research enterprises to new levels of achievement. ("Give me a lever long enough and a fulcrum on which to place it, and I shall move the world.") The project would begin with a billion-dollar gift: $500 million for a life sciences research foundation at Cleveland Clinic, and $500 million to go directly into clinical departments for patient care and clinical research – contingent on matching grants. The purpose was to optimize all clinical services to expand value-based medicine. The intent was strategic, to revitalize both our clinical and research enterprises. The recipients of these gifts would leverage this discretionary money for top-to-bottom innovation. It was essentially a permanent matching fund for progress. Eureka!

FIGURE 3.1

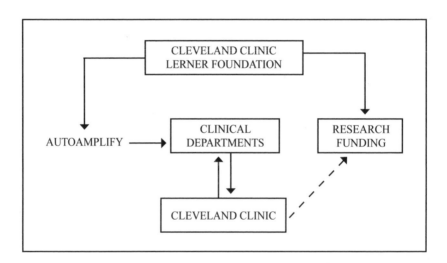

Archimedes seed money would guarantee research funding in perpetuity. By design, it would reinforce all departments, strengthen the academic mission, and attract matching donations. The interest on Mr. Lerner's billion-dollar gift would defray certain biomedical research costs and strategically fund clinical departments. On the research side, these monies would include initiatives in genomics/proteomics, medical informatics and stem cell research, along with money to attract and fund selected new biotechnology. Since medical center profitability tends to be cyclical and state funding is often diverted and generally diffused, a foundation to fund innovation across the organization would preserve and advance the mission. We even calculated the return on investment after hypothetical grants to each area of specialty medicine and programmatic research.

Adverse events spoil many plans, and Mr. Lerner's untimely death from brain cancer stopped Archimedes before it started. However, the concept is still valid. The viability of this method persists: Money fuels innovation and discovery, and that equals leverage for progress. If centers understood that matching funds were available to implement innovation, we still believe it would further stimulate creative thinking and attract further donations. Thoughtful investment is indispensable for academic success.

THE ACADEMIC HEALTHCARE SYSTEM

Multi-hospital systems used to have a record of being poorly managed, of breaking promises and offering no competitive advantage. The exceptions were the proprietary hospital systems, which were generally managed better than academic centers. The financially successful systems, whether for-profit or not, were those that were able to coordinate support functions across their operating units. The healthcare delivery system is now entering a new geographic dimension. The demand for services has led to the diffusion of specialty care out of the city and into the suburbs. Today, more and more people want to stay close to home for their outpatient and even inpatient care. It follows that academic medical centers recognized this community interest, established satellite clinics and acquired community hospitals. The formation of a new and complementary healthcare delivery system provides a continuum of care for the surrounding region. (More detail in chapter 10)

The objectives in creating a healthcare system are to advance community medicine and improve the practice environment for the network doctors. In general, the community hospital staff is composed of non-salaried physicians in private practice who are less aligned with the hospital compared with the academic physicians and scientists. The community hospital department structure is headed by elected chairmen often with defined tenure. Physician input is inconsistent. Quality is less easily improved. The community medical staff is mostly nonacademic and may not feel any close emotional bond to the academic mission. The staff is more used to competition than cooperation. Nonetheless there is growing recognition about the advantages of alignment. Rather than imposing rules, other than quality guidelines, the best approach is to work on alignment by communication, soliciting physician input, providing necessary equipment, building common (integrated) information systems, and improving the facilities.

Try to develop a collegiality in your system that is born of respect. Good relations between salaried staff and private physicians need constant cultivation. One of the biggest mistakes academic medical centers make is buying large numbers of physician practices – a huge credit negative. Money can't buy friends. But you get a better class of enemy.[43] As Warren Buffett said, "A fool and his money are soon invited everywhere."[±]

Academic centers and some larger hospitals are moving toward or have already adopted a staff model, which means that physicians generally practice in one location. We know that the moment doctors get in their cars, productivity falls. To restructure the organization, some hospitals are trying to eliminate the department/ division hierarchy by creating centers of excellence or institutes that unify medical and surgical departments. It has more potential in some specialties than others. The success of this endeavor depends on leadership of the new entity, the specialties involved, acceptance by the staff, and where they report and to whom. Structure determines overhead. Flatten the organization wherever possible. The risk is to turn small silos into big silos. Avoid a completely new geologic formation until thoroughly vetted.

THOUGHTS ON ACADEMIC MEDICINE

It is clear that the academic healthcare sector is becoming increasingly diverse and evolving in scope and purpose.[44] Visibility alone in tertiary care cannot prevail. The public is weighing in on what it expects from a great academic medical center. *U.S. News & World Report* uses equally weighted criteria in evaluating the best referral hospitals: clinical performance, specialty by specialty based on volumes and outcomes for selected procedures; peer evaluation, which mainly reflects the reputation of the physicians, their leadership in specialty societies, scientific publications, research grants, and a record of innovation; hospital infrastructure, which includes technology as well as nursing metrics such as nurse-patient ratios and Magnet status. In addition to the rankings, there are a growing number of report cards that evaluate hospitals and doctors in practice. Consumers are demanding to know quality information, and this will only increase as people pay more out of pocket. They are interested in transparent prices, quality and service. Angie's List and Consumer Reports have joined the list of rating services as have many health insurers.

It's great to be ranked nationally, but whether the academic health center is recognized or not, the important questions are these: Does the organization have both high volumes and the highest published favorable outcomes? Are scientists attracting more NIH grants each year? Does the scientific endeavor relate to diagnosis

---

[±]   Visitors to Warren Buffett's offices on the 14th floor of a plain-vanilla building on the edge of downtown Omaha are greeted by a small porcelain plaque inscribed with those words.

or treatment of specific conditions? Are the medical school professors rated highly by their medical students? Is the medical school performing in accordance with its mission? Interestingly, not every organization that is nationally ranked is even the best in its region. Is yours?

To address these questions, we wrote a credo to live by.± We believed that the *singular purpose of the Cleveland Clinic was to benefit humanity through the efficient, effective, and ethical practice of medicine, by advancing scientific investigation and medical education, by maintaining the highest standard of quality, and by honoring creativity and innovation. Each member of the organization is a guardian of the enterprise and is responsible for assuring that its name is synonymous with the finest healthcare in the world.*

To paraphrase an old saying, fame is what you can take from a great medical organization – character is what you give back.† Our mission was to assure that the academic organization should thrive far longer than the biological lives of its current staff. That will happen as long as the highest priority is patient care.

My wife, Dr. Bernadine Healy, wrote a classic essay on "The Art of Medical Care"[45] in which she summed up the art of medicine in four principles: Mastery. Individuality. Humanity. Morality.

> *Mastery* is expertise and wisdom as much as knowledge and creative thinking.

> *Individuality* is patient-focused and means searching for unique patient characteristics that may be at odds with established dogma.

> *Humanity* can be best explained by a quote by Dr. Charles H. Mayo: "When I am your doctor, I try to imagine the kind of doctor I'd like if I were you. Then I try to be that kind of doctor."

> *Morality* applies to the foundation of the doctor-patient relationship. The patient "turns over a measure of privacy and control to the doctor only because of need, creating an asymmetric partnership that demands physician integrity."

±   "Credo" is the first word in the Apostles' and Nicene Creeds. It means "I believe." J. Still wrote in his 1587 "Hymn agst. Spanish Armada": "We will not change owre Credo for Pope, not boke, nor bell; And yf the Devil come himself, wee'll houned him back to Hell." This sentiment speaks to the intrinsic, pervasive, and permanent characteristic of a credo. (Schwartz SI. *Credo, Conduct, and Credibility.* Bull Am Coll Surg 1997: 82(12); 8-13)

†   Fame is what you have taken, Character's what you give. (Taylor B. *The Poetical Works of Bayard Taylor.* The Riverside Press. Cambridge, MA: Houghton Mifflin Company 1864, p. 318.)

We know that professional interdependencies in a good medical organization make the individual physician wiser, more efficient and more secure. Physicians in a high-performance clinical environment act together and yet remain remarkably independent. It is this collective genius of an organization that differentiates one medical center from another. The practice of medicine will always be a cooperative movement of physicians on behalf of society. At the Cleveland Clinic we knew that every year we had to grow stronger in science, education, clinical acumen and the organized delivery of healthcare. These measures constitute a commonwealth of intellect, a republic of ideas, and the best example of physician-led healthcare.

CHAPTER 4

HEALTHCARE TRENDS, POLICIES AND PROPOSED REFORMS

None of us can have as much as we want of all the things we want.

— Justice Oliver Wendell Holmes
Collected Legal Papers
Harcourt, Brace and Company, NY,
1920

In the United States, we have many fortuities: incentives for entrepreneurialism, free market opportunities, superb graduate education, support for the disadvantaged, widespread philanthropy, volunteerism and a liberal democracy. Compared with the rest of the world, we have a low rate of unemployment, a mobile labor force and good returns on our investments in science and technology.[1] We have an intense spirit of freedom that stimulates competitiveness, ingenuity, and individualism. Our culture encourages free will, free people and free enterprise. Our pluralistic approach to healthcare and our support of medical science are unique to America. American medicine is one of the best examples of our culture and is an index of our civilization.[2]

Medical care in America has many positive attributes: minimal waiting time, choice of well-trained physicians, unsurpassed medical research and leadership in technology development. Every major American city has a hospital equivalent to the best in the world. Unfortunately, questions of finance overshadow the good news about American medicine. Our predicament is more than an entitlement issue or a debate about universal coverage. The problem in paying for healthcare and everything surrounding it is one of the major public financial challenges of our time. The large presence of the government that pays for an increasing share of U.S. healthcare also imposes costly regulations and unfunded mandates, which complicates the fiscal dilemma. Pluralism will be tested in the name of saving the economy.

Public programs now spend more than they take in. Pete Peterson calls it the vending machine government, which underwrites consumption for entitled interest groups and borrows from our children.[3±] From 2000 to 2005, federal expenditure for pensions and healthcare rose from $600 billion to $950 billion annually.[4] The unfunded fiscal commitments grow at the rate of $2-3 trillion each year and have soared from $20 trillion in 2000 to $46 trillion in 2005[5]... and the effects of aging on entitlements hasn't started yet.

Despite these numbers, we still devote rhetoric and resources to promoting a sense of entitlement. In other words: Ask not what you can do for your country, rather demand of it what it can do for you.[6] Healthcare is spoken of as a basic human right, like freedom of speech, freedom of assembly, and the right to petition the government. This sounds good but ignores the fact that human rights, as conceived by the founding fathers, are freedoms of action – not to claims of economic goods and services.[7] In other words, freedom to believe, to be free, to vote, to pursue happiness – not what you are "entitled" to possess.

THE FINANCIAL SITUATION

About 1 percent of America's sick population accounts for 30 percent of all healthcare expenditures. Five percent account for nearly 60 percent of spending. Extensive use of medical technology, new (and heavily advertised) pharmaceuticals, a changing mix of diseases, our affluence, decadence, and cost-concealing, employer-based insurance (the "moral hazard") all drive the demand for healthcare. Unfortunately, devices and pharmaceuticals are not subject to normal consumer price constraints because of insurance. Newhouse summed it up 15 years ago: "... the cause of increasing costs appears to be increased capabilities of medicine and is common to developed countries."[8] Specifically, our expenditures relate to overutilization, high pricing, amenities and administrative costs.[9] The medical training and the culture in the U.S. frequently lead to the application of high-level technology from cradle to grave. Because something *can* be done – something *must* be done.

±　"Anybody who can read and write and doesn't run for office, knows how to balance the budget." (Peter Drucker)

When President Johnson signed the Medicare Act in 1965, he reassured voters by saying that "an extra $500 *million*" of new spending would pose "no problem." In 2007, Medicare expenditure was $431 *billion* (HHS, 2007). Government payments for healthcare have expanded to 45 percent of total health spending,[10, 11] and they are projected to reach 50 percent by 2016.[12] By 2050 Medicare and Medicaid spending alone is estimated to reach 20 percent of the GDP.[13±] Our country's financial health depends, to a great extent, on the growth rate of per capita medical costs. If we continue along at the same rate, healthcare spending will squeeze out the majority of other federal programs. In view of these projections, beware of unfunded promises.

Future Medicare payments will be substantially affected by the increase in the absolute *number* of elderly people even more than their longevity.[14] We are near a negative cash flow for Medicare. Social Security will follow in ten years. But what is often unaccounted for are the differences in personal health spending across the country. Some variations are attributed to disparities in age and income, the number of doctors, and practice styles. Other factors include private insurance coverage, the generosity of public programs and mix of services used by a given population.[15] We need to study the more efficient regions and apply the lessons to higher cost areas.[†]

Despite escalating cost, the strengths of the American healthcare system cannot be ignored. Much of our outlay relates to real progress. Since World War II, Americans have spent a rising share of total economic resources on health and have enjoyed substantially longer lives as a result.[16] In the 1950s there were as many people in the hospital for hemorrhoids and hernia repair as there were for heart disease and cancer. In the past half-century, the mortality for cardiovascular disease has dropped by more than a third. During the 20th century, science and medicine added 26 years to our lifespan. If one lives to be 65, there is a 70 percent chance of living an additional 20 or more years. Technological and pharmaceutical advances for myocardial infarction, low birth weight infants, depression and cataracts have shown benefit well worth the cost.[17] The outstanding advances in healthcare over the past century have been as valuable as all other sources of economic growth combined.[18] However, there still is

---

±   For a detailed discussion of CBO's long-term projection of healthcare spending, see Congressional Budget Office, *The Long-Term Outlook for Health Care Spending*, November 2007. In the CBO December 2008 report, the increase in public spending is attributed to increases in per capita cost per case rather than the number of beneficiaries.

†   There are geographic variations in per capita spending on non-healthcare items, such as housing, food and transportation. And there are equally strong variations in rates of cancer, heart disease and diabetes, which are not easily explained. Interestingly, variation in spending also applies to the VA Healthcare System. Their variation is similar to that in Medicare, despite the fact that the VA system uses an explicit allocation formula to distribute funds to regions (*Geographic Variation in Health Care Spending*. Congress of the United States, Congressional Budget Office. February 2008)

a social gradient that relates to premature mortality.[19] The disadvantaged consistently suffer from more health problems than those who are better off. Low income, poor education and the occupations that go along with those conditions are all predictors of high mortality.[±]

Public and private budgets cannot support this growth in medical expenditure. Medicare spending has slowed in recent years because of changes in payment policy,[20] but the short-term lulls are expected to be replaced by cyclical surges. The system is not, as many have said, riddled with fraud and abuse. Instead, it is payment and regulatory complexity that add to expenses. The federal government and its numerous branches are involved in monitoring cost effectiveness (where they have a clear stake) in manpower, medical education, allied health, healthcare technology, and nearly every other field related to healthcare. If you give a small boy a hammer, suddenly everything he encounters needs pounding.[†] As Eugene McCarthy reflected, "The only thing that saves us from bureaucracy is its inefficiency."[21]

Congress has added to the problem over the years by trying to achieve universal coverage by means of very complex regulations.[§] Failed government regulation leads to more government regulations, many of which add cost. Rather than controlling monopoly, regulation creates monopoly; rather than promoting the public interest, regulation rewards private interests; rather than encouraging operating efficiency, regulation condones managerial slack; rather than reducing prices, regulation raises costs.[22]

Government regulation is necessary to guarantee a certain level of patient safety and to limit fraud. But most government directives are complicated, and compliance places a large and unnecessary financial burden on the healthcare sector. Ideally, Congress would undertake a periodic review of healthcare regulations, to debride

±   The five illnesses with largest contributions to rising cost are heart, pulmonary, mental disorders, cancer and hypertension. Of those five, mental disorders have the greatest increase in treated prevalence – about 50 percent more people treated between 1987 and 2000. The increased population in each disease category has increased about 20-30 percent in that time. Barr DA. *Introduction to U.S. Health Policy. The Organization, Financing, and Delivery of Health Care in America.* Johns Hopkins University Press, 2007.

†   In the present crisis, government is not the solution to our problem; government is the problem. From time to time, we've been tempted to believe that society has become too complex to be managed by self-rule, that government by an elite group is superior to government for, by and of the people. Well, if no one among us is capable of governing himself then who among us has the capacity to govern someone else? ...We hear much of special interest groups. Well, our concern must be for the special interest group that has been too long neglected... "we the people," this breed called Americans. (Ronald Reagan, First Inaugural Address, 1981)

§   For a good review of past health policy, read Etheredge L. *On the Archeology of Health Care Policy. Periods and Paradigms.* 1975-2000 Robert Woods Johnson Health Policy Fellowships Program. Institute of Medicine, Washington, D.C., March 2001.

the excess and resist new intrusions. Current and proposed directives should be subject to thoughtful evaluation. Do they restrict competition? Do they require excessive documentation and shift costs to providers? Do they constitute a barrier to efficiency? Are they irrational, political or anti-profit? Congress or its contract body should examine the size and budget of regulatory agencies in the healthcare sector. What was the agency's original mandate? Has there been a metamorphosis beyond that purpose? Over-regulation is more than an annoyance. It often blocks efficiency, contributes to the high cost of healthcare, and deserves reconsideration in light of cost and consequences.

Medicare and Medicaid gathered mass through eight administrations and 20 Congresses. Congress ignores the fact that expanding benefits does not control spending. To reduce expenditures, Congress knows that it has to control both price and utilization. Unfortunately, many of its policies have an unintended effect of penalizing creativity, productivity, access, and profit in healthcare. The cost of regulation is largely hidden. Ben Wattenberg calls Medicare "intergenerational transfer," wherein the young give dollars to government; the elderly receive dollars from the government; both get mad at the government and keep loving each other.[23]

FACTORS AFFECTING MEDICAL PRACTICE

Healthcare practice and expenditures may be viewed as a cascade of related factors. (Figure 4.1) Each variable causes a series of events that ultimately affects the practice of medicine. At the top are *demographics/trends*. Peter Drucker called demography the future that has already happened.[24]

FIGURE 4.1

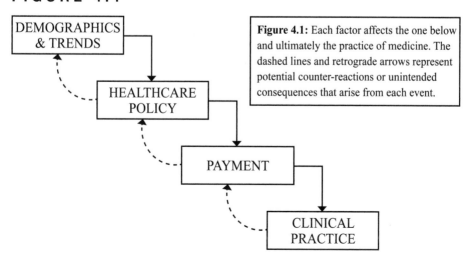

Figure 4.1: Each factor affects the one below and ultimately the practice of medicine. The dashed lines and retrograde arrows represent potential counter-reactions or unintended consequences that arise from each event.

Beginning in 2010-11, the aging of the population through sheer numbers will impact every aspect of our society.± The number of elderly will nearly double between now and 2030 (46 million increasing to 83 million, or 12 percent rising to 20 percent), and this will affect funding, hospital utilization and physician manpower.[25] Before 2000, the young outnumbered the old. That relationship is reversing, the same way that the number of urban dwellers now exceeds the formerly dominant rural population.[26] The older generation is healthier and wealthier than their counterparts in past years. They're better educated, more prosperous, and suffer fewer disabilities. Although functional limitations multiply with aging, increasing income appears to be related to a downward trend in the percentage of men and women with disabilities. Just as wealth predicts a longer, more active life, education predicts fewer physical limitations with advancing age.[27]

Demographics will affect *health policy* as the ratio of workers to retirees changes – 4:1 now, 3:1 by 2020, and 2:1 by 2030. Labor has already transitioned away from its large capital base. Today it operates in a world of part-time, temporary and contracted employees, where job turnover is frequent, and there is a high probability of change in the financing of employer-based insurance. Approximately a third of our population growth is driven by a surge of immigration, amounting to one million legal and an estimated one million illegal immigrants annually. In 2005, recent immigrants totaled approximately 36 million people, or 12 percent of the U.S. population.[28] The foreign-born are relatively healthy and although they have less health insurance, they are disproportionately low users of medical care.[29] Their estimated $37 billion impact on national healthcare costs is half as large as our non-insured citizenry.[30]

The problem of the uninsured is one of the most visible public issues – approximately 47 million people who at some time in the year are without coverage. About a quarter of those without insurance are foreign born (10 million are not citizens); and a third are young adults. Although another third have incomes above $50,000,[31, 32] that income does not assure health insurance affordability. In 2008, the uninsured received approximately $86 billion of services during the time they lacked coverage; they paid $30 billion out of pocket and the remaining $56 billion was classified as uncompensated care.†

±   Note the number of births in the U.S. was 4.3 million in 2006, which is the largest number since 1961. Deaths in 2006 were 2.4 million, or approximately 22,000 lower than 2005. (Macro Trends. Healthcare Industry News Summary. January 2008)

†   The number of households with annual incomes of less than $25,000 who lack health insurance has gone down steadily since 1998. (DeNavas-Walt C, Proctor BD, Smith J, *Income, Poverty, and Health Insurance Coverage in the United States: 2006,* Washington, DC: U.S. Census Bureau, 2007), p. 21, http://www.census.gov/prod/2007pubs/p60-233.pdf; Also see, *"Health Insurance,"* Health Insurance Coverage (Reports and Tables), (Washington DC: U.S. Census Bureau, Housing and Household Economic Statistics Division), (http://www.census.gov/hhes/www/hlthins/cps.html)

This figure may soar as unemployment rises during the latest recession. Under the Consolidated Omnibus Budget Reconciliation Act (COBRA), a laid-off worker may retain employer health insurance for 18 months. Now the continued paid premiums are tax deductible for the employer. The point is that there is a new class of the uninsured – the recently unemployed.

In addition to demographic and labor trends, there is a growing obesity problem that will affect healthcare policy. Kenneth Thorpe and colleagues estimate that 27 percent of real per capita growth in spending from 1987 to 2001 is attributed to increasing rates of obesity, highest among ethnic minority and disadvantaged children.[33] This is perhaps the biggest priority in wellness education at work and in the home.

Payment depends on demographics and policies. Provider payments are increasingly tied to the federal budget. The hydraulics of subsidizing low government payment by inflated prices on the private side is under great strain. (Figure 4.2).

FIGURE 4.2

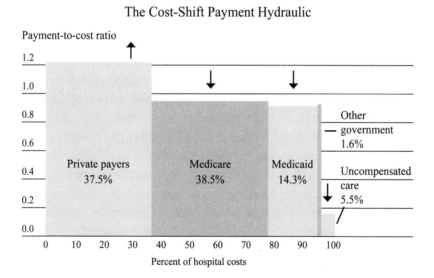

The Cost-Shift Payment Hydraulic

Figure 4.2: The payment-to-cost ratio changes slightly each year. The components of reimbursement are shown 1) by percentages of total expenditure; 2) by their respective payment-to-cost ratios. Specific payment / cost percentages are 129.4% private payer; 92.3% Medicare and 87.1% Medicaid.

Source: Modified from Lewin Group analysis of data presented in Lewin Group, Trendwatch Chartbook 2005: Trends Affecting Hospitals and Health Systems (Washington: American Hospital Association, May 2005).

The 1.0 line represents equal payment and cost. Since Medicare and Medicaid pay at or below cost, private payers make up the difference. In addition, there is uncompensated care, which is defined as the sum of free care for which the hospital does not expect payment and the bad debt that it does attempt to collect. Both are increasing. The way free care and bad debt are reported, it is not always easy to distinguish between them. Bad debt is an operational expense. Together, their collective impact is clear; uncompensated care is not free.[34] The government uses its market power to purchase services at below cost, which forces providers to shift costs to private payers, whose higher bills are often referred to as a hidden tax. It's really a shifting of revenues across payers.[35] "Real" healthcare premiums increase (as a proportion of wages) because healthcare expenses rise more rapidly than wages. Today, hospital financing depends on cost-shifting. If cost-shifting didn't exist, who would pay for underfunded public programs and the uninsured?

Because the government is the dominant insurer, private payers often use government's pricing as their own benchmark, and further reduce payments to providers through denials, delay in payment, and contractual nuance. In contrast to the provider's plight, the large commercial health insurers are highly profitable. They take their cost off the top and to stay profitable, they need only to raise premiums. Ten years ago the top ten insurers covered 27 percent of the membership nationally. Today the top ten health insurance companies cover 50 percent.[36] Policymakers who believe that they can reduce spending in Medicare and Medicaid by transferring responsibilities to commercial health insurers will be disappointed. When payment increases do not match inflation, history has shown that private health insurance firms either withdraw from the Medicare market or limit their offerings.[37]

All of these factors should be of concern to patients, because they affect the *clinical practice of medicine.* The romantic image of the solo practitioner whose armamentarium fit into a black bag is nostalgic. Today the biggest drivers of growth are new treatments and technologies, which account for half of new expenditures. Modern clinical practice is a complicated business, internally fractious, highly regulated, and less rewarding. From 1970 to 1995, the number of U.S. physicians increased by about 25 percent, whereas the number of administrators grew by more than 2,000 percent.[38] These numbers don't reflect the distribution of doctors, most of whom locate in areas of concentrated population. In the past 50 years, we have gone from a dozen categories of healthcare professionals to more than 220 categories today, including more than a hundred specialties.[39] The physician practice management industry has essentially collapsed. Primary care is no longer a growing specialty.[40, 41] Note the ratio of general surgeons to patients in the U.S. has also declined by 26 percent between 1981 and 2005.[42] It is clear that medicine is no longer the same wealth-building profession.

As Robert Louis Stevenson said,[±] "Everybody, soon or late, sits down to a banquet of consequences." The dashed lines in Figure 4.1 denote consequences. Past policies have produced unintended results. Medical specialties compete to gain added reimbursement in a hydraulic system where any advantage in one specialty is generally at the expense of another specialty. Decreased payments to physicians have resulted in less time spent with patients, personnel cuts, foregone amenities, limited access, and dated equipment, and, as we have seen, early physician retirement. Too often these policies end up hurting the very people that they were designed to help.[†]

The economy today and our budget policies cannot accommodate tomorrow's retirement boom.[§] Generational accounting also offers a bad prognosis for the Medicare beneficiary. The longer the government waits to administer a change, the harder it will be on future beneficiaries. In the past, a third of Medicare recipients also had employer coverage, but future retirees won't be able to rely on employer-sponsored plans to supplement Medicare. A new Medicare paradigm might allow people to fund their own retirement healthcare, perhaps through a medical IRA established in their working years with the government providing a backstop for catastrophic care.[µ] Whatever the solution in the private sector, defined benefits will likely change to defined contributions.[43]

WHAT'S WRONG WITH OUR PRACTICE OF MEDICINE?

It is useful to examine the features of U.S. healthcare and compare them to other developed economies. Although we have significantly higher healthcare expenditures per capita and the highest percentage of GDP devoted to healthcare, the *average real annual growth rate*, relative to gains in income, is similar to the Organisation for Economic Co-operation and Development (OECD) median.[44] The wide variation in

---

[±] Attributed to Robert Louis Balfour Stevenson (November 13, 1850-December 3, 1894), a Scottish novelist, poet and travel writer, and a representative of neo-romanticism in English literature.

[†] In 2007, 29 percent of people (up from 24 percent in 2006) with Medicare (11.6 million people) said they had trouble finding a doctor who would take their insurance. (Shute N. *Need a Doctor? Too Bad*. U.S. News & World Report, 2008: 144 (10); pp. 72-4).

[§] Financing broader coverage will require one or more fiscal initiatives: changing the employer tax exclusion, raising income taxes (or allowing the 2001-2002 tax cuts to expire), a value-added tax (VAT) or raising tobacco, alcohol and gasoline taxes. The consensus will probably be that further deficit financing is not a good idea. Whatever is done, reducing reimbursement is likely to be part of the strategy. Congress should concentrate on ways to better educate the public regarding wellness and provide incentives to own individual policies in return for lower premiums, catastrophic coverage and participation in cost-sharing.

[µ] See Goodman JC. *A Framework for Medicare Reform*. National Center for Policy Analysis. Policy Report 315, September 2008.

health spending among OECD nations is explainable by GDP per capita. America's high per capita GDP is enough to raise its per capita health spending above other OECD nations and accounts for 47 percent of the difference in per capita spending between the U.S. and the comparative countries.[45] The reasons for increased spending appear to be common among developed nations, and each country has a mixture of strengths and weaknesses in its policies.

In the past 20 years, U.S. life expectancy has increased three years, while disease, death rates, disability and hospital days have all fallen significantly.[46]± (see other OECD comparisons in chapter 5). It may be surprising, but compared with most OECD countries, we have fewer practicing physicians and nurses per thousand population, fewer medical consultations per capita, lower rates of hospitalization, fewer beds, shorter stays and less out-of-pocket spending (as a share of total spending). However, our health insurance premiums are higher and the U.S. spends significantly more on *administration*, nearly six times as much as the OECD average. Also, we have higher input costs for labor and capital.[47] Administrative expense has variously been estimated to be 15-30 percent of healthcare expenditures or higher. Social factors also fuel U.S. healthcare cost. Compared to OECD nations, the U.S. has significantly more† 1) teenage births; 2) abortions; 3) alcohol and drug abuse; 4) AIDS, tuberculosis, hepatitis; 5) murders; 6) reported rapes; 7) prisoners per 100,000 persons; 8) handguns; 9) family structure breakdown; and 10) litigation costs.

Healthcare is becoming the biggest growth industry in America. We are reaching the point where more Americans will be employed in healthcare than are employed in producing manufactured goods.[48] Despite our technical advances, we lag behind in adopting the electronic medical record.[49] All European countries have a broad generalist foundation comprising 70-80 percent of practicing physicians. In the United States these figures are reversed – 70-80 percent are specialists.[50] What appears to be a looming crisis may be greatly ameliorated by the growing number of nurse practitioners and physician assistants (currently numbering 150,000 and projected to

---

±   According to the CDC, National Center for Health Statistics, June 8, 2008, life expectancy climbed to a record of 78.1 years, up from 77.8 in 2005. Mortality also declined for 11 of the top 15 causes of death. Even deaths from accidents dropped by 1.5 percent. Alzheimer's surpassed diabetes to become the sixth leading cause of death in the U.S.

†   It appears to me that this is in fact what we in the United States have been doing of late. I proffer the thesis that, over the past generation, since the time Erikson wrote, the amount of deviant behavior in American society has increased beyond the levels the community can "afford to recognize" and that, accordingly, we have been re-defining deviancy so as to exempt much conduct previously stigmatized and also quietly raising the "normal" level in categories where behavior is now abnormal by any earlier standard. (Moynihan DP. *Defining Deviancy Down.* Am Scholar: 1993: 62 (1); pp. 17-23)

double by 2020).[51] But patient demand may still exceed physician supply. Economic factors are part of a long list of conditions that will be reshaping the practice of medicine in coming years.

Here are some other important issues:

- Medical school enrollment has not kept up with the growing population. The total number of students remained essentially unchanged between 1980 and 2000 at about 16,000 graduates, whereas the U.S. population grew by about 71 million people.[52][±]

- The United States was able to maintain an adequate supply of physicians because the number of entry-level allopathic <u>residency</u> positions (24,085 in 2006) greatly exceeded the number of graduates of U.S. medical schools (15,925 in 2006).

- Thirty-seven percent of doctors are in internal medicine specialties or primary care. Women account for 50 percent of physicians, but they comprise only 11 percent of surgeons. There is no evidence that women are going to be attracted to the demands of intense procedural specialties.

- The number of U.S. allopathic medical school graduates entering family medicine residencies has dropped by 50 percent. Of the internal medicine residents, only 20 percent go into primary care today. Since 1990, the number of colleges of osteopathic medicine has expanded from 15 to 25, with three additional branch campuses, and their total enrollments have more than doubled, from 6,892 students in 1990 to 15,586 students in 2007. In 2008, these colleges estimate they will graduate 3,463 students, and by 2015, the American Osteopathic Association projects that the number of osteopathic physicians will exceed 90,000.[53]

- Incentives for medical graduates to choose higher-paying specialty careers have been associated with the dwindling generalist workforce. Reimbursement rewards the narrow subspecialties more than the generalist.

[±] A more recent report from the Josiah Macy Jr. Foundation 2008 report, Revisiting the Medical School Educational Mission at the Time of Expansion (www.macyfoundation.org), medical schools are increasing in number and class size and are expected to graduate an additional 5,000 doctors each year by 2020. Schools of osteopathy are growing as well. The foundation report recommends changes in the admissions criteria and suggests ways to reduce the medical student debt burden.

- Currently, 25 percent of physicians come from abroad. International graduates entering residency may decline because of more strict visa requirements that have not yet had an effect.[±] This could be offset by a growing pool of applicants.

- Earning potential may fall with incremental reimbursement cuts. Changing lifestyles are already evident. Generation Y doctors (those born after 1980) are likely not to train or work so long or so hard. (The work-leisure trade-off.)

- New medical advances may improve outcomes, but do not necessarily improve provider efficiency. Productivity remains static.

- A third of doctors are 55 years of age or older. Younger doctors will be attracted to healthcare systems that have proven electronic patient records… effective records that provide interface between ambulatory and hospital practices.

- Medical groups are still small. Approximately 30 percent of physicians practice solo or with a partner. Fewer than 4 percent of all U.S. physicians work in practices with fifty or more other physicians.[54]

- A survey conducted by the American College of Physician Executives[55] indicates that nearly 60 percent of physicians have considered leaving practice earlier than the usual retirement age. They are tired of low reimbursement, loss of autonomy, bureaucratic red tape, patient overload, and loss of respect.

[±] The Education Commission for Foreign Medical Graduates (ECFMG) revised requirements for certification, which require graduates to pass a clinical skills test whereby applicants communicate in English with actors posing as patients. The exam difficulty, cost and travel expense has changed the pool of applicants. U.S. citizens attending medical school outside the U.S. or Canada have increased steadily and comprise 18 percent of 2006 applications. (Boulet JR, Cooper RA, Seeling SS, et al. *U.S. Citizens Who Obtain Their Medical Degree Abroad: An Overview, 1992-2006.* Health Affairs 2009; 28: 226-33). They do not perform as well on examinations, but are more likely to enter the U.S. workforce and practice in primary care activities compared with non-U.S. international medical graduates.

Inpatient admissions are trending down and were nearly flat in 2007. Yet, outpatient volumes have shown steady growth for the past 25 years.± As patients become more informed about readily available diagnostic testing and screening, they increase the demand for outpatient care.

The proliferation of minimally invasive surgeries, radiographic imaging, and interventional cardiac procedures is being accommodated by new outpatient facilities in the community. Even chronic disease management has moved away from the hospital and into community clinics. The core hospital services are gradually being eroded.

The overall distribution of medical services is far from uniform or appropriate to need. A large random survey of medical records found that only half of patients are getting the recommended level of basic care. Twenty-five medical conditions were analyzed for generally agreed-upon treatments or medications. Contrary to what many think, the study revealed underuse rather than overuse. Patients were being shortchanged on screening for cancers, other preventive medicine, antibiotics, serum lipid management, appropriate indications for imaging, and cardiovascular and diabetes management. As a result, there was substantial variation in quality of care scores. After evaluating 439 indicators of quality care, the conclusion was that *more* care should have been delivered.[56] Furthermore, the amount of appropriate care declined with age.[57] "Doing the right thing" for patients will significantly increase healthcare expenditures. As genomics leads to personalized medicine, finer-grained screening and treatment tailored to the patients' genetic profile will not be cheap.[58] The real question is whether the return on the added expense will yield commensurate higher survival or improved quality of life.

Whatever comfort we draw from evidence-based guidelines, much of medicine remains empirical. We are frustrated when patients don't fit into neat diagnostic categories for which standardized treatment yields predictable outcomes. But healthcare is an imperfect science and is practiced by an estimate of probabilities,

---

±   In the McKinsey Global Institute, December 2008 healthcare survey, U.S. costs and other parameters were compared with 13 OECD countries. Adjusted for per capita GDP (2006), the U.S. spent $650 billion more than the OECD average, of which two-thirds were attributed to out patient activity. Our greater expenditures in outpatient healthcare delivery relates to higher margins, physician judgment, technology, abundant supply, and price-insensitive buyers. U.S. admissions and length of stay are lower but our cost of supporting a patient bed day is double that of the OECD. The U.S. has an average bed occupancy of 66 percent compared with 75 percent in the OECD. The cost of physician visits is significantly higher in the U.S. despite the fact that disease prevalence here is slightly lower than peer OECD countries. The U.S. healthcare system appears to be more innovative and more convenient to use than comparative countries. (Farrell D, Jensen E, Kocher B, et al. *Accounting for the Cost of U.S. Healthcare: A New Look at Why Americans Spend More.* McKinsey Global Institute, December 8, 2008)

personal judgment and experience. Wennberg has exposed the enormous variations in testing, procedures and hospitalizations across the country.[59] His message is that more testing and procedures mean worse healthcare. His solution would be to put the markets that engage in over-treatment on a reimbursement diet. That is unlikely to happen by regulation. Instead, the way to add value is to educate physicians and patients. Vast uncertainty still exists in how to treat many medical conditions, and consumer information about providers is often confusing or not accessed. The *2008 Dartmouth Atlas of Healthcare* indicates that wide differences in healthcare costs for chronically ill patients who are dying are not driven by price, but by the quantity of total services rendered.[60]

Some of these flaws relate to the way medicine is organized. Physician and hospital incentives are frequently not aligned. Private physicians merely "rent" space in the hospital, and many provide little operational input into hospital management. It's easy to buy physician practices, but it's hard to integrate them into the hospital. In staff-model group practices like the Cleveland Clinic and the Mayo Clinic, integration is supported by the longstanding organizational structure and close interdependencies among professionals.

Ideally, patients would be best served if individual specialties were concentrated into regional centers. But it may be too late for this. Demand has driven the unplanned diffusion of specialty care into the communities. The 130 heart transplant centers across the nation are a good example. Some of these centers do only a handful of transplants a year, though it has been established that patients enjoy better outcomes at high-volume facilities with experienced practitioners. The economic inefficiency of the American healthcare system becomes disproportionately more costly as healthcare expenditures rise.

Good health is intimately tied to socioeconomic status and educational attainment. The educated person is more likely to seek medical advice on screening, counseling, immunizations and regular preventive examinations. The doctrine of prevention comes with its own fallacies, including the belief that preventive medicine is inexpensive and always reduces costs. Health improvement depends on personal responsibility and physician advocates. Providing all recommended preventive services could require up to 7½ hours a day of physician time.[61] Wellness will depend on how well we educate people and what incentives are provided for them to pay attention to their personal health. There's an old saying that genetics loads the gun, but environment pulls the trigger.

MEDICAL MALPRACTICE

As Rhett Butler said to Scarlett O'Hara in *Gone with the Wind*, "What most people don't seem to realize is that there is just as much money that can be made out of wreckage as there can from building. I'm making my fortune out of wreckage." The American tort system is the most expensive in the world – amounting to 2.2 percent of the GDP ($250 billion annually), which is more than double the combined rates of Japan, Canada, France and the United Kingdom. When access to court is easy, compromise is unstable.[62] The result is costly inefficiency, cumbersome procedures and inconsistent awards.

Lord Peter Levene, chairman of Lloyd's of London, pointed out that the cost of litigation is "pernicious, cancerous, and ruinous... the most significant drain on the economy, which among many things results in a poisonous atmosphere that discourages innovation."[63] The increasing number of lawsuits is not motivated by any increase in actual malpractice, but is driven by lawyers seeking contingent fees, the naiveté of citizen juries, and the fact that malpractice is pled as a tort rather than a contract.[64] Juries are moved more by the degree of a plaintiff's disability than by actual negligence.

Risks seem not to be predicted by patient characteristics, illness complexity, or even physicians' technical skills. Instead, risk appears related to patients' dissatisfaction with their physicians' ability to establish rapport, provide access, administer care and treatment consistent with expectations, and communicate effectively.[65] According to data from the U.S. Department of Justice, the Government Accounting Office, the Congressional Budget Office, and the National Practitioner Databank, 57 percent of malpractice trials involve claims of permanent injury; 33 percent of trials involve death. There is a 27 percent win rate for plaintiffs in large counties. Note that medical malpractice is governed by state, not federal, law. Every jury is different and decisions are widely inconsistent.[66] I can't remember who said this, but one healthcare administrator suggested that "the ultimate solution for eliminating all medical errors and all malpractice is for the institution to get rid of all the patients."

The total cost of the medical malpractice system, about $28 billion, represents 1.5 percent of total healthcare spending.[67] Nationwide medical liability cost amounts to about $3,500 per hospital bed annually. (AON Global Risk Consulting Hospital Professional Liability and Physician Liability 2007 Benchmark Analysis) However, legislative reforms and strengthened defenses have stabilized the frequency and severity of professional liability results.[68]

In addition to the more visible premium costs, the true cost of defensive medicine is spread across the entire profession. Unnecessary tests, extensive documentation, and intensified end-of-life care are done more to avoid suits and to satisfy the courts than for patient benefit. The lawyer's contingent fee system is an incentive for high settlement. Insurers unable to forecast the number and size of claims simply abandon the market.

To prepare for litigation challenges, the healthcare institution needs to integrate all risk management activities and learn from every bad event. Communication is the foundation of malpractice prevention. Unanticipated outcomes in which patients are harmed are best disclosed promptly and surrounding facts fully explained to patients and family. If compensation is appropriate due to an injury, settle immediately. A statement of sincere regret and formal apology are essential. The institution should provide disclosure coaching, and the responsible physician(s) must personally speak with the family of the patient.[69]

Litigation reform is difficult but not impossible. Since the legal profession essentially makes the laws, it is unlikely that contingency fees can be changed or even regulated. There are some excesses that can be controlled, however, such as duplicative litigation and punitive damages for injuries caused by approved products. State legislatures are trying various legal reforms, such as offsets to the collateral source rule, abolition of joint and several liability, and shortening of the statute of limitations. California has one of the oldest and most effective reform programs, the 1975 California Medical Injury Compensation Reform Act, or MICRA, which restricts non-economic damages to $250,000, limits attorney fees in medical malpractice cases, and does not allow product liability suits in cases of alcohol, cigarettes, or high-fat food usage.[70] Texas also has a $250,000 cap on non-economic damages.

Caps have blunted the growth in medical liability losses compared with states without caps. In Texas the number of medical malpractice cases filed in 2005 was down 41 percent from the average filings during six years before 2003.[71] Direct tort reforms almost always result in fewer cases filed as well as a decrease in malpractice premiums and lower premium growth. Recent publications based on the AMA's Masterfile Data have reported that non-economic caps and direct tort reforms generally have a positive effect on the number of physicians per capita in a state.[72] However, analysts have found that relatively strong tort law provisions can explain at most only one-fourth of the variation among states in the average loss costs.[73]

Outside the U.S., the majority of civil law jurisdictions use non-jury courts to hear medical malpractice claims. Neither France, Germany, nor Japan use civil juries. The requirement for a civil jury in personal injury cases was eliminated in England in 1883. The court has the power to order use of a jury but English case law clearly states that should be done (if at all) "only in exceptional circumstances." In Canada, any party may make a motion to declare a case "complex," allowing the judge to dismiss the jury and hear the case him or herself. Such motions are frequently granted in malpractice and product liability cases.[74]

Both Common Good and the Harvard School of Public Health propose *expert health courts* without juries. In their proposal, specially trained administrative judges would make decisions and write opinions, advised by neutral experts paid by the court. The injured party would receive 100 percent of their actual monetary losses including future lost income. But damages for pain and suffering would be paid according to a preset schedule depending on the injury.[75] Instead of a flat percentage of the award, lawyers' fees would be based on their time and investment in the case at hand. This plan is supported by a broad coalition, including providers, safety experts and consumers' groups like the American Association of Retired Persons, and six major hospitals including New York Presbyterian and Johns Hopkins have volunteered to participate. Trial lawyers oppose this plan because they insist that juries and only juries must make the final decision. Too bad. Civil juries were established to resolve disputes involving matters of fact. They were never intended to decide standards of medical care as a matter of law.[76]

UNIVERSAL CARE

When Winston Churchill entered the British army as a commissioned officer in 1897, he was a model for the Victorian colonial wars: cavalry boots, jodhpurs, pressed military tunic and choker collar. He was assigned to India and had to travel forty miles across a scorching plain and then up a steep winding road to Malakand Pass. He arrived disheveled, covered with yellow dust, and was then issued a tent, a seat at the staff mess and a tumbler to be used for whiskey. This presented a problem for him, because even at an early age, Churchill had long preferred the taste of wine and brandy, and the taste of whiskey turned his stomach. However, here in the barrens, he faced a choice of tepid water, tepid water with lime juice, and tepid water with whiskey. As he put it, he "grasped the larger hope."[77]

To grasp the larger hope, we must first understand the financial realities of medicine today. Though we live in an imperfect world, we are challenged to build the best and most attractive delivery system for patients, payers, purchasers and physicians. In our democratic society, American health policy is made through negotiated consensus among shifting coalitions.[78] In recent years, certain coalitions have been calling for a government-run, single payer, or "universal" healthcare system. Some believe that government-run healthcare would be simpler and less expensive.± So far, the easiest way to argue against this proposal is to point to results from nations that already have some version of universal coverage. While some do a good job of providing primary care, the advantage is offset by the need to implicitly (sometimes explicitly) ration care. These countries have their own operational inefficiencies and need to impose an ever-rising tax burden on their citizenry. Only government has as many tools to control costs: rationing, regulating medical fees, limiting access and controlling supply and technology. But these have the additional effect of stifling initiative, curtailing innovation, and postponing the discovery of new treatments and cures.

Government-run systems create low expectations, together with the belief that poor access is the price you pay for equal access.† There is not one government-run healthcare system that is considered adequately funded by those who have to deal with it.[79] The demand for more spending is inexorable.§ Canada does not allow purchase of private health insurance but reimbursement is based on fee-for-service. In contrast, citizens in the UK may purchase health insurance and 11-12 percent choose to do so.[80]

Canada exhibits other variants on the universal care theme, because only a quarter of it is financed by the federal government, with the rest being paid by the provinces and territories. Private insurance is allowed only for prescription drugs, eye treatment, dental care, and other services not covered by the Canada Health Act. In the U.S., we spend more on healthcare because we pay physicians more, use more resources per "event," and charge more for hospital care and pharmaceuticals.

Nationalizing healthcare doesn't stop cost from rising, nor does it guarantee ready access. And it will not diminish public expectations. According to Newhouse and Reischauer, "If the single-payer plan has benefits that are around the current average, roughly half of people with above-average coverage now will have less coverage under reform, something that they are unlikely to take kindly. And if the single plan is much better than the current average, costs explode."[81]

More medical care does not necessarily mean better health. Sir Douglas Black, a distinguished British physician, observed that there has been no significant change in

---

±   Americans rail against their government's weakness, paralysis, venality, and profligacy. Yet, it is the citizens who give their money and time to ensure that no changes can be made that are at the expense of their subsidy, their Social Security cheque, their tax break; it is mostly the voter's money that bribes the politicians; it is voters who insist that more needs to be done, but with lower taxes and without killing any existing programmes. *Voters, Blame Thyself,* The Economist, October 29, 1994: 333 (7887); pp.17-8)

†   Quoting Churchill, "Capitalism is the unequal sharing of blessings, while socialism is the equal sharing of misery." (http://www.winstonchurchill.org/i4a/pages/index.cfm?pageid=823).

§   What people want is not the satisfaction of their wants, but better wants. (Knight FH. *The Ethics of Competition.* Piscataway, NY: Transaction Publishers. 1997.)

the relative health status of the various occupational classes in Great Britain over the half-century that the National Health Service (NHS) has been doing its best to provide equality of access.[82] Healthcare insurance doesn't guarantee efficient or effective healthcare. This is also true in Europe despite a strong primary care presence.

Average life expectancy has little to do with healthcare spending. Life expectancy varies across occupations and socioeconomic groups. We know that the single greatest determinant of health status is education. James Smith, a health economist at the RAND Corporation, found that education is consistently linked to longer lives in every country where it has been studied.[83] Although wealth generally buys better health, education is more important than race and obliterates any effects of income. The unskilled, uneducated continue to fare worse as shown by higher mortality and morbidity. Differences between the rich and poor as to mortality are unchanged even in countries that have health insurance for everyone. All the industrial countries face a similar challenge: a relentless rise in healthcare expenditures, a widespread realization that expense trends are unsustainable and little political consensus about solutions.[84]

A *British Medical Journal* comparison of the British NHS and Kaiser Permanente concluded that the per capita costs of the two systems were similar. However, the analysis found that Kaiser provided its members with more comprehensive and convenient primary care services and much more rapid access to specialists and hospital admissions. After adjustments for differences between countries, the NHS cost was calculated at $1,764 per capita compared to a Kaiser cost of $1,951.[85] Kaiser had two-and-one-half times as many pediatricians, twice as many obstetricians-gynecologists, and three times as many cardiologists per enrollee as the NHS. After referral, waiting times to see a specialist were more than six times longer in the NHS. For nonemergency hospital admission, 90 percent of Kaiser patients waited less than three months; one-third of NHS patients waited more than five months.[86]

In our culture, a government-run system could be more expensive than our pluralistic approach because access (utilization) would expand significantly. Federal funding is no more sustainable than reliance on conventional employer-based health insurance. The single payer would have the power to achieve its cost-reduction goals by setting arbitrary prices, dictating practice standards, shifting payments, and restricting services.[87] Ask those who encourage the adoption of universal healthcare what's going to happen to overall quality, to access, to students going into medicine, when professionals are treated as employees, and as generalists substitute for specialists.[88] As Ronald Reagan said, "When you get in bed with the government, you're going to get more than a good night's sleep."[±] Universal care is a noble ideal, but the best and most sustainable solutions are through a reformed pluralistic system.

POLICY CONSIDERATIONS

What are the solutions? The best reform must achieve three goals: 1) preventing the deprivation of care caused by the inability to pay; 2) avoiding wasteful spending (controlling cost); and 3) permitting wide latitude in choice.[89] These are lofty goals in reform but what are the immediate priorities? To insure needy children; to cover catastrophic care as part of public and private insurance (no one should be financially ruined by illness); to make insurance purchase more affordable; to reduce the number of uninsured. Quality of care, fiscal transparency, and wellness are the foundation of any and all reforms.

Employer-sponsored health insurance, which benefits approximately 60 percent of American workers, may have worked after World War II, but employer coverage has many emerging negatives. The short list is that it compromises the business, it is increasingly unaffordable for small enterprises[†] and it leads to over-consumption.[§] By not taxing employer-based health insurance as income, the government creates open-ended tax expenditures, discourages economic self-discipline, locks people into jobs, and essentially subsidizes insurance for those whose employers provide it at the expense of those whose employers do not.[90]

The employer-based subsidy is defended on three grounds: 1) broad purchase; 2) advantage of aggregated purchasing; 3) risk pooling.[91] While the value of the tax exclusion for employer-based private insurance is greater for high income than for low income employees, there is no cap on or deductibility for the Medicare payroll tax. With increasing income, the Medicare tax is progressive.

The exemption of employer-paid health insurance from payroll and individual income taxes reduced federal and state revenues by $160 to > $200 billion. Employers do not share fiscal responsibility and do not pay for healthcare – they pass it on in the form of lower wages or higher prices. Real wages have been relatively flat for 30 years.[92] In the 21st century, insurance premiums have increased about four times greater than the growth in wages.[93]

±   Ronald Reagan. *What Ever Happened to Free Enterprise*. Ludwig Von Mises Memorial Lecture delivered November 10, 1977, Hillsdale College, Hillsdale, MI

†   Of the six million U.S. companies, 98 percent have fewer than 100 employees. Half of businesses that employ fewer than 10 employees have stopped offering coverage.

§   Employers pay on average 84 percent of premiums for single coverage and 73 percent for family coverage. (Henry J. Kaiser Foundation/Health Research and Educational Trust, *Employer Health Benefits, 2007 Annual Survey*. September 2007)

For decades, a myth has been perpetuated that people with the most means, whose needs are often less, consume the most care and those with the least means and greatest health problems consume the least care.± The facts are otherwise. When personal income is ranked and analyzed according to medical expenditure, healthcare spending is relatively *invariant* to income. In fact, expenditures per person is *highest* in the low income category and approximately equal in the top four income groups.[94]

FIGURE 4.3†

Annual Health Care Spending per Person in 2005 Dollars

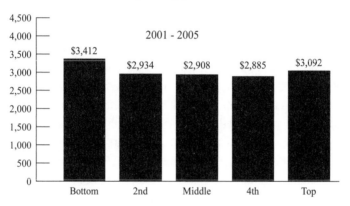

Income Divided into Quintiles

Tabulations by Gary Burtless, The Brookings Institution, from the 2001-2005 Medical Expenditure Panel Survey household files, September 2008.

As the above figure indicates, healthcare spending is highest in the low income category presumably because people with lower incomes have more serious health problems. This includes the aged who consume more health services. If health goods and services were distributed on the basis of need, spending would be higher in the lower part of the income distribution as is the case.

± Reiterated recently in *The World Health Report 2008 Primary Health Care – Now More Than Ever*. World Health Organization, p. xiv.

† Annual health spending per person includes expenditures on healthcare goods and services in the U.S. population including household out-of-pocket spending, expenditures that are reimbursed by insurance, and healthcare that is financed by other sources. Spending is converted into constant 2005 prices using the U.S. BLS estimate of the Consumer Price Index (CPI).

However, there is a strong relationship that links higher healthcare costs to worse insurance coverage. Higher healthcare costs in an area increase insurance premiums, which causes employers to eliminate coverage. Higher healthcare costs also drive up the cost of Medicaid and other government health programs, which leads state government to constrict eligibility requirements.[95] There is also a reported correlation between no insurance and higher mortality.[96] According to some experts, the absence of health insurance, by itself, is a more powerful predictor of impaired access to healthcare and poor outcomes than ethnicity.[97] However, this group tends to be poorer, less educated and has a higher incidence of preventable risk factors. The uninsured can and do take advantage of emergency departments and safety-net clinics for routine care. But when the need arises for expensive pharmaceuticals, specialist referrals, or surgical procedures, access is a formidable challenge.

Like any gambling enterprise, the insurance game is structured to favor the house. It doesn't protect lower income people with chronic diseases from the high cost of healthcare. Healthy people get a relatively bad deal unless they are aligned with a large group.[98] Approximately one in ten Americans is covered by individual (not group) health insurance, and the market hasn't increased in the past few years.[99] People who have an established illness may have trouble getting individual coverage. Also those who buy their own insurance get no tax relief unless their premiums exceed 7.5 percent of their adjusted gross income.

Insurance obtained through an employer is not portable (four in every ten workers change jobs each year), whereas insurance purchased by individuals is portable. If health insurance portability is desirable and if the tax law favors employer purchase, why don't employers purchase individually owned (and therefore portable) insurance for their employees? The answer: Federal law makes this impossible, or at least impractical. Although there is some disagreement on the point, lawyers generally interpret the Employee Retirement Income Security Act (ERISA) of 1974 as amended by the Health Insurance Portability and Accountability Act of 1996 (HIPAA) to say that employers can purchase only group insurance with untaxed dollars.[100] The difference in tax treatment effectively doubles the cost of traditional health insurance for those who must purchase it themselves. There will not be true portability until people can own their own policy. HIPAA guarantees that a new employer can't deny you insurance because of health status. However, it doesn't guarantee the same set of benefits as you had with your previous employer.

The overarching goals of healthcare reform are to reduce the rate of spending and at the same time decrease the number of uninsured. There is no one solution, but the solutions are likely to be incremental, and in order to be successful must not give more incentives to become uninsured. The sick and poor have to have better access to insurance. Personally, I believe we should offer a variety of public and private plans and not rely on a government-controlled, fixed-budget solution.

INVENTIVE CHANGE

"The country demands bold, persistent experimentation. It is common sense to take a method and try it. If it fails, admit it frankly and try another. But, above all, try something." [101] As of September 2007, eight states and the cities of New York and San Francisco have either enacted or are proposing health insurance reform. In April 2006, Massachusetts became the first state to attempt a universal healthcare coverage plan. In a preliminary analysis, they found that 20 percent of the uninsured in Massachusetts actually qualified for Medicaid but had never signed up.[±] Another 40 percent were young people who earned enough to purchase insurance but chose not to buy it. The Massachusetts solution requires all residents to obtain insurance, and plans are to make insurance more affordable through higher deductibles and co-payments and fewer mandated benefits. They call this the "personal responsibility principle." Early results indicate that the number of uninsured has decreased to 2.4 percent and pharmaceutical costs are significantly lower. True, close to half-a-million more people are now insured but 60 percent are enrolled in Medicaid or tax-subsidized plans. Consequently, physician visits are up. If private insurance is not purchased, state initiatives create new entitlements to be paid for by increased taxes. Deregulation is rarely discussed. No one is prepared to address the increased demand for access that is likely to occur when coverage expands. So far, spending has increased and compared with the national average, the per-capita cost in Massachusetts is high.[102]

From a legal standpoint, only about half of the 260 million Americans with health benefits have state-regulated health insurance or HMO coverage. The other half has self-insured benefits that are not regulated or taxed by the states as insurance. In this "unregulated" group, 100 million have self-insured employee benefits paid by employers or collectively bargained funds. [103] Therein lies an opportunity for this self-insured population to drive healthcare change. Based on the Wennberg variation analysis, there would be a significant cost savings if selected medical conditions were treated by provider teams who have better than expected outcomes. Informing

---

±   One in four Americans – about 12 million people – who don't have health coverage are eligible for Medicaid and the State Children's Health Insurance Program (SCHIP) but aren't enrolled, a new report shows. (National Institute for Health Care Management Foundation.) This includes 6.1 million children, or 64 percent of all uninsured children. (*1 in 4 Uninsured are Eligible for Aid but Aren't Enrolled.* National Institute for Health Care Management Foundation, Washington Post, April 25, 2008).

patients about the best regional physician teams (for their specific condition) would be a great innovation in the private market. Since patients have an incentive to spend less, they could take advantage of the Porter/Teisberg team approach to patient care. (See chapter 5) When observed outcomes are better than expected outcomes, expenditures are lower. The best provider teams (lower cost, better outcomes) could be rewarded more from the savings for exceptional results. *That would be the ultimate in pay-for-performance.*

Twenty years ago, Lester Thurow observed that while no one is ever willing to come right out and say it, the long-run aim is to return the system to the point where a large fraction of healthcare costs comes directly out of the individual's pockets.[104] Corporations, insurers, and pharmaceutical manufacturers are all trying to pass risk (cost) onto the consumer wherever they can. This trend cannot be stopped by further regulation or even by mass movement to a government-run healthcare system. Consumers are still going to have to take control of and make decisions about their healthcare expenditures. The consumer has finally reached the crossroad – either take control actively by educated self-interest or become a passive participant and assume the risk allocated to you.

All the stakeholders look at healthcare reform based on their own economic interests. People are far more likely to respond to economic incentives than social engineering. High-deductible plans constitute a transition from employer-based to individual-based insurance. The cornerstone of a consumer directed health plan (CDHP) is a health savings account (HSA).± The easiest way to understand HSAs is to describe them as "health IRAs,"[105] or better yet, a 401(k) only for medical expenses.†

Eligible individuals and their employers make tax-free contributions to the HSA, which is portable. The HSA is available only to people who purchase high-deductible health plans, who are not covered by other health insurance, and who are not enrolled in Medicare or claimed as a dependent on someone else's tax return. HSAs allow people with high-deductible plans to invest pre-tax money to cover out-of-pocket medical costs. In fact, there are *triple tax savings*: pre-tax contributions; investment grows tax-free; medical withdrawals are tax-exempt. HSAs give consumers an economic incentive to stay healthy. It is estimated that HSAs could reduce spending by approximately $40 billion, or 6 percent of total private health spending.[106]

±   Created in the Medicare Prescription Drug Modernization and Improvement Act, December 8, 2003, and improved in the Tax Relief and Health Care Act of 2006. There are variations that depend on ownership and portability. For this discussion, we call them all HSAs.

†   We are early in an era of a more activist government. Will this be the end of CDHP? It may take another form, but individual responsibility and cost-sharing will likely prevail even with universal healthcare. It's too expensive for the government to cover all costs.

The only randomized trial pertaining to individual cost-sharing was conducted by RAND.[107] Cost-sharing reduced overall use of medical care, but there was no difference in change of use between effective and ineffective care.[108] When free care was compared with a large cost-sharing policy, utilization declined as cost-sharing increased, but at a declining rate. Comparing free care with 25 percent coinsurance or deductible reduced the use 20 percent; but a 50 percent coinsurance plan decreased spending only about 25 percent; and the 95 percent coinsurance plan, about 30 percent.[109] Free care did not improve health habits, physical functioning, or mental health for the average person.[110] Free care for the "sick poor," however, did result in better visual acuity for people with poor vision and better control of blood pressure for low income hypertensive patients.

High-deductible or cost-sharing plans are criticized on the grounds of complexity, lack of price transparency and narrow coverage. Since an HSA benefits the healthier, generally younger population, their enrollment would change the conventional insurance market. Those with more serious conditions would then have to pay higher premiums because the risk pool would have changed. That is precisely the reason why the health insurance industry should be reorganized to improve access and affordability. (See Appendix I)

Further analysis of healthcare reform is beyond our scope or intent. However, the table below summarizes principles that are likely to work and opposites that are unlikely to bring about practical reform.

TABLE 4.1

LIKELY TO WORK	WON'T WORK
restructure insurance purchase	ideological solutions
encourage health insurance	total free-market or total government
means tested for affordability	mandate employer insurance
tax subsidies (credits)	continued defined benefits
multiple insurance options	more incentives for over-consumption
cost-sharing plans	perpetuate cost insensitivity
guaranteed renewability/portability	price controls
continue state initiatives	unfunded mandates
promote wellness	ignore catastrophic coverage
more consumer information	
support evidence-based practice	

There is no one solution. Complete government coverage is unsustainable without enormous state and federal tax increases. The government role should be to continue Medicare and to support the disadvantaged. Even then some cost-sharing will be required. We need to call an "ideological truce" and acknowledge that any proposal for achieving broader coverage will have some downsides. The objective of reform begins by making people aware that many illnesses are preventable. We have a huge public health problem ahead because of deviant lifestyles and apparent ignorance about wellness. Also, health insurance mandates for employers or individuals should be discouraged. Such mandates would bring about an "unprecedented expansion of government power." [111] Mandates are virtually unenforceable without a new and costly infrastructure. Instead, the most practical approach is to target waste. Clean up costly state mandates; eliminate complex insurance purchasing (see Appendix I); reduce the regulatory burden on providers and insurance companies; revise tax codes that contribute to the unaffordability of individual health insurance. Step up the efforts to make medicine safer through better and continuous education for doctors and patients. Develop an integrated and secure electronic patient record nationwide. *Concentrate on keeping people healthier, not just providing broader coverage.* These measures won't solve all the problems, but they will improve the financial dilemma that causes our political gridlock.

To many in the healthcare profession, the ongoing debate about healthcare reform is a frustrating distraction. In the past, doctors didn't go into medicine to learn policy, study economics, or to pay attention to cost of care. Cost and quality are new dimensions to their responsibilities. Unless physicians become active participants in these matters, medicine will fail in its humanistic mission. Practicing doctors don't have to get mixed up in arcane policy issues, but they are duty-bound to know the full impact of their decisions on the care of the patient. Armed with this full-service knowledge, the doctor is better prepared to exercise humanism in the form we dreamed of when we got our first white coats. Healthcare still provides a vantage point from which physicians see and even participate in scientific discovery and in the acceleration of progress. We serve mankind like no other scientific endeavor. If all that weren't enough, we actually help people. Medicine is part of real humanism that has few equals.

THE BUSINESS OF MEDICINE

*... that finance is given a place ahead of work and therefore tends to
kill the work and destroy the fundamental of service. Thinking first
of money instead of work brings on a fear of failure and this blocks
every avenue of business – it makes a man afraid of competition, of
changing his methods... that the way is clear for anyone who thinks
first of service – of doing the work in the best possible way.*

— Henry Ford reflecting on what he first learned about business
   Ford H., *My Life and Work*
   Doubleday, Garden City, NY, 1922

After appointing new division leaders in medicine and surgery, we decided to
give them exposure to leadership in other professions. We arranged interviews with
notables in sports, business and the arts. The insights were fascinating, but I most
remember Cleveland Orchestra conductor Franz Welser-Möst. After an exceptional
concert in Severance Hall, we had a private dinner with the maestro. He raised his
glass and said, "*You know, gentlemen, we are in the same business: the business of
perfection.*" As physicians, we know that perfection is based on knowledge, experience and dedication, and is frequently elusive. But we also know that we are in the
business of results. Each of us, no matter where we practice, has three responsibilities: quality, cost and performance. Physicians are often resistant to accept the

responsibility of cost. However, price drives cost[±] and that alone forces us to think about value and efficiency.

During this modern period, advances in science and technology have improved the value of healthcare and have forced us to change *how* we practice medicine. In the early 20th century, resources and empirical knowledge were limited; therefore, much more time was devoted to supporting patients and their families. By the 1960s, specialty medicine gained prominence. A whole new generation of doctors trained in the last quarter of the 20th century contributed to remarkable progress throughout medicine, often at the expense of bedside relationships. No surprise that many people became disillusioned with the 20th century doctor. They complained about the automaton who lacked the compassion of the (largely ineffective) family doctor of yesterday.

The high cost of healthcare is related to the success of medicine, not its failure. Patients are happy to insist on state-of-the-art care, and suppliers are all too happy to provide it.[1] Although nominal healthcare spending in the United States has increased about 10 percent per year during this period, the expenditures overall have provided progressively better value. A report from the Lasker Foundation concluded that improvements in health for the past 30 years account for 50 percent of the gain in our standard of living.[2] Harvard economist David Cutler also found that increased consumption of new and more expensive drugs and other innovative technologies generated longer life, more productivity and lower healthcare costs, which, together, offset the cost of pharmaceutical research and consumption.[3] Lichtenberg estimated that new drugs may account for as much as 40 percent of the increase in longevity from 1986 to 2000 worldwide.[4] Since healthcare accounts for a large gain in life expectancy, many of the expenditures should be viewed as a credit, not a debit.

Aging brings new fiscal consideration. As we grow older, there is a higher cost of healthcare per year of life gained. In other words, the value of healthcare decreases as we age.[5] However, we have to look at *active* life expectancy, not age alone. In

---

± One reason for the popularity of price controls is the confusion between prices and costs. Prices are not costs. Prices are what pay for costs. Where the costs are not covered by the prices that are allowed to be charged, the supply of goods or services simply tends to decline in quantity or quality, whether these goods are apartments, medicines, or other things. Politicians who say that they will "bring down the cost of medical care" almost invariably mean that they will bring down the *prices* paid for medical care." The actual costs of medical care – the years of training for doctors, the resources used in building and equipping hospitals, the hundreds of millions of dollars for years of research to develop a single new medication – are unlikely to decline in the slightest. Nor are these things even likely to be addressed by politicians. What they mean by bringing down the cost of medical care is reducing the price of medicines and reducing the fees charged by doctors or hospitals. (Sowell T. *Basic Economics: A Common Sense Guide to the Economy*. New York, NY: Basic Books, 2007).

many countries, the number of older *disabled* people is trending down, presumably due to progress in healthcare.[6] A longer life free of disability will make a person feel better, but extended life will not reduce overall Medicare costs. Each patient is still a cost center.

CHANGES IN THE PRACTICE OF MEDICINE

During the past decade the evolution is notable.

THEN	–	NOW
Clinical autonomy	–	Public oversight
Demand	–	Supply considerations
Acute care	–	Wellness and prevention
Primary treatment	–	Chronic disease management
Planning	–	Finance first, then plan
Defined benefits	–	Defined contributions

Clinical autonomy is disappearing as public oversight gains momentum. For a long time there seemed to be no law of supply and demand in medicine. As demand increases, expenditures rise, and supply becomes more tenuous. Today physicians don't want to work the same long hours as their predecessors; nurses are in short supply; labor costs increase faster than reimbursement; new technology is expensive; and some surgical specialties are less attractive because of stress, litigation and length of training. Beyond acute care, the fact that wellness may prevent disease is finally accepted. Also, primary treatment is evolving into coordinated chronic care. In future hospital planning and development, the era of build it and they will come is long past. Financial planning precedes any major project. Employer-based insurance is changing as more risk is transferred to the employee.

Doctors are not becoming less important, but they are becoming incorporated into the American regulatory state – and losing a certain amount of freedom in the process. They are angry and bewildered about reimbursement and compliance, and many find it difficult to keep fully abreast of developments in their fields. As patients reach 65 years of age, the number of doctor visits begins to increase. In the Medicare population, the "dispersion" of patient care among multiple physicians limits the effectiveness of pay-for-performance that relies on a single retrospective method of assigning responsibility for patient care.[7] In one year the typical Medicare patient sees seven different doctors, including five different specialists working in four different practices.[8] Generalist physicians report that roughly four separate problems are addressed at each office visit for elderly patients and that even more issues are addressed for patients with chronic illnesses such as diabetes.[9] For a hypothetical 79-year-old woman with five medical conditions, current clinical practice guidelines would support the use of 12 medications.[10, 11] Media reports, Internet information and advertising influence patient expectations. As more administrators and legislators monitor their activities and patients become more knowledgeable, doctors feel they have less control over their professional lives.

Hospitals operate in an environment characterized by elaborate rules and requirements: laws, regulations, normative expectations of professional organizations, and peer pressure.[12] I don't know of any other profession that is more subject to officious meddling by unqualified authorities. Medical professionals must submit to intrusion into everything from clinical decision making to their own compensation on a scale that any other profession would consider imperious and insulting. Americans have no caps on spending for food, clothing or housing, nor are there limits on remuneration for attorneys, entertainers, journalists, athletes—or health insurance executives. In spite of its steady progress, medicine is enmeshed in a culture of blame fueled by government regulators, politicians, lawyers, and the media eager to scapegoat it for social, political and economic ills. Our profession is heavily regulated. Get used to it.

Service organizations tend to have performance problems because they are not strictly commercial businesses. The demand for medical care is irregular and unpredictable. Patient needs are idiosyncratic and no two patients are alike. There is no law of supply and demand (rising price doesn't curb demand), and there is insufficient competition among providers. Productivity gains in medicine are preferentially captured by patients and suppliers rather than by providers. Productive efficiency of healthcare has not improved because it is a service business (despite more technology).[13, 14±] Physicians spend about the same time with patients today as in the recent past.

The fact of the matter is that we are not in the business of business; we are in the business of medicine. The business of medicine is a changed life: advice that saves a life, treatment that adds quality to living, and sometimes just making the final days comfortable. And this business is best conducted with input from physicians who are totally aligned with the medical center wherein they practice. In academic health centers, the synergy among doctors, hospitals, research and education has the potential to strengthen the individual physician and to establish an ideal practice

---

±   Baumol's law states because healthcare is a labor-intensive service industry, productivity lags behind manufacturing sector productivity, causing costs in service-related markets to rise over time. Service industries do not benefit from labor-reducing technologies to the same extent as manufacturing. Doctors have to see one patient at a time, whereas in a factory a technological breakthrough can markedly improve output, often with less labor.

environment. Some would say this amounts to surrendering individuality to the organization. Not at all. Medical interdependencies enrich the clinical experience and make the individual physician wiser, more efficient and secure.

Money is a commodity; talent is not. The aligned physician group has unity of purpose, manages their support team, and serves as a repository of knowledge, and yet, the individual physicians can remain remarkably independent. It is the collective genius of an organization that distinguishes one medical center from another.

We live in a peculiar era: The brokers, the money changers, and the payers are in charge – not the provider, or even the receiver of healthcare. There is no parallel in law, architecture, the arts, or in other professions or even in most industries. Commercialism in medicine is relentless and, if it persists, will erode trust between physician and patient, and economics will drive ethics even more than it does today.[15] Medical operations must earn a margin above costs to assure the continuing improvement of services, but this is a qualitatively different margin from that pursued by a public company. For the company, maximizing profits is and should be the only goal. For a medical institution, profit is not an end in itself, but the means to an end. Money is necessary for success, but profit is not the sole reason for the academic enterprise.

The cost of medical care is not reduced in the slightest when the government imposes lower rates of pay for doctors or hospitals. There will still be just as many resources required to build and equip a hospital or to train a medical student. Countries that impose lower prices on medical treatment have ended up with longer waiting lists to see doctors and with less modern equipment. Because of an inadequate supply of doctors willing to practice medicine under these conditions, a substantial proportion of the doctors in Britain have come from less developed countries with lower quality medical training. Costs have not been lowered for the same medical care. Lower prices have been paid for lower quality treatment.[16]

U.S. HEALTHCARE

Of the approximately 5,700 U.S. hospitals, 49 percent have fewer than 100 beds; about 35 percent have from 100 to 300 beds; 11 percent between 300 and 500; and only 5 percent have more than 500 beds.[±] Most of the academic health centers fit into the largest bed category. Allegedly 2,000 of the nearly 3,900 acute care hospitals make little or no profit. The top tier of 500 to 1,000 hospitals is consistently profitable, has good credit ratings and claims a substantial share of the market. And then there's everybody else.[17]

±   American Hospital Statistics, 2006. (2008 Health Form LLC, an affiliate of the American Hospital Association)

Americans played a key role in 80 percent of the most important medical advances in the world, including half of all new major medicines developed, over the past 30 years.[18] Nevertheless, the World Health Organization (WHO) ranks the U.S. healthcare system as 37th in the world, "slightly better than Slovenia." We are penalized for not having "universal" healthcare.[19] ± After accounting for the unusually high fatal injury rates (non-natural causes) in the United States, the life expectancy is as high here as in other OECD countries.[20]

The U.S. is criticized for low-quality care, defined as higher death rates for diseases amenable to medical care.[21]† Many of the cross-national metrics are inaccurate because of definitional issues. Our higher administrative costs in the U.S. relate to customer service, compliance and case management. We have good, if not the best, access and a short length of hospital stay. In a comparison of five countries (Australia, Canada, New Zealand, England and the United States), the U.S. ranked either best or second best in just over half of the 21 categories. It was first or second in three of the nine survival indicators for breast cancer, cervical cancer and leukemia in children less than 16 years of age.[22] We have the lowest mortality for colon, breast and prostate cancer.

Despite the "polls" showing the U.S. as ranking the worst in satisfaction about healthcare, individual perceptions regarding personal health status are remarkably consistent around the world. These perceptions of personal health correlate strongly with respondents' income level, both globally and regionally.[23] In every region the wealthiest quartile of respondents is most likely to offer favorable responses and the bottom quartile, the least likely. The WHO report ranks the U.S. number one in the world in responsiveness to patients' needs in choice of provider, dignity, autonomy, timely care, and confidentiality.[24]

± For an in-depth review of the WHO methodology (and its ideology) read Whitman G. *WHO's Fooling Who? The World Health Organization's Problematic Ranking of Health Care System.* CATO Institute Briefing Papers, February 28, 2008.

† The Organization for Economic Cooperation and Development (OECD) collected data from 30 industrialized nations regarding 21 different health outcome indicators (Mattke S, Kelley E, Scherer P, et al. *Healthcare Quality Indicators Project: Initial Indicators Report.* Paris, France; Organization for Economic Cooperation and Development 2006.) No country scored consistently high or low on all 21 indicators. Most countries scored well on certain indicators and other areas need improvement in all countries.

THE BUSINESS OF MEDICINE

A not-for-profit medical center, however altruistic, needs to think and behave more like a business in order to survive and improve. But this is to a large extent playacting. No business would put up with the many impractical, unprofitable, and irrational activities that must go along with the mission of the academic medical center.

The differences between many commercial businesses and the business of medicine may be listed as follows:

1) Healthcare is consistently labor intensive and capital intensive;

2) The majority of cost in providing hospital services relates to facilities, equipment, labor, and overhead that are not easily flexible. Cost increases in medicine are often greater than in other businesses and relate to polypharmacy, surgical procedures and supplies;

3) Medical information technology lags because of software cost and maintenance, no private or public support, unappreciated savings, the cost of ambulatory and hospital interfaces, logistic disparities, referrals in and out of the system and other interfaces for laboratory medicine, post-acute care, radiology and anesthesia;

4) There is more profit incentive in business (largely because of shareholders) and higher margins compared with hospital care±;

5) Compared with business, our revenue cycle management is far too complicated and inefficient;

6) Payers don't reimburse healthcare providers accurately or on time;

7) Personal medical debt is paid last. It seems harder to manage a patient's credit risk than a customer in commercial business;

8) Healthcare is increasingly regulated, which adds to cost;

9) There is a significant premium for science and education;

10) Healthcare does not deal with sales management in the same way as a conventional business. All of the skilled labor and the various support systems in a hospital or a doctor's office are the "sales force." The exceptions are administrators or physicians who are out trying to recruit physicians to join a system, but they are not selling a product;

± The latest (2005) hospital total margins averaged 3.7 percent (American Hospital Association), which is significantly lower than any category of large commercial business.

11) In corporations there tends to be more access to capital, more money to buy talent, more emphasis on production, sales, market share and profit, and in some of those businesses, less expenditure for compliance or quality;

12) Governance differs in that trustees in healthcare are not paid and have less performance-driven incentive compared with corporate directors. Corporate boards are smaller; directors receive payment; and they are more intent on monetary performance in comparison with large, voluntary, unpaid and more passive healthcare boards.

Having listed these major differences, my personal opinion is that commercial business is a lot tougher than the business of medicine. In the real business world, profit is all-important and personnel often have less security. Shareholders are more demanding than patients.

Although the healthcare enterprise is not exactly like a for-profit business, it is still a business, complete with management, finance, delivery and intangibles. Each of these elements depends on investment and performance, and each is subject to the economic risks of the business world. We have learned some lessons from the real business world. Our financial success depends on our level of debt and our free cash flow. Management isn't minimizing risk; it's maximizing opportunity at reasonable risk.[25] We have to hire only the best personnel for direct patient care. Throughout this book, we emphasize that problem solving alone is not progress.

A for-profit business can also learn a few things from nonprofit healthcare. Concentrate on the core mission and don't stray too far from your field. Specialize wherever possible. Develop interdisciplinary communication. Encourage discussion before decision. Develop policies from staff ideas, not by administrative fiat. Good leadership always encourages innovation.

In a follow-up to his best-selling book, *Good to Great*, Jim Collins dissents from the view that the primary path to greatness in the social sectors is to become more like a business.[26] Instead, what non-profits need is greater discipline. By that he means disciplined planning, disciplined people, disciplined governance, and disciplined allocation of resources. In the good-to-great framework, a great organization delivers superior performance, makes a distinctive impact in the community, and achieves lasting endurance. Gary Hamel adds his observation that what matters most today is not a company's competitive advantage at a point in time; instead, the greatest advantage is the capacity to evolve, i.e., its evolutionary advantage over time.[27] Strategies materialize over years, and short-term losses often must be tolerated while systems are modified and departments grow to profitability. According to former Gillette CEO Jim Kilts, "If you achieve just about median performance year in and year out, you will be number one over five to ten years. If you seek to be number one year in and year out, you will do things that wreck the business. People get this wrong all the time."[28]

Not-for-profit does not mean "no margin." The financial drivers of academic medicine remain profitability, asset productivity, and capital structure. But the medical center, unlike a for-profit business, can't shed its "unprofitable" customers. It would be easy if every patient required only high-margin surgery. As it is, these highly technical surgical specialties subsidize many less-profitable medical services. You might be tempted to load your facility with high-tech, high-profit gadgets, but conscientious management demands that you balance a good return on investment by serving genuine medical need. Conventional business puts profits to use in securing the mission, paying debts, financing growth, and paying shareholders. The not-for-profit medical center uses its margin for capital equipment, new construction, pension contributions, debt payment and future investment.

As the nation faces the prospect of more healthcare for the elderly, we may see more regionalization of some tertiary and all quaternary specialties. The majority of elective surgical procedures will be conducted in specialty hospitals or institutes within a hospital or in ambulatory surgery centers, some with two to four days extended stay. There will be more high-tech imaging everywhere outside the hospital, including compact units in group practices. Remote patient monitoring (management) and other forms of telemedicine will facilitate follow-up and will help to reduce readmissions. And, there is likely to be a proliferation of competitive retail and company clinics and other methods of convenient access. Retiring at the end of 2004, I missed the wave of less expensive retail clinics that have been set up in various discount chain stores, grocery stores and pharmacies.± Fees are generally discounted and the drawing card is convenience. The question is whether the academic center should make that strategy part of its regional primary care group. This trend is here to stay and it could conceivably be a good source for referrals. Success depends on low operational cost, fast turnaround and customer satisfaction.

BIOMEDICAL INFORMATICS†

The healthcare players are not yet well connected by electronic networks that are routine elsewhere.[29] The informatics chasm between the healthcare business and other industries is enormous. It is estimated that no more than 15-20 percent

---

± ...expected to grow to 3,000 within 5 years. (Kaisernetwork.org March 13, 2007)

† A science that deals with biomedical information, its structure, acquisition, and use. (Stead WW. Personal communication).

of U.S. medical institutions use an electronic record system.[±] By contrast, during the past 10 years, more than $20 trillion worth of goods and services have been bought and sold over the Internet. Our healthcare industry is fragmented, and a lack of coordinated informatics contributes to it. This liability is also hindering the development of quality management and quality improvement in healthcare, both of which run on data.[30] Sorry to say that our legacy institutions "...are jumbled mixtures of multiple business models, struggling to deliver value out of chaos, incorporating indecipherable systems of cost accounting, excessive overhead, pervasive cross-subsidization, and an unacceptable amount of variability and medical error."[31]

Forty-plus years ago, Simon Ramo wrote that the computer is the foe of [this] disorganization and chaos.[32] Today, informatics in healthcare is essential both for competition and for strategy – if strategy involves widening the regional practice and offering greater value to the community. Digital information provides greater accuracy, speed, communication and better practice management. The patient gains an understandable personal health record and more efficient access. The payer should have access to valuable quality metrics, effect a faster and more accurate provider transaction, and reduce the back office hassle. The hospital or group practice administration benefits from all of the above, not least by the opportunity to reduce the manpower related to revenue cycle management and quality assurance.

We outlined differences between the healthcare business and conventional businesses. There are also differences in informatics between healthcare and other businesses. The rate of discovery in the biological sciences and in new healthcare technology accelerates very rapidly. Most commercial businesses handle fewer inputs and outputs than their counterparts in healthcare. Most industries deal with physical systems that are more consistent with the laws of physics, whereas most of healthcare deals with biological systems. Variation is evidence of an error in the manufacturing process. Biological systems are inherently variable; they evolve through random changes in DNA sequence and survival of the fittest. Biological risks are not yet known. Other industries are able to isolate change and stage their introduction into routine production more systematically than can healthcare.[33]

±   The latest survey found that 4 percent of physicians reported using a fully functional electronic record system and 13 percent a basic system (DesRoches CM. Campbell EG, Rao SR, et al. *Electronic Health Records in Ambulatory Care - A National Survey of Physicians.* N Engl J Med. 2008: 359 (1); 50-60).

Researchers at the Commonwealth Fund report that industrialized countries have widely different levels of acceptance of health information technology.± According to a 2006 survey, only 28 percent of the U.S. primary care physicians use the electronic medical (health) record compared with 79 percent in Australia, 89 percent in the United Kingdom, 92 percent in New Zealand, and 98 percent in the Netherlands.[34] An electronic medical record is used by 100 percent of Danish physicians to access medical databases and issue prescriptions, order laboratory tests and track results, send referrals to specialists, physical therapists, or any hospital in the country, and chart consultation notes and hospital discharge summaries. Patients can access their health records and check not only their personal health information but also see who else has viewed their records.[35] In the United States there is no universal patient identifier that enables ready authentication of the consumer across the healthcare system. New approaches to establishing identity and trust are needed.[36]

Slow adoption of the electronic patient record is related to cost, interface problems, complexity, training time, and down time.† Senior doctors are especially unmotivated to adopt an electronic record. A fear of failure rightly exists among hospital informatics personnel. Medical chief information officers are generally vendor dependent, don't have experience in technical development and have fewer resources compared with industry. The cost of a fully implemented patient electronic record is very expensive and may amount to more than $200 million for a hospital of 500 to 1,000 beds and its outpatient facilities. Consultants are often biased toward one system or another, making it difficult to trust their choices. Other decisions are complicated by institutional politics and cost. The benefits of having a comprehensive inpatient repository are lost as administration dithers with budgetary constraints. In addition, installing an electronic record for the thousands of mid-sized and small hospitals is still hugely expensive and will consume further outlay once in place. Many hospitals wonder whether the expenditure is worth it and so they delay, thinking that they will get more for their money later on. Over-investment

---

± Five objectives for interoperable computerized medical records: First, patient records should support patient care and improve its quality. Second, they should enhance the productivity of healthcare professionals and reduce the administrative costs associated with healthcare delivery and financing. Third, they should support clinical and health services research. Fourth, they should be able to accommodate future developments in healthcare technology, policy, management, and finance. Fifth, they must have mechanisms in place to ensure patient data confidentiality at all times. (Dick RS, Steen EB, editors. *The Computer-Based Patient Record. An Essential Technology for Health Care*. Washington, D.C.: National Academy of Press, 1991).

† Barriers cited in the literature include purchase price, installation cost, acceptance, maintenance expense, interoperability issues, concerns about security and privacy of personal health information.

in healthcare information technology (IT) generally results from poor choice of products, a lack of acceptance by the staff, or unusually high maintenance costs – some of which is attributed to customization. Electronic record systems often elicit a chorus of moans from doctors and nurses. In our experience, doctors complain for six months and then can't live without it.[±]

The Markle Foundation found that 91 percent of Americans believe that patients should have access to their complete medical records, and about two-thirds of those polled believe that the access, especially test results, should be online.[37] In theory, patient access to their personal health records should also avoid duplication, educate the patient and ensure that the correct information is always where it needs to be – with the patient.[38] In the future, patients will "own" their records. The personal health record, or PHR, is a secure electronic repository that enables a patient also to share information with multiple healthcare providers or others at their discretion.[39] Kaiser Permanente is now making PHRs available as a free service to all members. The Kaiser PHR, called My Health Manager, offers access to the member's electronic health record, lab test results, and immunization records. Other functions include online appointment scheduling, online prescription refill requests, information about eligibility and benefits, and secure messaging with clinicians.[40] An unintended consequence of HIPAA is a slow down in the adoption of personal IT solutions, because HIPAA threatens legal action if privacy is perceived to be unprotected.[41]

The interface between group practice outpatient records and the hospital repository has been slow to develop, primarily because the IRS made it illegal. Encouraging community physicians to link to the hospitals' databases were seen as a form of kickback for referrals. This impediment was removed in May 2007, when the IRS created a safety zone for these transactions. The provisions are that the hospital must have access to all of the records created by a physician using the hospital technology, make its technology available to all its medical staff physicians, and provide the same subsidy to all physicians.[42]

Paper-based information storage and retrieval is fraught with lost records, duplication, delays in diagnosis and treatment, an increased risk of medical errors

---

±   In a survey of electronic records functionalities in major clinical units, respondents from approximately 3,000 hospitals indicated that only less than 2 percent of U.S. acute care hospitals have a comprehensive electronic records system, i.e., present in all clinical units, and approximately 8 percent have a basic system, i.e., present in at least one clinical unit. Computerized provider-order entry for medications has been implemented in 17 percent of hospitals. Larger urban hospitals and teaching hospitals were more likely to have electronic records systems. (Jha AK, DesRoches CM, Campbell EG, et al. *Use of Electronic Health Records in U.S. Hospitals*. Published at www.nejm.org March 25, 2009 (10.1056/NEJMsa0900592).

and a storage burden. The end result is poor service, increased length of stay and higher cost.[±] But current electronic records systems are far from perfect. Geared toward transaction processing, they do not synthesize new information from disparate sources. The Vanderbilt University informatics group is sponsoring a systems approach to practice. Instead of data processing around specific practices, they link decision making information into work processes. This "closing the loop" approach offers doctors and nurses a process-control dashboard showing where clinical correction is needed while there still is time to act prospectively. Although this support will not eliminate variability in practice, this tool augments the practitioner's memory by making information consistently and rapidly available throughout the practitioner's workflow.[43]

According to Dr. William Stead, a pioneer in decision support, such systems will inevitably supplant expert-based practice. Human memory-based medicine is increasingly unreliable. The complexity of biomedical information and technology already overwhelms the individual expert's cognitive capacity.[†] Specialization (sometimes defined as knowing more and more about less and less) is not the answer, because it fragments care. And fragmented care is the opposite of the personalized, "holistic" medicine that is promised by genomics and systems biology. Even if it were not doomed to be replaced by computer memory, we would want to move beyond reliance on human memory alone. Other industries have shown that a standard process is the key to consistently producing the desired result. There is no reason to believe that healthcare can be an exception to this rule.[44]

Most healthcare chief executives have marginal experience with information technology and rely on staff consensus or consultants in choosing an electronic medical record. Be aware of unanticipated costs. Some vendors will undercharge at the front end and make it up by installation fees and add-ons. The chosen electronic record has to produce value for clinical medicine, business, research and education. At the outset, consider the outpatient practice and the hospital repository as a unified record. There should be a common IT architecture across the system. Standardize and integrate across all "business units." If individual patient records are a component of the system, the customer has to be satisfied with enablement and ease of usage. Understand the IT budget and their spending trends. The pay-me-now-or-pay-me-later mantra is the IT leverage on budget. A good chief information officer is cost-conscious and figures out how IT can improve revenue generation and how to get

---

±   A multi-hospital study has recently shown that hospitals with automated notes and records, order entry, and clinical decision support had fewer complications, lower mortality rates and lower costs. (Arch Intern Med 2009: 169 (2); 108-114)

†   In 2007, there were more than 670,000 new articles indexed in MEDLINE (U.S. National Library of Medicine, Key MEDLINE Indicators, http://www.nlm.nih.gov/bsd/bsd_key.html.

projects done on time at or below budget. Having said that, all service requests to IT have to be funded. The clinical and research departments must understand that IT is not free. Personally, I don't know the optimal table of organization for IT, but duplication is the downside of decentralizing IT.

The inability to establish base requirements for comparison with vendors' products is a consequence of marginal technical experience. The system requirements of the academic medical center must be satisfied before buying and installing an integrated electronic patient record. The gap between what is available and the necessary requirements has led some healthcare organizations to build their own electronic medical record. Most of these homegrown systems have addressed a more narrow aspect of patient care or provide functions in complex or data-intensive environments that cannot be met by the general medical records system (such as clinical pathology laboratories, cardiac catheterization suites and other imaging facilities). Care must be taken to see that such new systems do not further fragment healthcare IT, which can happen if transaction, workflow or device systems are not integrated with the overall medical record system. Among the successful endeavors to build more comprehensive and integrated systems is the work of Mark Smith, M.D., and Craig Feied, M.D., at the Washington (D.C.) Hospital Center.

Their installation was created because of department demands. An important system requirement was that it had to be facile at integrating information from multiple sources. They believed that the best design is modular and should incorporate all data fields. According to Smith (personal communication), he and Feied learned some valuable lessons during the three years they spent designing, developing and using a comprehensive yet surprisingly nimble information system that ultimately was purchased by the Microsoft Corporation.[45]

1) Data are data, which means that there should be no distinction between administrative, financial and clinical data. Integrate at the outset.

2) One cannot foresee all the value of the data delivered. You don't know what people will use data for until you supply it *and* the user doesn't know what they will use it for until they have it.

3) More data are always better. The adage that in the absence of action, information is overhead doesn't apply. It is better to have data than not to have it.

4) Don't waste your time on completeness; avoid over-design. Introduce multiple small rollouts, any of which could fail, and not jeopardize the success of the whole project, compared with one comprehensive rollout, which (after installation) may be problematic and obsolete.

5) Content is king – a variant of the 80/20 rule, i.e., 80 percent of the benefit is in access to some type of information that was not available before.

6) Sunshine the data. When you display the data, change will effect itself in an organization. Hidden information is the enemy of organizational efficiency – e.g., in an emergency department, doctors can spend 40 percent of a clinical shift looking for data instead of talking to patients and thinking critically about their problems.

7) Information is the 15 percent lever – i.e., the trick is to find the right 15 percent and effect the right change such that the remaining 85 percent of the system is levered to flip and self-organize in the direction that is wanted. An example of this is bed assignments in emergency departments (EDs). Four different hospital services are involved – admitting, nursing, environmental, and the ED. Admitting must know which beds are empty and clean. Nursing controls information about which patients have been discharged. This information is transmitted to environmental services whose staff clean the room and notify admitting after they have done so. Hidden knowledge is the problem everywhere. In some hospitals, not yours of course, nurses have even been known to hide empty clean beds from admitting.

8) No design by committee and no training. This is unconventional wisdom to design by a small group who know the content and realize that it should be so simple that it requires no training. If it requires training, it's too complicated. If the system is good, people will use it.

9) Employ the patterns and the aggregation of data. Add generic display tools and pattern recognition aids and you will discover a lot of things that you did not know were happening. A good example would be the mistakes in the registration procedure.

10) Build modularly. Avoid monolithism. If the system is modular, you can throw away parts that are outdated or not working. If you have a monolithic system: a) it takes a long time to design and will be out of date by implementation; b) it takes years to amortize cost; c) it takes time and money to change a monolithic system.

Of these ten "lessons" Smith believes that the three most important principles are: 1) avoid over-design; 2) assure that content is king; 3) always sunshine the data.

Researchers have a major stake in healthcare delivery. Their work depends on acquisition of discrete clinical data.[46] Data is a strategic asset and the priorities are reimbursement, communication and quality assessment. Structured reporting will produce values for variables, i.e., data extractable for all of the above plus research initiatives. Today we have multiple workflow silos of often idiosyncratic information. Tomorrow, data integration will add to evidence-based practice and "comparative effectiveness"; however, privacy and security are prerequisites.

The next breakthrough in clinical informatics will be the integration of financial services into the patient record. Today's billing is less about the transmission of financial information and more about the submission of voluminous clinical detail. The next iteration of the revenue cycle will be different: 1) charges will flow to claims as a natural by-product of the care delivery process, which reduces late and lost charges; 2) clinical data will flow to claims as a by-product of the electronic medical record without requiring health information management intervention; 3) clinically relevant detail will be incorporated on bills, without interfaces between disparate systems – registration, health information management, and patient accounting.[47] All of this will be easier when health insurers and banks align to facilitate patient-provider financial transactions. We may be a long way from insurance reform (standard contracts, community rating, Internet benefit comparisons and purchasing), but as high-deductible plans become more popular, increased out-of-pocket spending will call for more bank transactions. A clinical event captured on the electronic record can assign a claim, aggregate the charge (depending on the insurance benefit) and bill for services. This integration could make revenue cycle management as we know it today totally obsolete and should save enormous administrative costs. (See Appendix II for my proposed flow sheet and advantages to all participants.)

Carr[48] believes that information technology has become a commodity that is necessary for production but "insufficient for advantage." This may be true for many commercial businesses but it is not yet the case in healthcare. Improvements in record storage, ordering accuracy, quality monitoring, research and education – all possible with the electronic medical record – constitute a significant competitive and quality advantage for healthcare systems. As IT is further commoditized by low-cost processing power, by multifunctional generic capability and by hundreds of millions of people on the Internet, it's likely that commercial business and healthcare will purchase fee-based web services from third parties "similar to the way they currently buy electrical power or telecommunication services."[49] All the codes, clinical records, data integration, operations and financial interfaces will be contracted over the Internet at greatly reduced cost. This is where the path turns.

CREDIT RATING

When not-for-profit hospitals need funds to make capital improvements, they use their income, or turn to fundraising and borrowing. A few have revenue from other related or non-related businesses. In 501(c)3 medical institutions, interest rates are favorable and even better with a good bond rating. Bond rating adjusts the medical center's credit rating up or down depending on current income, equity related to debt and estimates of the organization's future capability. The credit community judges hospital management and operations according to cash flow. In tough economic times, the rating agencies will exercise greater scrutiny. They have now integrated quality into their methodology. The analysts don't care about your reputation; they can't amortize goodwill. They are indifferent to organization, structure, promises, past investments, alliances, doctors or scientists (however prominent), or even reimbursement trends (payer mix), except as part of new regulations affecting the entire industry.

As the economic picture worsens, downgrades are increasingly likely. It's not so much that competition for insured patients has worsened, but overall weak financial performance relates to rising unemployment and related (increasing) bad debt expense. Emergency department volumes continue to rise. Patients are deferring elective procedures. In the financial market, losses from investments, the variable rate debt structures, the lack of liquidity and support of large capital investments will be primary factors in downgrades.

Many hospitals will review affiliation opportunities and even divest system assets when performance falters. Long-term debt will be restructured, expenses slashed and strategic capital plans reassessed. Now is the time to really communicate with aligned physicians. Don't hang crepe. Accentuate the strengths of the organization, the options chosen and why, and show them the best methods of mutual cooperation.

Moody's Investor Services summarizes the faults of failed hospitals:[50]

- An excessive board and management focus on "mission over margin," which often contributes to recurring operating losses and excessive reliance on investment income.

- A combination of undisciplined capital spending with little or no oversight from the institution's board (and no attention to return on investment).

- A weak market share caused by an unclear clinical "niche," which results in institutions losing negotiating power with managed care plans.

- An inability to recruit physicians, which affects patient volume.

- A lack of planning or adjustment to overcome local area economic fluctuations.

- An inflexible or failed approach to adapt to Medicare and Medicaid funding and policy changes.

The not-for-profit hospital bond rating has been revised down from stable to negative. New factors that do not bode well for the sector include flat hospital admissions, forecasts of declines in Medicare and Medicaid reimbursement, more bad debt from a weaker economy, skilled labor shortages, equity market losses, and risk from variable rate debt.

MEDICAL PRACTICE MODELS

Regina Herzlinger of the Harvard Business School is among those who believe that despite astonishing advances, healthcare is inefficient, ineffective, and consumer unfriendly.[51] She's right, with a few caveats. We have an impractical culture in the United States that leads to a lot of expensive technology applied at the end of a natural lifespan. Because something can be done, the patients or families often insist on it. We can't change our culture, but we can explore different and more efficient methods of practice.

Enthoven and Tollen[52] believe that the ideal model for healthcare delivery would be an integrated delivery system where the appropriate care is managed by a team that relies on evidence-based practice, electronic patient records, and the best medical equipment. These authors believe that insurance risk – adjusted prepayment, which rewards physicians for keeping patients healthy – is a better method than fee-for-service coverage. Fee-for-service indemnity coverage compounds the moral hazard inherent in all health insurance by paying providers more for doing more, whether or not more is likely to benefit the patient.[53] The potential advantages of prepaid group practice are: lower rates of hospitalization, lower resource use, and more efficient practice. Theoretically this includes better quality management, more coordinated care, and improved preventive care. I like the team idea, but capitation has a checkered past. People have figured out that prepayment gives the provider incentive to do less or select less ill patients. Children's services may be an exception for preventive and behavioral care not reimbursed under insurance plans.

Porter and Teisberg[54] maintain that the most fundamental and unrecognized problem in U.S. healthcare today is that competition operates at the wrong level. It takes place at the level of health plans, networks, and hospital groups. Instead, what is needed is competition based on results. Competition should relate to prevention, diagnosis, and treatment of individual health conditions, which ultimately remodels healthcare policy and payment for disease system management. The solution is to create a distinctive strategy in each practice area. They favor a system in which patient care services are organized into integrated practice units that compete to treat specific patient conditions. In this patient-centric approach, all the services that treat a certain condition would be under one roof, thus reducing patient shuttling. The nation would be served by regional centers for specific diseases or organ systems. They believe that organizational and payment change represents the best opportunity to reduce healthcare costs and improve efficiency. Otherwise, competition that does not improve value is zero-sum competition. Examples of zero-sum competition include cost shifting, increased bargaining power, restricting patient choice, and reduction of costs by restricting services. However, results-based competition depends on information provided to the consumer about service, outcomes and prices.

Their integrated practice unit concept may be ahead of its time except in the academic centers or larger hospitals where there is more alignment of physicians and department interdependencies. Ideally, we need to combine the procedural and "cognitive" specialties and vest authority, responsibility and accountability into a flexible, responsive, scientific and economic unit. This will come about sooner rather than later. In organizing this team approach, be aware that the majority of older patients have several chronic conditions that are often unrelated. About 93 percent of Medicare spending is on the 75 percent of beneficiaries with three or more chronic conditions.[55]

Former Supreme Court Justice Sandra Day O'Connor gave an interesting perspective on the Porter/Teisberg idea: "Let me tell you my dream," she said. "To have consultation with all the experts available at the same time who've already looked at everything and they are all in the same place and there to help you through the process." The surgeon, the radiologist, the oncologist, the plastic surgeon, nurses, specialists, psychologists and so on – everybody there to help you through the process of what to do. "I think that would be terrific," she said.[56] I agree and certainly for diabetes, oncology, neuroscience and specific cardiac conditions *interdependent* doctors in close proximity will facilitate care and patient well-being.

These two new and better ideas about structure are both headed toward integrated delivery systems and integrated practice units. Obstacles, which are not insurmountable, include the fact that the vast majority of healthcare today is provided by private practice physicians, a third of whom practice solo. Instead of an integrated clinical group that would respond to major chronic diseases, medical care is currently fragmented and based on a loose doctor-to-doctor referral system. I have confidence that the next generation of providers will align to effect these new ideas.[±] As Porter and Teisberg point out, this will also entail new responsibility for consumers to become knowledgeable about wellness and to act more responsibly.

These proposals are stimulating new thinking about better ways to coordinate care. As mentioned previously, *The Dartmouth Atlas of Healthcare* (2006) has shown enormous regional variation in the prevalence of treatment across the country.[57] The *Atlas* differentiates between what it calls "high-cost" hospitals, which treat patients more intensively and spend more Medicare dollars, and more efficient "low-cost" hospitals. It shows that elective surgery rates are about the same in high- and low-cost regions. However, there are local spending differences that relate to the prevalence of acute care hospitalizations: Miami and New York City have over-built acute care beds in comparison with Minneapolis and Portland, where there are fewer hospital beds and less utilization. Commercial health plans have focused on controlling price rather than controlling utilization. Growth in specialist visits and intensive care stays are increasing in high-cost regions. One of the major areas of waste lies in the high and unwarranted intensity of hospital and physician services, especially in the last months of life. [58] As chronic diseases predominate, we don't provide good coordinated medical care. In emergencies, patients head for the local hospital; for minor illness, they visit their family doctor. But for chronic conditions, there is less coordination between their primary physician and specialists. Effective coordination of care results in better and cheaper treatment.[59]

INTEGRATIVE FACTORS

Gordon Brown summed it up this way, "In health, price signals don't always work; the consumer is not (yet) sovereign; there is a potential abuse of monopoly power; it is hard to write and enforce contracts; it is difficult to let a hospital go bust; and we risk supplier-induced demand."[60] All true, but a number of integrative factors are converging and they will profoundly affect providers, payers and patients. This cluster of trends amounts to a discontinuity. Here is a forecast of factors that will affect healthcare over the next 10 years.

[±] A specialty that delivers more effective medicine that reduces the volume of services is currently penalized because reimbursement to all specialties increases with added volume. Specialty-specific conversion factors would provide an incentive for self-regulation to determine the best practices based on data from outcomes-focused registries. This change in methodology would reduce competition and fragmentation of specialty medicine. (Mayer J. *Is There a Role for Our Profession in Solving the Problems of the American Healthcare System.* Ann Thor Surg 2007: 84; 1432-34).

FIGURE 5.1

Payment reform
consumer-driven plans
reform tax code
community insurance
rating
portability – fewer state
mandates
payment linked to quality
state experimentation

Informed Consumerism
standardized quality data
transparent pricing
wellness
healthcare navigator
second opinion programs
medical record ownership
personalized medicine
(genomics)
comparative effectiveness

Integrative factors in healthcare

Financial Services
payer/banking alignment
point-of-service collection
self-pay management
smartcard access for
medical records and
collection
EMR claims/billing
pay for performance
incentives

Clinical and Business Intelligence
integrated electronic
medical records
web-based scheduling
telemedicine – remote
monitoring
network-based wireless IT
supplies ~ inventory ~
charges interconnected
hospital workflow redesign

At the top, *payment reform* is the key issue. Consumer-driven healthcare means shared responsibility. Changing the tax code will give further incentive to buy high-deductible policies by giving premiums and out-of-pocket payments favorable tax treatments.[±] Insurance will be easier to buy, and payment to the provider will relate to quality. The regulatory changes that create tax-advantaged health savings accounts will give employers more incentive to switch from benefits to defined contributions. No matter where you live in this world, consumers (patients) are going to have more incentives to take better care of themselves through the desire to save money.

± Deductions are subtracted from taxable income. Credits are subtracted dollar for dollar from taxes owed.

Governments, employers, and insurance companies can no longer bear the full cost of coverage. Individual responsibility for some share of medical expenses may prove to be the most powerful reason to become knowledgeable about personal health in order to avoid costly serious illness later on in life. The informed consumer will have a great impact on the healthcare market. For practicing physicians, shared responsibility means higher patient expectations.

Financial services will expand to accept the tax-advantaged health savings accounts. This convergence of health insurance and the financial services industry will add value from a wide range of available financial services, improved automation in the revenue cycle and greater efficiency in the transaction. Consumers gradually will accept high-deductible plans and use credit and debit cards for transactions of personal expenses. This will require business partnerships between payers, banks, providers and employers. For the provider, new financial services mean more automaticity, which can be served through the electronic patient record. In doing so, the provider will decrease revenue cycle cost and accelerate more accurate collections. (see Appendix II)

The third integrative factor in modern healthcare is called *clinical and business intelligence*. It requires adoption of standardized electronic medical records with ambulatory and hospital interfaces and incorporation of financial services in the patient record. Health insurance purchasing and appointments will be transacted more efficiently through the Internet. We need to make processing a claim or getting healthcare information as easy as buying a book from Amazon.[61]

The fourth component, *informed consumerism*, means greater patient sovereignty. Today, people spend more time researching a new TV set than they do selecting a physician. Awareness is not informed consumerism. We rely more on coverage than information. Patients have little incentive to shop for high-quality, lower cost healthcare. One survey found that only 12 percent of Americans study the cost or quality of healthcare.[62] Even among those with heart disease, 42 percent sought no information on their medical condition or treatments.[63] As understandable information becomes available to the consumer, patients will become more knowledgeable and they should demand higher quality. Their cause is strengthened by the Centers for Medicare and Medicaid Services (CMS) who recently announced a sweeping policy to stop paying hospitals for "preventable complications." The CMS position rests on the principles that payers should pay more for the treatment of conditions that require more resources and for conditions that the provider could not reasonably have prevented. More should be paid when evidence-based or consensus-based best practices are followed, but reimbursement should be less or not at all for low-quality care. Naturally, the last will be the most contentious because of risk variability.[64] A policy of not paying for hospital infections sounds good, but immune compromised patients, transplant recipients, and those receiving chemotherapy should be excluded. What is not known is whether the policy will engender risk avoidance.[65]

As patients face higher deductible insurance premiums, they need to know out-of-pocket cost up-front. Most hospital personnel cannot handle price inquiries and instead direct the patient to various representatives or worse yet to recorded messages. Ideally, this could be done electronically at registration, but telephone inquiries must also be handled accurately by trained personnel. Instead of requiring hospitals to calculate charges, another approach to transparency is to allow hospitals to charge a certain percentage above the Medicare rate, e.g., to disclose that their private charges are 110-130 percent of the Medicare rate. This would simplify price transparency because the patients then would have to compare only one price.[66]

Informed consumerism embraces the concept of wellness, which is based on health improvement and elimination of preventable conditions. The whole patient experience must be made more navigable and effective therapeutically. These improvements rely on a more informed patient who has a heightened consciousness of his or her personal health status. For serious illnesses, they should seek second opinions. Owning your health record will be the norm. Advances in genomics will lead to "personalized" diagnoses and treatments.

These changes in modern healthcare pose two questions: Will it be more prospective? And second, will it moderate escalating healthcare consumption? It's unknown today whether patients who have greater responsibility for their healthcare will take a personal interest in preventive care. Will patients make decisions based on price and quality information? Will they be able to navigate the complexities of consumer-driven healthcare? All of these questions go back to personal responsibility and incentives to purchase healthcare insurance. So far, there is little evidence that public reporting of outcome data has had a significant effect on patient decision making, nor has it affected the rate of hospitalization. As more patients move to high-deductible health plans, this is bound to change. The informed consumer who requires expensive diagnosis and treatment will ask more questions, seek more second opinions, and pay more attention to provider ratings. Competition among providers may not significantly lower cost, but it should reduce adverse outcomes and improve service. Finally, what will patient sovereignty mean for providers? Consumer satisfaction is not a proxy for quality, profitability or even consumer loyalty. Study after study shows that what patients value above all is good communication from their doctors and hospitals.[67]

Like politics, the business of medicine can make strange bedfellows. It involves a complex web of relationships and motives that may distract us from the highest ideals of our profession. So we must never forget that the goal of every hospital is to be the best place to receive care, the best place to practice medicine, and the best place to work.± This is the intellectual capital where value in medicine resides. Value respects and honors patients and protects their interests and privacy. Sometimes, the best specialty medicine is the most expensive healthcare initially, but frequently it becomes the least expensive treatment over time, and thus a better value. Value in medicine is far more important than money to the patient, but cost seems more important to society. It is difficult to put a price on hope, wisdom, skill and compassion.

±   Fred DeGrandis, personal communication

STRATEGIC PLANNING

To build may have to be the slow, laborious tasks of years.
To destroy can be the thoughtless act of a single day.

— Winston Churchill
Churchill WS. *The Unwritten Alliance:*
Speeches 1952-1959. London: Cassell, 1961, p. 320

Strategic planning is an exercise in futurity. ...Be careful, as the Irishman said, "What has futurity done for us?"[1] Well, maybe nothing, unless the plans produce favorable results. In fact, some believe that "giving up the illusion that you can predict the future is a very liberating moment."[2] My view on strategic planning, or intent, or architecture, or thinking, or whatever other derivatives that come to mind today, is this: Without a plan, the organization is apt to bounce from crisis to crisis and miss the opportunities. Strategic planning is a thought process, the goal of which is to find opportunity and act on it. The plan sets the course.

Strategic planning is making choices. It is a process designed to support leaders in being intentional about their goals and methods.[3] A strategy is a commitment to undertake one set of actions rather than another, and this commitment necessarily describes an allocation of resources.[4] In any profession, plans depend on the current business model or design, the environment or market, prevailing policies and the organization's mission. A sound culture precedes a great strategy. Led by the chief, the executive group should do the planning... even to the point that the leader writes the first drafts. One person, however, can't drive the strategy. However conceived, the plan has to be both descriptive and prescriptive. It doesn't tell you exactly what to do but it should provide direction. The longer it is, the less likely it will be followed or even referred to.

Some in leadership hire consultants to do their strategic planning. Consultants may be useful for an overview of the healthcare sector. Some believe that consultants can facilitate and focus discussion among the planners. But using a consultant deprives you of the experience of self-analysis and creativity that may be the most valuable part of the process. Many chief executives lateral this activity to a planning committee and then approve the finished document. A committee often doesn't have the knowledge or experience and may not receive proper direction. I would bet that most of those plans are not followed. One of the reasons that leadership and governance should craft the strategic plan is that they alone have the responsibility of making the plan work. Detached personnel and consultants generally do not make it happen.

As the plan is drafted, broad input and healthy debate, even dissent, is essential. The process has to stimulate extensive discussion. Ingenuity comes from encouraging bottom-up thought and driving top-down initiatives.[5] This plan, if followed, will be the course of action for the next several years. The plan must be well-financed, all resources accounted for, estimated risks clearly understood by knowledgeable and influential participants, and internal consultation widely sought to finalize the drafts. Luck is where preparation meets opportunity.[6]

Rumelt believes that most corporate strategic plans have little to do with strategy.[7] They are simply three-year or five-year rolling resource budgets and a rough projection of market share. Calling this "in-the-box" instrument a strategic plan creates false expectations that the exercise will somehow produce a coherent strategy. Likewise, best practice benchmarking may be important for improving operating efficiency, but organizations seeking to distinguish themselves should draw the line at mimicking a competitor's strategy.[8]

Peter Drucker wrote extensively about responsibility and follow-up.[9] The first problem, as he sees it, is that planners and implementers are rarely the same people. One group (often outsiders) plots the strategy, hands it off to a second group, and then goes home. Plans go to the bottom of an operating manager's desk drawer, and that's the end of them. Second, goals and incentives may be misaligned. People may be rewarded for doing something different from what is needed. A third problem is a lack of continuity in key management positions. People who should follow through on a matter at a critical juncture have been promoted or have moved on, and their successors lack the knowledge, commitment and passion to do what is necessary. Finally, the problem may be poor communications. The people who have to execute the plans may not know what to do or they may have received confusing or conflicting directions.

PREPARATION

Planning is part of the responsibility of leadership and is the precursor of effective strategy. At the very least it is an exercise in authority. Vision isn't about knowing where the company is going. It's about knowing where the *industry* is going.[10] If you don't understand the profession, the market and the mission, you are not fit for leadership. Strategic planning is turning vision into a realistic document that addresses priorities, methods of implementation, expected results and value.[±] To take charge of planning influences your peers, emphasizes the importance of planning and is one of the best examples of proactive leadership. Whatever strategy is adopted, it has to be actionable and result in practical goals. As Herb Kelleher wrote to Southwest Airlines employees in the early 1990s, "The number one threat is us. We must not let success breed complacency; cockiness; greediness; laziness; indifference; preoccupation with nonessentials; bureaucracy; hierarchy; quarrelsomeness; or obliviousness to threats posed by the outside world."[11]

Why plan at all? Because healthcare is changing perhaps more rapidly than any other profession. Remember, it is not the strongest of the species that survives, nor the most intelligent, but rather the one most adaptable to change.[12] Steve Muller, a former president of Johns Hopkins University, said it this way, "Change is here, like it or not. More change is in view. Change breeds doubt. Doubt kindles choice. Choice is opportunity, opportunity to do better or worse."[13] Given those choices, we would all choose better. Direction is about creating the future rather than resurrecting the past. To do that, planning has to be based on the strengths of the organization. In our case, we were fortunate to be able to take advantage of our excellent model of medicine – the interdependencies among specialties, the coordination of experience, and the collegiality born of a respect for accomplishment.

Ideally, a strategic plan is crafted to reshape the field that you are in. Everyone agrees that the current healthcare system is bloated. Attention to cost is achieved through greater process efficiencies and improved coordination of care. The most creative plan will reshape the market. The other platforms mean that you are adapting or following. An example of *shaping* would be the development of a new healthcare system that the Cleveland Clinic accomplished in the 1990s. We organized and integrated hospitals and ambulatory care throughout the region. An example of *adaptation* would be the conversion from paper to electronic records. *Following* is what we tend to do in the patient accounts area by unstandardized contracting,

---

± As Liddell Hart wrote: "A plan, like a tree, must have branches if it is to bear fruit; a plan with a single aim is apt to prove a barren pole." (Hart BHL. *Strategy* New York, NY: Frederick A. Praeger, Inc., 1954).

trying to collect cash up-front, chasing payments, and attempting to reconcile monies received from payers. We have no choice but to follow the rules for compliance. The practices of yesterday, however, such as expanding the campus, may not work in the future because of the current economic situation that affects all professions.

In reviewing the opportunities, it is equally important to assess what you should not be doing and why. Does the organization require radical change? Most hospitals, and you might say the same for businesses, don't require radical change unless they are failing. The question is, change to what – better, not worse. Planning is not all about promoting change, but knowing what to do.[14] For years we pushed every service to adopt a philosophy of "better to best" but one has to be careful, because better can be the enemy of good. It depends on what resources are required and whether massive organizational change produces the desired return.

As you strategize, keep in mind that quality *per se* is not a strategy. Quality is a given. In the value equation of quality/cost, the numerator involves correct diagnoses, proper treatment, good outcome and consistent, good service. The denominator of the equation is the cost over time. The objective is to reach the proper balance, keeping overuse and underuse to the minimum and reducing misuse to the irreducible minimum. Value across a healthcare system depends on cost, quality, and turning sound plans into reality.

In the healthcare business, there are numerous methods to improve performance. At the outset, are you getting the most out of hard and soft assets? As a point of departure, be sure that these matters are addressed either in the plan or the tactics:

- profitless growth
- improved supplier relations
- service complaints
- poor lines of business
- physician performance by service
- gaps in your electronic health record
- yield from translational research
- wellness programs for employees/patients
- services that could be expanded or repositioned

In the early 21st century there are some policy issues that a plan should take into account: What are the estimated changes in public and private reimbursement? Assuming the worst case, how would you increase productivity to offset declining reimbursement? Productivity depends on efficiency. Start by understanding and improving the process of healthcare delivery. Any methods to improve patient throughput by workforce remodeling and reduced administrative expense are worthy of consideration. The convergence of electronic health records and financial services would be at the top of my list for efficiency. These comments are by no means complete. They serve only to begin the discussion.

An organization can satisfy demand through new services and facilities. Where are the unmet needs? What factors constrain demand? What services could be expanded or moved? Success is increasingly dependent on an electronic patient record to tie it all together. How can you further encourage innovation, especially in organization and process? Where can scientific investigation gain greater return? Does medical education need reorganization? Do you have the best teachers? Good strategy must be based primarily on logic, not on experience derived entirely from intuition.[15]

Greater value implies greater efficiency. The enterprise must produce greater benefits for the same cost or the same benefits for a lower cost. Sustained competitive advantage is an economic concept – the culture must have positive economic consequences and it must be different from your rivals'. Barney and Clark[16] believe that the differential culture must be "imperfectly imitable." In other words, if rivals try to imitate the culture, they will be at some disadvantage.

BEGINNING

Where does planning start? As an English proverb says, "A good beginning makes a good ending." If you're new to the organization or if you are writing a first strategic plan, start by reviewing the organization's history from the founding through recent times, and above all, understand the accomplishments. This gives the staff a good perspective on change and the potential for growth. This is where we are now, and these are the lessons we have learned along the way from the previous and current strategies. In a new administration, one of the first goals of communication is to understand the strategy. Our product is medicine. Research and education are equally important, but you exist first and foremost to take care of patients. Otherwise, forget clinical medicine and transform the organization into a research foundation.

Before the executive group engages in strategic planning, remember what Warren Buffett calls the "institutional imperative"[17] : As if governed by Newton's first law of motion, an institution will resist any change in its current direction; just as work expands to fill available time, corporate projects or acquisitions will materialize to soak up available funds; any business craving of the leader, however foolish, will be quickly supported by detailed rate-of-return and strategic studies prepared by the troops; the behavior of peer companies, irrespective of whether they are expanding, acquiring, setting executive compensation, or whatever, will be mindlessly imitated.

Don't write a supercilious document with lofty impractical goals, a tome that will collapse of its own weight. Heed the foibles of this sequence as recorded in 1922 by psychiatrist Walter Menninger,[18] who circulated a memo he had seen:

> In the beginning was the plan
> And then came the assumptions
> And the assumptions were without form
> And the plan was completely without substance
> And the darkness was upon the face of the workers
> And they spoke amongst themselves saying
> "It is a crock of s---, and it stinketh"
>
> And the workers went unto their supervisors and sayeth
> "It is a pail of dung and none may abide the odor thereof"
> And the supervisors went unto their managers and sayeth to them
> "It is a container of excrement and it is very strong
> Such that none may abide by it"
>
> And the managers went unto their directors and sayeth
> "It is a vessel of fertilizer and none may abide its strength"
> and the directors spoke amongst themselves saying one to the other
> "It contains that which aids plant growth and it is very strong"
>
> And the directors went unto the vice presidents and sayeth to them
> "It promotes growth and is very powerful"
> And the vice presidents went unto the president and sayeth to him
> "This new plan will actively promote the growth and efficiency
> Of this company and these areas in particular"
>
> And the president looked upon the plan
> And saw that it was good and the plan became policy

The point is... don't approve plans that are not ingenious. Because you are the chief, your colleagues are apt to follow. Complain loudly until someone provides a plan that makes sense and can be followed.

There are many formats for planning. A plan is not an encyclopedia. When it is finalized, be sure that it encompasses 1) the reality of your position; 2) advantages and disadvantages of the organizational model; 3) market changes; 4) where you want to go (in the intermediate term); 5) how you're going to get there; 6) the investment required and a source of funds; and 7) prioritized tactical execution. Address the traditional scan of strengths, weaknesses, opportunities and threats. Today, contingencies are more complicated. Do you have contingencies to deal with pandemics, terrorism, catastrophic litigation, natural disasters, loss of key personnel and economic downturn affecting reimbursement?

Michael Porter introduced the concept of generic strategies: cost leadership, differentiation and focus.[19] Building a system requires capital, but savings can be realized by consolidating certain operations, patient financial services, and contracting. Although the investment is considerable, *cost* improvement will be realized later on through a unified electronic health record. *Differentiation* is gained by imbedding quality standards in the new system. Find a competitive advantage in each specialty. The question is whether you can transfer your reputation including all the intangibles to a larger system. Don't dilute your image. After the initial *focus* on building the system, decentralized leadership at the local level will succeed when the vision is clear and good communication exists between the academic center or the principal hospital and the community hospitals.

In the preliminary assessment divide your analysis into inside and outside. On the inside, determine whether the table of organization (structure drives strategy) is optimal for today and tomorrow. The strategy has to match the financial picture. Performance includes productivity, quality and service. Payer issues fall in between your inside and outside analyses. How have you fared in past negotiations? How are your payer categories changing, and are you a price taker or an effective negotiator? Are your payer contracts fairly standardized? Do you really know whether the received payment is accurate?

On the outside, focus attention on demand and competition. Know the ratio of medical:surgical admissions and their trends. Find out where regional demand is underserved. Map your key services as they relate to the market. A two-dimensional diagram can be constructed with the major services, such as neuroscience, orthopedics, cardiac, urology, etc., horizontally across the abscissa. On the ordinate, scale either volume or market share. If you can ascertain market share accurately, that will suffice. Take the first service and record its market share in the region compared with the major competitors in that specialty; then do the same for the other services. If possible, go back each year for five years to see how the service has grown or shrunk in the market.[20] Now you have a service comparison of where your organization stands in the region.

Now that you have asked the right questions and analyzed market share by service, focus on the socioeconomics of your service area. Patients and personnel face a weak economy. How will they react? The answer is mixed. While capital is problematic, the labor pool may actually improve. Good doctors may be easier to recruit. The obvious downsides include increased bad debt, fewer elective cases and reduced Medicare and Medicaid reimbursement. The short-term future may not look good, but it will be easier to manage if you plan for contingencies.

You may be tempted to look for business overseas. We looked hard at some international opportunities but none was quite right, mainly because of the cost and potential management time that would have been required. Global competition is not necessarily bad but needs sizable capital investment, preferably by the host government or investors. Beyond culture and language, family relocation and distant management also are important considerations. Other issues are the same as in regional expansion – transfer of reputation, recruitment and competition. There are some attractive distinctions, however, and becoming an international healthcare resource continues to be an ambition of leading academic medical centers.

THE PLAN

In 1990, our first plan started out with a vision statement: We wished to achieve a distinctive competency in every specialty; to never have an unsatisfied patient; to deliver comprehensive care; and to develop a worldwide market for specialty medicine. We believed that adhering to that vision was realistic and doable and, more than that, necessary. Why? To have *distinctly competent specialties* is essential for referral and reputation. Not only for patient value but also for our academic reputation, which attracts the best staff. To build your practice, it's more than being busy – it's differentiation – it's being the best.

To never have unsatisfied patients is not an empty goal – it means service has to be exemplary. Patients want both process and substance, the base of which is communication. If medicine is devolving into a commodity, market share will be increased by the best outcomes, innovation and service. Patients expect a good result and they do not want to put up with lousy service in order to get it. Service requires continuing education of personnel, clear information to patients and a coordinated clinical process. An informed patient can readily appreciate outstanding service and intuitively recognizes competence, integrity, compassion and good organization.

As for *comprehensive care*, 18 years ago we did not have a strong primary care network. Specialty care was expanding throughout the community hospitals. We had to strengthen our referral pattern through a new delivery system. Finally, a great academic healthcare center should attract a *worldwide patient clientele*. If the medical organization is truly excellent, people will come from far and wide for second opinions, diagnosis, treatment and follow-up.

Because we had advanced medical and surgical specialties, a global referral practice was in place and easily fit into the vision. In the earlier years of our organization, there were few non-profit multi-hospital systems, no serious for-profit threats and no need for a delivery system apart from the main hospital and outpatient clinic. Looking back, the timing was right to plan and build a comprehensive health system. And, we had a first mover's advantage that we exploited to the fullest. Strategic planning was necessary to validate the vision, and that "exercise" culminated in an optimal integrated delivery system. Progress is made by exploiting opportunities, not just by solving problems. All one can hope to do by solving a problem is to restore normalcy.[21] If your plans include developing a new health system today, you are late but it is not impossible. Remember, there are all sorts of entry barriers in new markets. If you are late (getting into the market), you have to be better.[22±]

±   To read a comprehensive study of strategy and operations, see Kaplan RS, Norton DP. *The Execution Premium: Linking Strategy to Operations for Competitive Advantage.* Watertown, MA: Harvard Business Press, 2008.

FIGURE 6.1

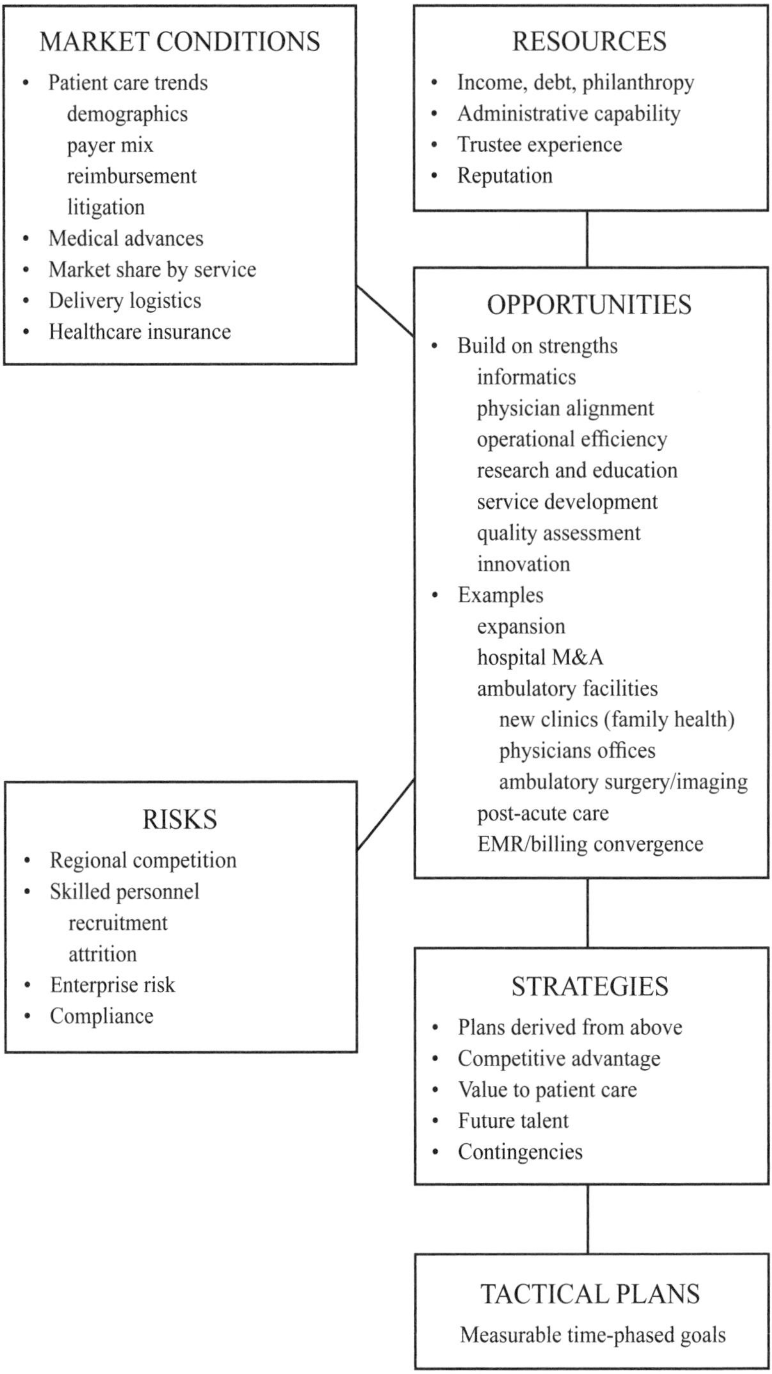

MARKET CONDITIONS	RESOURCES
• Patient care trends demographics payer mix reimbursement litigation • Medical advances • Market share by service • Delivery logistics • Healthcare insurance	• Income, debt, philanthropy • Administrative capability • Trustee experience • Reputation

OPPORTUNITIES

- Build on strengths
  informatics
  physician alignment
  operational efficiency
  research and education
  service development
  quality assessment
  innovation
- Examples
  expansion
  hospital M&A
  ambulatory facilities
    new clinics (family health)
    physicians offices
    ambulatory surgery/imaging
  post-acute care
  EMR/billing convergence

RISKS

- Regional competition
- Skilled personnel
  recruitment
  attrition
- Enterprise risk
- Compliance

STRATEGIES

- Plans derived from above
- Competitive advantage
- Value to patient care
- Future talent
- Contingencies

TACTICAL PLANS

Measurable time-phased goals

Figure 6.1 is only one of many formats for strategic plans. Create your own. They all stress an overview of the market, a study of the organization, and the options or opportunities ahead. Strengths and weaknesses are part of internal analysis. Opportunities and threats (the uncertainties) relate to the external world. The threats are more than competitors; they also are dissatisfied patients. The self-analysis includes what you are doing right and wrong. In our case, we wanted to capitalize on our strengths, our non-profit status, our brand, our staff model and our operations. However, there was no system approach to healthcare delivery anywhere in the region. Building or acquiring facilities in surrounding communities risks referrals from private practice physicians who see any new entrant as a competitive threat. As trust is built over time, we believed that damaged relations would improve. We anticipated the move from acute to chronic care and added primary care staff. In all areas of our mission, there were huge opportunities… and we had the resources.

If your organization has a superb, engaged staff, excellent specialty reputation, and the necessary financial resources, success is not guaranteed but the probability is greatly improved. In our case, the new direction was regional health. Not an easy task. First we had to build strategically located clinics. Next, we had to develop a large primary care base – starting with more than 200 new doctors. Then we positioned outpatient surgery, laboratory medicine, and radiology in these outlying areas. Acquisition of community hospitals followed, but the coordination of care between outpatient clinics and the hospitals was more difficult (see chapter 10).

One of the first decisions is to estimate how many years forward the written plan will serve. The uses of planning forecasts are amusingly illustrated by economist Kenneth J. Arrow. When Arrow was serving in the military, one of his jobs was to compile long-range weather reports. He and his statisticians found that the forecasts were no better than numbers pulled out of a hat. Consequently Arrow asked his superiors to be relieved of this duty. The reply was: "The commanding general is well aware that the forecasts are no good. However, he needs them for planning purposes."[23] We fared better than Arrow's forecasts when we wrote our first strategic plan. However, we couldn't see more than a few years ahead. Subsequent plans could predict out to five years with reasonable accuracy. Our plans were based on how long we thought it would take us to accomplish specific goals (creating a delivery system, expanding outside Cleveland, developing certain specialties, building new facilities, and consolidating administrative activities).

Some leaders are reticent to personally engage in strategic planning, because things are going well and any new strategy could be risky. The objective in strategic planning is to exploit the opportunities that are available at reasonable risk. A review of 750 of the most significant business failures in the past quarter century reveals that half may have been avoided and resulted from flawed strategy rather than execution.

Examples would be unsuccessful mergers, optimistic borrowing, staying the flawed course, overestimating capabilities, betting on the wrong technology, and so on.[24] In healthcare, as in many other businesses, the foundation of successful strategies is based on existing talent and good recruitment. If the attrition rate of the staff is high, you can have the best strategies in the world and it still will be difficult to implement plans fully.

In strategic planning every medical organization should ask: What is our value proposition? The majority of academic medical centers have unique value that they can offer throughout the community. The plan should include better access through new facilities. Develop information about wellness and how to navigate the healthcare maze. A large healthcare system must give priority to leadership and career development, continuing medical education and training updates for all skilled personnel. The opportunities for learning should be given equal weight to healthcare delivery.

One obvious fact we didn't appreciate until the early 1990s was that people didn't want to travel downtown for routine healthcare – they preferred to stay in their communities. An academic organization that wants to meet this demand by expanding into surrounding communities is taking on a big job. It should be prepared to invest money thoughtfully in every hospital it acquires or fund other strategies such as building surgical and imaging centers, medical office buildings, healthcare clinics, and post-acute care services in or around community hospitals. The national market for brand healthcare is expanding, but for the most part, healthcare strategy is still a local matter.

Our multiyear estimates were reasonably accurate, but we didn't predict the impact of some of the reimbursement changes. Financial forecasts hinged on an average 3-5 percent profit, which was not always easy to achieve after expansion, new construction and academic expenses. In the early years, we established clinics that were staffed largely by primary care physicians. We added the imaging and outpatient surgery facilities based on demand. We chose their locations for their prominence, visibility and ease of access (near freeway exits). We either built new facilities or acquired relatively new buildings. As an outpatient strategy is designed or expanded, the first order of business is to figure out where the initial draw is. What you learn may surprise you. In later stages, you can expand your marketing to contiguous areas. After factoring in referrals to specialists and selectively adding specialty lines, we realized a profit in each of those satellite operations, on average within the first three years.

DIFFERENTIALS

When asked to build competitive advantage, most healthcare executives assess what the competitors do and strive to do it better. Their strategic thinking regresses towards competition. This can lead to imitation rather than innovation, and it earns only incremental improvement.[25] Successful strategy is rarely a copycat one.[26] That is not to say that you should not have a good understanding of your competitors' organizations, practices and resources. Your rivals' vulnerabilities may provide good ideas, even a new direction.

In healthcare this is not too hard to figure out. You need to assess the character of your competitors. Are your competitors passive or aggressive? If they fall into the latter category, what is their next move – almost always it is local expansion or acquisition. They could be recruiting your talent for development of a highly competitive service or business. Remember, they have the same interests as you: to seek or create demand, accelerate access, improve the quality metrics, market value and grow most services internally and by outreach. Do they have the resources and management capability to do so? If your competitors are passive, your strategy could awaken them and you have to anticipate their countermoves. Competitiveness must be thought of as a relative comparison of growth rates, or benchmarking of performance to assess how well each participant has done in developing the capabilities for innovation and growth, and not about the mutual potential for damaging one another.[27] Don't let yourself become so obsessed with your competition that you can't see them clearly or learn from them. In other words, don't underestimate your opponents, but don't waste your time "hating" them.

Jeff Bezos suggests that rather than focus on the competition, his people should "Be afraid of our customers because those are the folks who have the money. Our competitors are never going to send us money."[28] If you're falling behind a competitor, you want to ask not only, "What are we doing wrong?" You also need to ask, "What are they doing right?" Having several assumptions for each forecast is a good way to conduct operational and financial planning and, certainly, it's good for discussion. In particular, what is realistic? Where do you get the resources, which in healthcare come largely from profit, borrowing and philanthropy?

Competitive advantage is a description of today and tomorrow, not of yesterday.[29] Differentiation means providing value that competitors can't duplicate, at least for a while. Table 6.1 reviews some differentiating factors. The real differentiation is whether you can craft a plan and carry it out in the allocated time. The *Yes* column lists proven methods that have the potential to set your medical center apart from other medical organizations. The *No* column summarizes the deficiencies that detract from value.

TABLE 6.1

DIFFERENTIATING FACTORS

YES	NO
Authentic leadership	No strategic plan
Deserved reputation	Follower
Clinical quality/service excellence	Price taker
Aligned and valued staff	Reduced capitalization
Continuous innovation	Widespread outsourcing
Timely decision process	High cost structure
Operational effectiveness	Undistinguished reputation
cost control	Rising uncompensated care
capacity management	Disingenuous marketing
continuous improvement	Performance trending down
Selective regional growth	Unaligned physicians
Outstanding research/education	Referrals out-of-network
Integrated informatics	Low quality/service rankings
Strong negotiation team	
Abundant resources	
Successful philanthropy	
Government and private grants	

In healthcare, you cannot compete on price because prices are determined either by Medicare, Medicaid, or commercial payer contracting. However, you can compete on efficiency, quality, and service. The academic medical center can't be the low-price provider because of education and science responsibilities. Similarly, price discrimination is not a competitive feature today. Competitive advantage cannot be achieved by trying to outsource key operations or by reliance only on cost cutting or reduced capital investment. Also, dependence on one or two highly technical specialties is dangerous. Legitimate efforts to reduce uncompensated care may be beneficial but it depends on the incidence of uninsured patients. There are ways to increase productivity on an assembly line, but in a service organization, individual physician productivity reaches a certain level and there is not much more you can squeeze out of doctors without adversely affecting their practice. Physician extenders and the electronic medical record will improve efficiency significantly.

The single greatest competitive advantage for any large organization is sound collective judgment and speed in decisions and implementation. Many believe that providing the most value for the lowest cost is the formula for success; instead it is the best value for the lowest cost in the least amount of time.[30] To say it another way, competitive advantages tend to fade because distinctive capability declines or the markets in which that capability is applied shrink or become less valuable.[31] Since competitive advantage is likely to be short-lived, a healthcare organization should strive for permanent *comparative* advantage. Virtually all hospital or health system plans have to address aging facilities, expanding informatics, contiguous physician office space, improved access and process, all in an era of changing consumer demands. The real question is whether the advantages provide greater access to better healthcare.

There is a whole literature on behavioral economics explaining why executives back bad strategies.[32] Overconfidence, inflexibility and unappreciated real costs top the list. An aversion to any risk may result in unwillingness to seek opportunities at reasonable risk. Another flaw termed "anchoring" is especially dangerous if one is anchored to past performance and assumes the future will be the same or better. Most business consultants will advise killing poorly performing strategic experiments early rather than suffering the sunk-cost effect, which throws good money after bad. However, healthcare is much more of a long-term proposition than a conventional commercial business. As you plan, avoid the herding instinct. The best example of that was the rush to *buy* doctors' practices. And finally, there is the glitz or vanity flaw in which strategy is swayed by publicity more than substance. Don't bulldoze ahead without wide review of the plan.

PHYSICIAN INPUT

Strategic thinking at the department level and input from doctors is valuable, but you have to engage them. Don't send them an e-mail and tell them to write back if they have any ideas. Start by reviewing the trends in the percent of revenue, expenses, and profit that each department contributes to the organization as a whole. Then give them a worksheet to think about (Table 6.2).

Let the department deliberate these essentials and then meet with them as a group.

TABLE 6.2

BASELINE ASSESSMENT	LANDSCAPE	PLAN
Financial position	Competitive analysis	Reorganization
Academic contribution	Market	Innovation
National ranking	Demand	Expansion
Quality/service	Personnel	Controls
Space utilization		Investment objectives
Location of services		Resources required
		Action proposed

In every academic center, there are fiefdoms with their own priorities that are not necessarily in step with the overall strategy. There are some great doctors and scientists who don't think much beyond the next day or beyond their personal academic pursuits. Part of leadership is to encourage the department head to manage proactively and think strategically. This is not a poll or a budgeting exercise or a new project. You should expect fresh ideas. We used to tell our staff, "This is your Clinic. Act to improve it."

For each specialty, ask the chair about what the competitors are doing in the regional market. Show them the trends in market share. What could we be doing in your specialty and is it worth it? Are we good enough to expand and, if so, what do we need?

Be sure that leaders in clinical areas understand the value of a good annual professional review, which can differentiate performance and productivity. A good review will determine the challenges that affect performance. Does your specialty department have distinctive competencies that separate it from the competition? When the department is not optimal, individuals will cite various operational deficiencies that allegedly decrease efficiency in practice. Those charges have to be addressed if you expect progress. If you are not the best, why are your competitors better?

The executive team doesn't know the department as well as the chair should. A planning exercise engages the department members to think about where they are today and hope to be tomorrow. The staff is used to working, not planning. Give them an overview of impending change. Then, start with the baseline assessment, where they stand in the landscape and finally where they would like to be in five years. Ask the department for a growth plan and what resources it will take to get there.

"We are not doing so well," you hear. I say you are not thinking hard enough or you have a lackluster staff. If that is the case, it is probably your fault. Perhaps politics got the best of leadership. Dissidents should be tolerated, but you should demand constructive skepticism. The point is, if a plan failed, learn from it before you start over. Expunge the word *can't* – *shouldn't* and *wouldn't* are acceptable – but *can't*, such as we *can't* stretch that far so we *can't* get the data or we *can't* recruit, are unacceptable excuses. Instead, demand fresh ideas and persistence.

COMMUNICATION

After the strategic plan is reviewed and debated and becomes a complete document with tactical plans and timelines, the essentials should have been put together well in advance by your communications team. Determine what you want to release publicly and what you want to reserve for internal consumption only. Some of the information in the plan will be proprietary. There should be plenty to offer the public about operational improvements, financial forecasts, system recapitalization, service expectations, academic strategies, and institutional philanthropy. You especially want everyone to know your plans to benefit the community and advance public health. Governance should understand every detail of the strategic intent. In communicating future plans, you have an opportunity to remind your audience about the history of the organization as you explain the reasoning behind your strategy. At the Cleveland Clinic, our excellent marketing director devised a clever accordion-fold document summarizing our culture, history, achievements and direction. This was an educational and useful tool for philanthropy.

One activity that is almost always overlooked is *follow-up*. In most healthcare organizations, there is little emphasis on tracking the results of big plans and initiatives, seeing if they worked or not, and why. If initiatives are outsourced, what are the financial and service implications? Which plans were scrapped and for what reasons? How well were the goals and timelines met? The chief executive is ultimately responsible for follow-up, but for assistance in this I often considered setting up a special office or designating an individual solely dedicated to tracking down trends and goals. (I would have done it, except for the fact that the chief administrative officer for our Board of Governors was masterful at organizing follow-up information.)

Keep the board of trustees informed, but in the case of a new strategic plan, it's best to do it in stages.[33] Discuss the changing competitive landscape and the financial and organizational resources available for future development. For every problem, there are opportunities. Remember, finance first; then plan. Map out the future priorities and their rationale and include returns on these investments. The discussion should be as interactive as that of the executive team. When the board understands the issues and the "business" of healthcare and sees progress in the document presented, they may well add to the process. My advice, however, is not to let trustees initiate or control the process. If anyone among the trustees doesn't like the plan, ask for a detailed refutation. Dialogue between the chief executive and the board of trustees and their acceptance are essential for the rollout of a successful strategic plan.

FINAL THOUGHTS ON STRATEGY

It is apocryphal that if you don't know where you're going, you may wind up someplace else. People who have the responsibility for an entire organization must have their receptors on at all times. In scanning the spectrum of daily activities, the leader must be able to zoom in on areas of opportunity or risk. The near-term future is your responsibility. I like George Stalk's method of "open files."[34] He has categorized the files as 1) faint signals – could be a strategy, but right now is too early; 2) watch list – potential strategies but the competitive advantage is not yet clear; 3) hallucinations – provocative issues that are far out and may not materialize. Regardless of uncertainty about direction, there are some who believe that the formal planning process is a waste of time. Remind them that leadership of an academic medical center is an endless search for new opportunities, and the strategies can be self-replicating. Planning is part of learning. The only competitive advantage… is [the] manager's ability to learn faster than his competitors.[35] And, institutional learning is more difficult than individual learning.

Remind your colleagues about the advice from Judge Learned Hand: "We accept the verdict of the past until the need for change cries out loudly enough to force upon us a choice between the comforts of further inertia and the irksomeness of action."[36] You want to plan before change becomes irksome. It can be a very rewarding and thoughtful exercise. If done properly, it brings people together. The strategic plan provides visibility for the intended action and makes leadership responsible for delivering those actions. An expeditious plan is essential. Time is also a strategic weapon and is the equivalent of money, productivity, quality and innovation. Managing time has enabled many corporations to reduce costs, upgrade technologies and offer a wider array of products. These companies are time-based competitors.[37]

Any academic medical center looking to the future has thought about growth through merger or acquisition. Yet for the moment, the era of not-for-profit hospital acquisition is temporarily winding down. Any merger today really has to fit a deliberate strategy. And, the post-merger integration is more important than the steps in alliance. If the academic institution ventures into the community, the first challenge is merging its culture with that of the community hospitals. If the academic institution plans on starving the acquired hospital, the acquisition will ultimately fail and the private practice physicians will go elsewhere. Management consultants have long recognized that mergers and acquisitions are not a strategy in themselves. Adding hospitals or clinics with no plan to capture additional growth or to create further synergies can be a flawed strategy.[38] The aims of alliances are to gain competitive advantage through contracting leverage and building critical capabilities. A good healthcare system can increase the rate of innovation. Don't forget that each community hospital in the system should have a plan, perhaps not a formalized plan, but a plan about how to grow its business and add value in healthcare for the population they serve. The objective is to better respond to market and technology changes,[39] not create a larger bureaucracy.

The reasons why some hospital alliances are not successful is that they: 1) focus on short-term financial results rather than long-term strategic objectives; 2) lack trust; 3) have an uneven commitment and an imbalance of power; 4) fail to inform mid-level operatives of goals or fail to involve them; 5) don't have clear expectations; 6) have no mutually accepted performance measures.[40]

A blind allegiance to growth can also waste a lot of money. Growth by itself may add revenues but it can also induce market share conflicts that end up costing more than the organization gains in true profit. Is the spending level conspicuous, and does the intended growth result in greater patient value? Growth by itself is the scoreboard; it's not the game.[41] In healthcare the "game" is how to consistently add value wherever the organization assumes responsibility.

Strategic planning helped the Cleveland Clinic achieve major growth from the 1990s through the turn of the century. We spent about $1.5 billion in building and acquiring new facilities, and about a third of those funds each came from income, philanthropy and debt. In addition, we invested $700 million in the acquired community hospitals. In 15 years our leadership team organized and recruited new physician, science and administrative leaders; established a family health center network of 14 clinics; acquired nine hospitals; built a new emergency facility and an operating room pavilion that included a minimally invasive surgery education center; developed gastroenterology and urology centers, research and eye institutes, a cancer center and two hotels; built two integrated clinics and hospitals in Florida; and designed (external architecture) a heart institute. A new college of medicine was created for the education of physician scientists. In addition, two large office buildings that formerly were industrial headquarters were donated to the Cleveland Clinic. All of these measures increased our market share significantly (see Appendix III).

Our acquisitions were simultaneously offensive and defensive and followed the plan. The purpose of growth in the community was to introduce the Cleveland Clinic performance measures, to satisfy our plan for more comprehensive care and to preserve and advance the community hospitals. We exercised our plan rapidly because we believed that "the most effective defense is to prevent the battle altogether."[42] The implementation of these plans resulted in an "intrinsically inimitable" strategy, at least for awhile. If you have a good team and the resources, your healthcare organization can achieve this performance or exceed it.

There are numerous principles of enduring success. The time-tested ones include: 1) exploit before you explore – i.e., exploit existing assets and capabilities before you develop new ones (exploitive activities are generally local and market-driven); 2) diversify the business portfolio; 3) remember your mistakes; 4) be conservative about change. Great companies very seldom make radical changes.[43] Major organizational change rarely creates value. "The company should redesign only if there is compelling evidence that the current structure is suboptimal and can't address this shortcoming less invasively."[44] For academic medical systems, concentrate on innovation, selective growth, and process experimentation – all of which entails risk. A strategy is not based on hope. Strategy is what you work for to achieve real progress. "There is no security on this earth... only opportunity."[45] That is why good planning is essential. However, all your collective brain power is wasted if nothing happens afterward.

OPERATIONAL MANAGEMENT

The best advice I ever got occurred at a breakfast meeting in Dallas with a group of business leaders. One of them, a plain-spoken, self-made, street-wise guy, came up and said, "When everything gets really complicated and you feel overwhelmed, think about it this way. You've gotta do three things: First, get the cow out of the ditch. Second, find out how the cow got into the ditch. Third, make sure you do whatever it takes so the cow doesn't get in the ditch again."

— Anne M. Mulcahy, Chief Executive Officer
Xerox Corporation

Leadership of an academic medical center differs from that of a typical community hospital. The reasons are that academic centers have a larger healthcare delivery system, higher case mix, the responsibility of research and medical education, and more salaried medical staff. Regardless of these differences, managerial activity in all hospitals, large or small, relates to productivity, revenue and cost. To that base today, we add quality, innovation and consumerism... and the urgency to make it happen.

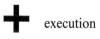

| productivity revenue cost | ▶ | productivity revenue cost | + | quality innovation consumerism | + | execution |

Managing productivity means optimizing schedules, appointments and procedures. Added efficiency is contingent on expanded and integrated informatics, real-time cost management, and discipline in the deliberative process. The trends toward wellness, prevention and chronic care will require more emphasis on primary care, geriatrics and nurse practitioners. Innovation in process and structure depends on how well the institution invests in leadership to encourage free thought, debate, and experiments. Consumerism is unstoppable. Recognize that the patient is the sovereign consumer. Educate the patient and welcome symmetry in the patient-provider relationship. Strive for a "healing hospitality" that blends clinical care with guest services. A new culture should develop around quality and service. As medicine moves toward commoditization, you will need to distinguish your medical center by outstanding service, coordination of care, and superb outcomes. Therein are the great opportunities for operational management. Strategic opportunism is as important as strategic alignment.

Drucker, a generation ago, explained management in terms of five functions: 1) setting objectives; 2) organizing work (which includes planning and assigning responsibility); 3) motivating and communicating; 4) measuring (and following up); and 5) developing people.[1] The leadership team is expected to see this broad perspective. It's up to you to uphold the mission of the enterprise and set performance standards in accordance with the mission. The scope of the mission may be broad, but the value to the community concentrates on patient care.

According to the 80/20 principle, business should focus on the most profitable segments for fastest growth.[2] Healthcare can't do that to the same extent as traditional business. If we did, many internal medicine specialties and post-acute care activities would be markedly downsized. In healthcare, unprofitable services may require cross-subsidization rather than elimination. In fact, only highly technical, acute care specialties actually make money. When all costs are accounted for, less than a dozen specialties are profitable, and fewer yet if laboratory medicine, anesthesia, and radiology are excluded.

Healthcare is a pure service business. Our shareholders are our patients. Our product is a clinical outcome. Our patient takes the profit in the form of good health. However, medicine depends as much on operational innovation as business does and perhaps more. Financial performance in the medical sector is largely a function of health policy, the patient-payer mix, managed care contracts, and operational effectiveness, which includes physician performance. What the public and elected officials need to understand, however, is that "not-for-profit" shouldn't mean "money-losing," and that a hospital system provides the best value to its patients, community and local taxpayers when it can achieve a margin over expenses.

All businesses require proactive management. At the Cleveland Clinic, our operational principles were: 1) to protect and advance the mission; 2) to promote honesty and integrity as a basis of our culture; 3) plan, decide, communicate and act; 4) recognize individual and group success; 5) honor creativity and innovation. You may draw on past experiences, but only the future is manageable. "I saw great businesses become but a ghost of a name," wrote Henry Ford, "because someone thought they could be managed just the way they always were managed, and though the management may have been the most excellent in its day, its excellence consisted of alertness to its day, and not in the followings of yesterday. Life, as I see it, is not a location, but a journey."[3]

Even the most confident industrialist, however, would be challenged by the business of medicine. Hospitals are not ruled by the conventional logic of either business or science. To start with, there are the numerous inefficiencies relating to highly variable patients and payments. Skilled workers cost money and there are few alternatives to expensive professionals. Nurses and some technicians are in chronic short supply. Waste is still evident, beginning with poor correlation between the inventory and charges. Generally, hospital management does not know the precise cost related to specific diagnoses and treatments. The electronic health record is not yet standardized or integrated. Payer contracts are even less standardized. As reimbursement declines relative to cost, large academic centers depend more than ever on philanthropic support. Many elements of the hospital administration are entrenched and change-resistant. Drucker made the observation that much of what we call management consists of making it difficult for people to get their work done.[4]

Since medicine is now subject to more economic risks, many precepts from commercial business apply to healthcare management: 1) managing is not an act to minimize risks; good management looks for opportunity at reasonable risk; 2) a complex organization is best managed by decentralized authority, but everyone has to be responsible and accountable and have clarity about goals; 3) hire only the very best people regardless of entry level (If you don't hire the best managers, mediocre people will invariably hire mediocre people. I learned a long time ago that mediocre people gaining the majority are huge risks to any organization because they will eventually change the culture.); 4) focus on potential, not just problems; if you're only solving problems, you're doing something wrong; 5) good management is based on accurate information… continuously refine the reporting systems (The American humorist H. Allen Smith[5] suggested that of all the worrisome words in the English language, the scariest are "uh oh." If you don't have the right information, you can't manage anything.); and 6) finally, keep looking for opportunities; the reasons for competitive advantage are usually temporary.

RETURN ON MANAGEMENT

Management is not just passive, adaptive behavior; it is taking action to get the best results consistently.[6] You've heard of return on investment. You should insist on return on management, which is the ratio of productive energy released to the management, time, and attention invested.[7]

Applying this principle to medical management yields the following:

High Return on Management	Low Return on Management
project follow-through	ill-defined goals
improve key metrics	politically correct performance
compliance with regulation	no accountability
new ideas every day	chronic indecision
no fear of failure, only fear of poor service	complacency

Leadership and management have to understand priorities, set the course, communicate the plans, and make it happen. Management depends on key diagnostic measures, accurate data and compliance with regulations. Good management thrives on employee input. One study at a high-tech multinational firm found that over half the employees believed it was unsafe to say what was on their minds.[8] Feedback should be two-way. High return on management includes a good plan and follow-up, independent thinking, new ideas, no fear of failure – only fear of poor service, bad outcomes and not remembering failures. Create "a culture that is very hostile to complacency."[9]

Low return on management comes from lack of common sense, no input, and the inability to remove inefficiency in the process of care. Clear your mind of "can't." *Shouldn't* and *wouldn't* may be advisable under certain circumstances, but not *can't*. A low return on management includes the inability to plan and deliver, falling back on politically correct performance, having no accountability, indecision, and the toleration of mediocrity. Most mismanagement is related to bad execution, not getting things done, procrastination, and not delivering on commitments.[±] You have to find people who are smart, ambitious and understand that the goal is to have good ideas that improve the process of medicine. A high return on investment begins at the top. Knowing where the organization is going is the one task the leader cannot delegate.[10]

Clevelander Frederick C. Crawford, president of Thompson Products (which later became TRW), declared that he never thought of management as a science; he thought of it as common sense. A company, he said, is not bricks and mortar or money and finance. It's people. Successful management, therefore, is getting above-average effort from people over the long run. In his industry, Crawford believed that "you should not award an MBA to anyone until he or she spent a year as a factory worker."[11]

He delivered these maxims in 1933.[12]

- Choose not between good and bad; choose between better and best.

- Freedom is but the right to discipline one's self.

- Time is the most valuable thing in the world and the most wasted; it can't be stored.

- Whatever you're doing, do with all your heart, soul, and energy… average Americans exert themselves only to 75 percent of their potential. But average Americans will team up with inspirational leadership and rise above the average.

In 2005, Towers Perrin conducted a poll of 86,000 employees[13] that concluded that "the vast majority of employees across all levels in an organization are less than fully engaged in their work. Fourteen percent around the world are highly engaged, 24 percent disengaged and everyone else is in the 'tepid middle.'"[14] Training or observing methods offsite requires understanding and follow-up and

---

±   The top 10 low-value uses of time: 1) Things other people want you to do; 2) Things that have always been done this way; 3) Things you're not unusually good at doing; 4) Things you don't enjoy doing; 5) Things that are always interrupted; 6) Things few other people are interested in; 7) Things that have already taken twice as long as you originally expected; 8) Things where your collaborators are unreliable or low-quality; 9) Things that have a predictable cycle; 10) Answering the phone. (Koch R. *The 80 / 20 Principle: The Secret to Success by Achieving More With Less*. New York, NY: Currency Doubleday 1998).

preferably a change in practice. Otherwise, nothing will happen and personnel will continue where they left off.

The best managers (all must be leaders) have a strong emotional bond to the organization. They are enthusiastic about their work and are committed to creating an engaged staff. This is best achieved by eliminating bureaucracy, supplying necessary equipment and tools, and providing clarity of organizational purpose. Support your team, individually and collectively.

Those in supervisory positions can not just go along to get along. Don't put anyone in a supervisory job who couldn't do the work themselves. In one manufacturing company, personnel were asked how they learned their jobs. Out of a list of seven possibilities, "from my supervisor" ranked next to last. (Only company training programs ranked worse.) Often supervisors do not translate company policies into practice. They also may not enforce the right of every employee to frequent performance reviews or to career counseling.[15] Weed out everyone who is unresponsive to counsel... however, first be sure that their view of the situation is heard, respected, and investigated. Not to know is bad, but not to wish to know is worse.[16]

Ineffective management is generally attributed to one or more of these characteristics: passivity or complacency; no common sense; no sense of urgency; little knowledge beyond budget; fear of any confrontation; change resistant; doesn't walk the landscape; and not a problem solver. An even bigger deficiency is the lack of understanding purpose, which corrupts the priorities and decision making. These and other signals of incompetence are detailed in many publications.[17] The losers' 10 commandments are reprinted in Appendix IV. There is also a phenomenon known as the e-mail manager – one who has little direct contact with staff or personnel. Instead, they send out frequent missives on virtually everything, much of which is inconsequential, or worse, they chastise people through electronic mail rather than discussing the issues directly with the people involved. When feasible, two minutes of corridor conversation is often better than a dozen back and forth e-mails.

When personnel behave like apparatchiks,± it may be attributed to no supervision, intimidation, fear of failure or lack of training. All these can be remedied by

±   The Circumlocution Office was (as everybody knows without being told) the most important Department under government. No public business of any kind could possibly be done at any time without the acquiescence of the Circumlocution Office. Its finger was in the largest public pie, and in the smallest public tart. It was equally impossible to do the plainest right, and to undo the plainest wrong, without the express authority of the Circumlocution Office. If another Gunpowder Plot had been discovered half an hour before the lighting of the match, nobody would have been justified in saving the Parliament until there had been half a score of boards, half a bushel of minutes, several sacks of official memoranda, and a family-vault-full of ungrammatical correspondence, on the part of the Circumlocution Office. (Dickens C. 1857, *Little Dorrit*, I, Ch. 10. Harper & Brothers)

mentoring, by changing the supervisor or occasionally by replacement of the individual. Accountability requires effective communication, two-way feedback and follow-up. Tell the employees: Your boss isn't responsible for managing your career – you are. To reach your potential, you need to know yourself.

When operational management fails or incurs high cost, the organization may try to off-load responsibility to an outside vendor. Theoretically, outsourcing is supposed to lower cost, gain better and more consistent service, provide specialized experience, increase productivity, improve space management and reduce risk. The most frequent targets for outsourcing include housekeeping, food, laundry, mail services, security, pharmacy, parking, printing, maintenance contracts, freight management, storage, and even patient financial services. On the clinical side, emergency medicine, radiographic interpretation, laboratory testing, and anesthesia are increasingly bid out. However, outsourcing can come back and bite you. You incur the cost of outsourcing, and you still have the responsibility.[18] One cannot outsource risk. The management of outsourcing entails more, not less, accountability and responsibility. Also, it's not a good idea to outsource a function that constitutes a competitive advantage.

Competition is a loaded word in healthcare. We are aware of how other hospitals perform, but mainly as a management benchmark. We prefer to form complementary relationships that strengthen our market position and provide greater value to the community. Competitors are not our enemies. The enemy of every hospital is its infrastructure. You can always reduce cost by blindly chopping away at things; but the best means to reduce cost is by improving efficiency and addressing waste. Most waste falls under the categories of waiting, processing, duplication of effort, billing overproduction, inventory management, underutilized personnel, and poor logistics.

One of the most important lessons that I have tried to convey to the staff is not to worry about what your competitors are doing. Concentrate on getting better yourself. Where can you improve quarter to quarter and year to year, starting with all aspects of quality down through operations? That doesn't mean that you don't keep an eye on what other academic centers and community hospitals are doing, but view their trends, not snapshots. Learn from them. Over time, if someone is taking your market share overall, or in a particular specialty, that has to be addressed. You'll find that there is always a good reason. Most likely it is your poor service, bad results or delayed access. Insist on good results, new ideas, and dedication to the tasks at hand.

PERFORMANCE

Today major sociopolitical forces are transforming medicine – bureaucracies of every description, the rise of consumerism, changes in health insurance and a growing volume of government regulatory and legislative intrusions, all of which call for disciplined management. Healthcare organizations tend to be hierarchical, resistant to change and slow to implement. Although Toyota is a different business, some of its management principles apply to healthcare. The three Ms are useful reminders of the perils inherent in any business organization: *muda* stands for non-value-added or wasteful activities that should be eliminated; *muri* refers to people and equipment and their inefficiency from over- and under-utilization; and *mura* means unevenness, which results in irregular performance.[19] From Toyota we learn that strategy and management decisions should be based on a long-term philosophy. Concentrate on refining the process of moving patients efficiently through their outpatient and inpatient appointments. Grow leaders who thoroughly understand the work and the culture. Become a learning organization. Don't worry about finding problems; look for them. Every defect is a treasure – as long as you make the correction and it doesn't recur.

Greater size leads to bureaucracy that stifles innovation. Charles Lindbergh's flying across the Atlantic alone was less of a feat than if he had flown across the Atlantic with a committee.[20] The current Toyota chief executive officer worries most about "big company disease,"[21] the symptoms of which include pitfalls in staff growth: silos, apathy, disrespect of organizational priorities and poor cross-communications. Sound familiar? Part of Toyota's company lore is the need to develop "T-type" people. These are personnel who intensify and deepen their knowledge of their jobs (symbolized by the vertical stroke of the T), and who also learn other jobs (symbolized by the cross bar).[22] Toyota rarely weeds out underperformers, focusing instead on upgrading their capabilities. "Cut all costs, but don't touch any people." A favorite saying of a former Toyota chairperson is "Reform business when business is good."[23]

In healthcare, apart from a lack of good connectivity, there are huge inefficiencies in current ambulatory and hospital practice: one patient at a time; one room for one doctor. Basically we have a 9-hour (elective) hospital day, daytime scheduling, and the weekend effect (slowdown). In processing, our challenges include telephone appointments, paper records, significant duplication, charts held only by providers, and variable charges, co-payments, and deductibles. Don't ask people to address these problems without providing the knowledge and means to meet the goal. That means you need to provide performance data (trends), feedback, and time for implementation. Solving the root problems means get-up-and-go-and-see-for-yourself so that you as the leader really understand the problem. Revenues down? Layoffs are the last resort. Loyalty is not about putting the comfort of your people first; it's about putting their welfare first.[24]

In hospitals, there are many operational factors that retard growth. Without superb clinical outcomes and consistently high patient satisfaction, you will face strong competition and referrals out-of-network. You may have weak marketing (clinical program visibility) or be handicapped by poor recruitment, which may be traced to disgruntled doctors on your staff. Growth can be significantly improved by better capacity management. There are many "growth factors" that relate to operational capability. They won't solve themselves without managerial attention and consistent follow-up.

Physicians are among the world's hardest-working and most talented professionals. However, physicians also have to be accountable. If the organization has a staff model wherein employed physicians are paid a salary, that salary has to be correlated with collection for clinical services rendered. In clinical medicine, a good rule of thumb is that a physician's salary should support 2½ times the collection adjusted for pure "cognitive" (non-technical) specialties and for research and education responsibilities. Trends in process efficiency depend on how effective the organization is in making it easier for doctors to see patients. When is the last time you asked doctors for feedback on the efficiency of their clinic office (if it is associated with the hospital)? Chances are that medical records and capacity management are high on the list. The doctors may tell you there are not enough outpatient rooms, poor nursing assistance or inexperienced front desk personnel. At the same time, physicians tend to resist overbooking to adjust for cancellations or no-shows. They frequently repeat their patient complaints about long waiting time for ancillary services, especially radiology and lab medicine. These occurrences are real and contaminate the practice environment. You have heard it all. Now do something about it.

Revenue growth is the primary driver of long-term performance.[25±] Other important metrics include trends in *new patient activity,* market share by specialty, revenue cycle metrics, cash collected as a percent of net patient revenue, and returns on endowment investments. All are critical. In the healthcare business, the red flags that warn of a stall in progress are: 1) over-development of unprofitable services; 2) failure to innovate; 3) decline of measurable quality and service; 4) poor

---

± There are metrics in virtually every area of operations, finance and clinical care. Some of the key volume drivers are difficult but still measurable: 1) reputation based on results; 2) the right composition of services; 3) cleanliness of facilities; 4) high utilization of the latest equipment; 5) staff quality; 6) effect of quality on insurance contracting; 7) perceived ease of access; 8) hospital leadership; 9) patient and personnel satisfaction; and 10) favorable publicity.

human capital management; 5) inept (indecisive) leadership/governance; 6) low physician/nurse satisfaction; 7) running out of cash; 8) losing market share – even in one specialty. Jack Welch said there are three measurements to live by: employee satisfaction, customer satisfaction, and cash flow.[26]

REVENUE-DRIVEN COST

In healthcare, a dollar charged is far from a dollar earned, but a dollar saved is a real dollar "earned." The leaking bucket example (Figure 7.1) demonstrates where money leaks out of the institution. Every seasoned hospital administrator can think of even more holes. Fixing these leaks offers a huge opportunity to significantly reduce costs.

FIGURE 7.1

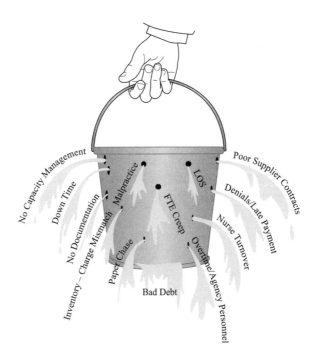

Groucho Marx said that a hospital bed is a parked taxi with the meter running. The majority of costs for medical services are related to daily equipment, labor, and overhead, all of which are fixed. Hospitals that hope to save costs by reducing services will generally save only variable costs. Unless declining consumption allows the hospital to reduce personnel and space and to limit capital expenditures, restriction of medical services has minimal influence. In other words, savings will be small unless beds are closed, staff dismissed, and physical resources liquidated.[27] The greatest areas of revenue enhancement and cost management relate to: 1) automating the revenue cycle; 2) simplifying and standardizing payer contracts; 3) improving operating room throughput; 4) coordinating (and reconciling) along the supply chain; 5) decreasing medical liability; 6) improving labor efficiency, wage index productivity, and production standards; 7) integrating the electronic health record for clinical medicine, operations, and research; and 8) reducing administrative overhead. These operating issues are the key to survival.

Of the direct revenue opportunities, the medical/surgical supply chain offers great potential. According to the Healthcare Financial Management Association,[28] the average hospital receives 10-20 percent of its reimbursement from charge-sensitive managed care contracts. Clinical inventories represent the majority of inventory dollars. Operating room inventory constitutes about 65 percent of the hospital inventory value. Measures that effectively enhance potential revenue and reduce cost for high-value supplies include:

1) automated inventory and charge master reconciliation;

2) no vendor interactions except through the material management office;

3) high-security areas for expensive inventory;

4) capital assets tracking (life cycle management);

5) selective reduction in variety of medical and surgical implantables;

6) collaboration with suppliers to reduce expired products and to improve rebates and credits;

7) periodically updating the charge master[±] and using input from clinical departments.

Supply management depends on purchasing at the right price, standardizing the inventory nomenclature, and, like all other aspects of operations, listening to the staff. Be sure to query doctors about their "advisory" relationships with vendors. Obtain all disclosures before contract talks. Group purchasing is less valuable on the high end of supplies. Reverse auctions are especially good for commodity purchases.

[±]   UB 92 and 1500 forms – professional and technical components

In my experience, we have fewer collaborative supplier relationships compared with other "industries." Japanese automakers call this knowledge-based sourcing, i.e., collaboration to lower cost and raise performance. Collaboration with suppliers for low-volume, high-cost devices and pharmaceuticals may have benefits if your system is large enough to be heard. But it has to be genuine and not just a negotiating ploy. To help supply chain managers, there are tools available, such as the Advisory Board Company's Spend Compass, which enables hospitals to find cost-savings, benchmark group purchase pricing and maximize rebates.[29]

An elementary solution to high device cost is to reduce the variety of surgical devices or appliances. Be careful. It can be done as long as you are aware of the caveats. A range of products may be beneficial for specialty training. Special types of devices may be age- and gender-specific. There is a learning curve after conversion to new products, and misadventures may result. The eliminated companies may have been the most innovative. You may suffer from adverse publicity about a "closed shop," which could affect recruitment and competition. For these reasons, procurement on price alone is not always justified.[30]

Currently, few hospitals automatically track inventory as it enters or leaves the procedure room. High-cost, low-volume devices and pharmaceuticals are not perfectly accounted for or even billed accurately. Most hospitals still depend on their personnel to document charge entry, procedure times, and patient identification. Conversely, manufacturers depend on distributors and salespeople for product location and usage. Reconciliation of consigned inventory by the vendor and the hospital is problematic. In the present state, there is little real-time electronic record data, and most inventories rely on barcoding. Radiofrequency identification will eventually play a major role in reconciling purchases and changes as well as in tracking assets. All of this data will enter the electronic patient record. The advantage is automated accuracy without human interaction.[31]

Medical operations at the department level are a huge area for cost management and revenue enhancement. Shore up communications first. Every clinical department meeting should start with a performance and quality improvement agenda item, e.g., trends in infection rate, patient and personnel satisfaction, objective outcomes and practice standards. One of the most amazing aspects of human nature is that physician leaders frequently do not communicate to their respective departments despite intensive briefing on a project or direction. Many department administrators are not analytical, too subjective, and prone to manage by anecdote. However, if working physicians, nurses and other personnel are given information regarding a problem, they will almost always help solve it. The doctors have to get involved with important issues in their department, namely documentation, access, service, cost and productivity. Physician managers may use a continuous improvement dashboard or the balanced scorecard [32] to assess performance. Dashboards for continuous improvement are readily available and important for day-to-day management. Look through that windshield and modify the metrics as times change. Whatever methods used to chart progress, accuracy and trending are essential.

Net patient service revenue is driven by the mix of staff appointments. New patient visits and surgical volume are strong predictors of patient service revenues. Because total operating cost is influenced by length of surgery, especially for complex procedures, the administration has to investigate the cost benefit of unproven new procedures. Efficiency is gauged by throughput and labor cost. Decreasing labor cost per visit is a real sign of improved efficiency. In our experience, nurses and nurse clinicians respond favorably to rotational assignments. Cross-training refreshes managers and personnel.

Of the leading indicators used to track performance, I believe that the number of *new patients*[±] is the most important sign of progress. New patients are the enthalpy (new energy) that battles entropy (dissipation, loss and failure). Price may drive cost, but in a service industry, management also drives cost. The number of people involved in hospital patient care, divided by the total number of people on the payroll, provides an interesting statistical trend. Look at personnel (FTEs) per average daily adjusted census, FTEs per available beds, and FTEs per operating volume including and excluding emergency department cases. As you drill down to the key metrics, determine whether your infrastructure is correct for the size of the patient volume or if it's top-heavy.

CONTINGENCIES

One of our operational tenets was to practice "preventive management." You cannot anticipate problems unless you understand the consequences of intended regulatory change and you know the trends in your organization's performance. The former depends on signals from federal or state sources; the latter depends on your operational discipline.

Some people in your organization will have measure-phobia born of experience. They've taken valuable time to collect data, only to see bad managers use it as a weapon, or simply not use it at all. You, on the other hand, can show the staff how metrics align strategy and mission, and use your metrics to drive operational improvement. The Advisory Board termed the aversion to enacting unpopular necessary changes as "a culture of conservatism." [33] Examples are failure to cut

---

[±]   New patients per staff is an even better indicator. Never events should be included in the balanced scorecard.

administrative cost, to close unprofitable facilities, and to consolidate programs after mergers.

Risk assessment may lead to operational changes that significantly reduce future cost. Reducing risk requires continuous attention and should involve trustees. Many of them have experience in *enterprise risk management* from their own businesses. Some areas of risk concentration in healthcare are listed below.

- disaster training for workforce
- contingency plans for pandemics
- updated human resource policies
- litigation about property tax exemption
- pension and other reserves fully funded
- medical/legal review team for malpractice
- plans for interruption of water, power, etc.
- safety of internal and external transportation
- annual review of strategic and operating risks
- financial consequences of an economic downturn
- prescription and pharmaceutical dispensing errors
- regulatory compliance in government reimbursement
- selected CPR training and protocols for cardiac emergencies
- back-up for billing and other informational technology services
- security for patient records, network access for applications and inventory
- adherence to high standards for air circulation in surgical suites and patient rooms

The second law of thermodynamics is customarily stated as "A system left to itself will tend toward a state of maximum entropy."[34] How does this apply to healthcare risk? Prevention is the best risk manager. Hire only the best staff, encourage active practices, provide an optimal environment for success, measure and publicize achievement, insist on accountability and emphasize clear communication between staff and patients. Raise standards by stimulating the best, not whipping up the laggards. Become a learning (and improvement) organization. Peter Senge popularized the concept in The Fifth Discipline: "...where people continually expand their capacity to create the results they truly desire, where new and expansive patterns of thinking are nurtured, where collective aspiration is set free and where people are continually learning how to learn together."[35]

IMPROVING CLINICAL OPERATIONS

Here is something interesting from our 1943 Cleveland Clinic *archives:*

1) Discharges occur too late in the day.
2) With the present nursing staff shortage, we can't place beds in the corridors to accommodate admissions from the emergency ward.
3) The waiting list for beds has to be prioritized.
4) Every vacant bed is not always ready.
5) Ambulatory patients should be informed of the possibility that they will have to wait for their appointments.
6) All doctors should notify the hospital by noon the day before discharge that their patient is to leave the next day.
7) The current occupancy rate is 95 percent.

Miss Abbie Porter, Superintendent of the Hospital, wrote this memorandum pointing out that we were under great pressure and had to send away as many as eight patients per day. Some patients had already paid in advance. She wanted to open 17 more beds that had been closed. She realized that with the nursing shortage, this was difficult. After 65 years, these problems didn't go away for us. Do they sound familiar to you?

Healthcare is a unique business. All problems directly or indirectly affect patient care. We constantly deal with the power of suppliers, declining government reimbursement, tougher surveillance, increasing uncompensated care, and now more point-of-service collection.

Periodically a number of questions should be discussed by the management team:

1) What is our comparative advantage and how can we improve?
2) How can we implement decisions faster? How can we simplify the process?
3) Do we have the right metrics to measure productivity?
4) Where do we spend money above budget: fixed costs, IT investment, consultants, etc.?
5) How can we better educate our patients?
6) Does our group purchasing offer the best pricing?
7) Where does our capacity management process break down?
8) Are long-stay and post-acute care cases managed optimally?
9) How can we better market quality?

10) What are the reasons for unprofitability in each area, e.g., staff attrition, denials, deteriorating clinical services, bad outcomes, poor customer service, low-volume services, long length of stay, escalating bad debt? The sticky point here is that losing money in a sizeable percentage of the patient base is often related to uncompensated care. A hospital can't fire the patients or divert them. Unfortunately, doctors in private practice can refuse to see them.

Hospitalized patients are constantly surrounded by compromises, most of which don't have to occur. Examples are inordinate waiting time, closed services on weekends or added stay because of indecision or poor coordination. Improving access involves improving the diagnostic process, working relentlessly on throughput and reducing all procedural complications. The goal today is to keep as many chronic care patients out of the hospital as possible, and to manage them in their homes whenever possible. This allows the outpatient and inpatient facilities to concentrate on acute care, which includes shortening the waiting time for elective procedures.

THE PHYSICAL PLANT

The Advisory Board has published some important reminders about inpatient facility planning.[36] 1) Hospital facility expansions are often premature if not unnecessary; executives should be skeptical about need to expand today; 2) Rigorous projection of facility needs depends on technology and practice change as well as demographics; 3) Anticipate the downstream impact of expansion, e.g., emergency department expansion and access to imaging or ICU days and bed utilization, which may strain inpatient resources; 4) Plan for interventional procedure flexibility, e.g., strategically placed shell space and pre-wired expansion capability are key considerations for accommodating future changes in volumes, mix, and technology. I would add that recruitment of surgeons will require added operating room capacity, the extent of which depends on the specialty. One of the biggest mistakes is to scrimp on infrastructure, e.g., cheap HVAC, inadequate air handling, lower electrical standards and poor wireless capability. In our experience, two other often overlooked features would benefit from more nurse input. The first is location of workstations, including physician work areas, and the second is storage space.

Hospitals should strive to create general purpose procedure rooms and intensive care units. The same applies to basic science laboratories. Because current inpatient room construction is complicated, try to achieve consensus about square footage, noise, visibility, multiuse and access to natural light. The best way to reach agreement is through three-dimensional design modeling. If new facilities are planned, factor in layout and design for patient comfort, privacy and safety (including patient visibility).[37] Consider ceiling lifts in selected areas and robots for supply deliveries. Healthcare facilities should attempt to eliminate hazardous materials in all areas of healthcare operations. These measures start with environmentally friendly cleaning products and include rubber floors free of polyvinyl chlorides, which eliminate waxing and stripping with potentially toxic products. Better measures to dispose of medical waste are highly sought after.

New construction is moving toward greater safety through design. To redesign the customer experience, Kaiser has created more comfortable waiting rooms, effective way-finding signage, and larger exam rooms with space for three or more people and curtains for privacy.[38] Other improvements include sound-absorbing tiles, special lights, bathrooms closer to the bed, and non-slip flooring. The Mayo Clinic strives for goals in the design and operation of its facilities that relieve stress; provide repose; reduce background noise; offer positive distractions; convey caring; communicate respect; symbolize competence; minimize the impression of crowding; facilitate way-finding; and accommodate families.[39]

My bias is to avoid fast track, which means construction begins before the design is completed. That may work in small projects or for modest renovation, but fast track generally leads to more change orders. Poor healthcare facility design is implicated in medical human error.[40] The new physical environment features single patient rooms. Although private rooms can initially cost more to build, their savings in long-term operational costs can offset the initial investment. Patients tend to recover faster in private rooms, they are less susceptible to disease transmission, and they are more likely to receive the correct medication because potential confusion with a roommate is eliminated. In addition to convenience for the patient and hospital personnel, there is evidence that infection rates are lower in private rooms, noise is reduced, equipment access is improved and overall privacy improves patient satisfaction.[41] Other innovations include the light that won't go off until caregivers wash their hands in front of the patient; window blinds interposed between glass panes to reduce dust and infection; individual rooms for neonatal intensive care; and nurse paging by vibration to eliminate overhead noise. New construction depends on wireless integrated information systems, clinical monitoring, paging and image transfer.[±]

Value mapping minimizes handoffs and transfers and thereby reduces fatigue. The most modern hospitals provide Internet access for patients and families and for nursing personnel and the hospital security staff. A great deal of time and money is spent on air handling in the operating room but airflow and purification are not yet standardized on general patient floors. The time will come when improved air handling will be part of modern hospital construction, and despite the cost of electrostatic cleaners and HEPA filters, the system should pay for itself by reducing the incidence of nosocomial infections.

HEALTH SYSTEM OPERATIONS

We have learned valuable lessons from the 20th century. System integration is difficult without physician alignment. Beyond group practice, the best way to "align" individual private practice doctors is through personal communication and seeking their input. Healthcare is subject to increasing business risks; however, change to a "business" should assure that the medical environment remains conducive to success for patients and staff. As medicine progresses from art to science, doctors increasingly rely on efficient operations. The executive team must explore every way to help them.

The principal non-medical issues for the provider are cost, organization (reports and communication) and payment collection. The other factors of quality, access and uncompensated care are linked to those three issues. There may be more problems today, but there are also more opportunities. Here are some broad priorities that relate to operational management:

- Exploit the electronic patient record. There are a number of lower cost ambulatory records and repositories available today that can improve efficiency, information exchange, safety, accuracy, and quality metrics. The electronic record is the key to improved quality,

---

[±]   Green building is no longer a niche market in healthcare. *The Green Guide for Health Care* is an open source document for non-profit healthcare that integrates environmental health principles and practices into the planning, design, construction, operations and maintenance of facilities, new and old. Sponsored by the U.S. Green Building Council, it will help organizations interested in pursuing third-party certification from Leadership in Energy and Environmental Design (LEED). The LEED green building rating system provides standards for environmentally sustainable construction, the goals of which include clean air, toxic chemical and waste reduction, carbon neutrality, and water balance.

reduction of administrative waste and facilitation of billing. In academic medical organizations, the electronic record should connect throughout the enterprise, including business functions to the consumer as a personal health record and to research.

- Improve physician alignment. This is easier to do if the organization already has a staff model. If not, build a large primary care base throughout the community. Primary care physicians need incentives to stay in the field. Attract the most capable physicians and inspire them to common goals. The best doctors will help to market quality. Invest in physicians and their leadership.

- Engage the health insurance companies and banks in a collaborative effort to produce an insurance card that automatically completes registration benefits, recognition and access to their personal health record. This smart card serves as a debit or credit card for healthcare services and may be linked to an HSA account. A good electronic medical record will soon be able to convert services into claims and bills that can be transmitted to the payer through a virtual clearinghouse. This partnership with banking and insurance will guarantee payment of out-of-pocket expenses for the qualified card member who uses the card for co-payments and deductibles. (See Appendix II)

- All personnel should be encouraged to innovate. Use open sources to receive solutions for administrative and organizational problems. How to redesign the current workforce model should be the highest priority.

- If your organization is a large referral center, improve hospital access through a centralized transfer office rather than having outside physicians attempting to contact individual services. Physicians in the community are less apt to manage extremely ill patients today, especially on off-hours or weekends.

- Emergency Department (ED) visits are increasing and will likely increase because of primary care referral, the uninsured and underinsured, deinstitutionalization of psychiatric patients, the lack of coordinated care for the underserved community, and extreme weather conditions. Stationing a patient advocate in the ED helps patients who may qualify for public support. The ED may generate the majority of inpatient cases for some services.[±]

- Stay abreast of technology advances in order to move procedures safely to the lower cost outpatient sites in the community.

- Be prepared for rate adjustments, Recovery Audit Contractors (RAC),[†] no reimbursement for certain complications, and consequences of conversions to ICD-10. As policy solutions evolve, have plans in place to deal with more uncompensated care.

- Address the cost structure as it relates to deployment of personnel, selective outsourcing, energy cost, leasing, and monetizing assets. Scrutinize all expansion carefully for accurate returns on investment.

- Devote more attention to alternative revenue sources, namely philanthropy and endowment investment.

- Personnel education should focus more on efficient office practice and excellent service. Physicians-in-training should be taught about health policy issues and healthcare finance, especially the cost of care that they render, including wellness. Teach medical students and staff about advantages of patient empowerment and why they should not resist informed consumerism. Pay attention to human resources: focus on leadership, recruitment, training, and the work environment. Emphasize measurement, action, and follow-up.

- Objectively review all forms of research regarding their return on investment, the clinical application of the translational investigations, and the use of space.

±   For more information, see: *The High Performance ED: Optimizing Capacity and Throughput to Meet Ever-Growing Demand.* The Advisory Board Company, 2008; and, *Hospital-Based Emergency Care: At the Breaking Point.* National Academies Press, Washington, D.C., 2007.

†   In a three-year demonstration project in five states, the RAC program identified more than $1 billion in overpayments and recovered nearly $850 million from inpatient hospitals. In 2008 alone, the average recovery per audited hospital was more than $900,000 (*Finance Watch.* The Advisory Board Company. January 2009).

- Catch the wave of enlightenment about keeping chronically ill patients *out of the hospital.* The challenge is follow-up, but there will be remarkable advances in telehealth, both for testing and examination. Concentrate first on diabetes and heart failure. Build on follow-up activities from a select number of conditions.

- Be dedicated to your mission, which is to take care of patients in the best possible way. All this other stuff, complicated as it is, is really a means to an end.

In summary, years ago we wrote out management tenets that probably are still valid today.

- Our product is medicine.
- Hire only the best people.
- You are in charge of quality.
- Resources go where treated best.
- No one owns space.
- Practice prevention in management and medicine.
- Motivate the motivators.
- Affirm, don't deny.
- Remember every mistake.
- Make things happen.

Create your own tenets and solicit input from the management teams. People like to work for a cause and to have a structure on which they can depend. Remember, management is about human beings. Its task is to make people capable of joint performance, to make their strengths effective and their weaknesses irrelevant.[4]

C H A P T E R   8

THE LEADERSHIP TEAM

My success, Andrew Carnegie suggested, may be found in my proposed epitaph, "Here lies a man who knew how to enlist in his service better men than himself."

— John K. Winkler
*Incredible Carnegie: The Life of
Andrew Carnegie (1835-1919)*
Vanguard Press, 1931

In the late 1970s when I was performing cardiac surgery, I had operated on a potentate who was recovering satisfactorily. Afterwards and true to human nature, his entourage was falling all over themselves in purposeless activity, the results of which lengthened the hospital convalescence. The overall care resembled Brownian motion flowing around and through a gaggle of ministers, doctors and other client-age. I grumbled to a friend of mine who was of the same nationality as the patient: Why does this have to happen? Who in his retinue is making all these requests? Why not treat the king as a normal patient? "Dear boy," my friend replied, "don't you understand? There is no king; the king is the people around him."

Ah, that's true, and it's also true for many businesses. Some of them, as a result of a bad team, fail or never reach their potential. The chief executive, in charge and responsible, has to assemble the right team of people upon whom he or she will rely for advice, ideas, experience, and results. Successful businesses thrive because of skilled, dedicated personnel in all ranks, and an organizational culture refined over the course of time. Drucker classified different types of teams: 1) An assembly line or a surgical team: The players play on the team, but they don't exactly play as a team. Each has a fixed position. 2) A symphony orchestra: The players perform as a team, plus they follow the same score. 3) A tennis doubles team: Only the team performs; the individual members contribute.[1]

Academic medical centers resemble a combination of a surgical team and a symphony orchestra operating in a closely networked system. The players follow a "score," which is the overall performance; and there are the "fixed positions" like clinical medicine and related academic activities, operations, finance, and human resources that, in the end, work together for a common purpose... the patient's good health. The incontrovertible fact is that in today's world of medicine, the care of the patient, sick or well, is a team effort. Each doctor has his or her own support team, and the members of that team reinforce each other's work. The culture[±] found in the best teams is based upon mutual respect, a sense of urgency, loyalty to the organization, and a shared determination to accomplish planned goals. Don't forget, the "customer" is part of your management team.

At the Cleveland Clinic, our structure would be described as decentralized management with central control of values. To achieve this model, planning, execution, and physician alignment is essential. Large medical organizations depend on a group of experienced executives, lay and medical professionals who contribute to central management. The operational elements critical to success include: 1) the best leadership at every level; 2) attention to the intangibles; 3) recognition of individual and group success; 4) intolerance of inaction and bad execution; 5) insistence on outstanding clinical results and service; 6) encouraging and rewarding innovation; 7) reinforcing the philosophy of the culture through communication. The biggest threats to any non-profit organization are the egalitarians who prefer governance by a privileged few who preach that everyone is equal regardless of ability (except them). This gets back to the warning that mediocre people gaining a majority will change the culture. The symptoms of failure are accusation, blame and criticism. When respect is lacking and replaced with cynicism and sarcasm, it has already happened. The end result is generally chronic inertia, no plans and lower productivity. I have always preferred meritocracy. No rank without merit.

±   Culture is variously defined as a collection of values, attitudes and beliefs. "...these definitions have reflected a static view of culture as the distinctive set of beliefs, values, morals, customs and institutions which people inherit... [whereas] more recent approaches to culture in anthropology provide a more dynamic perspective... viewing culture as a process in which views and practices are dynamically affected by social transformations, social conflicts, power relationships, and migrations." (Taylor JS. *Confronting "Culture" in Medicine's "Culture of No Culture."* Acad Med 2003: 78 (6); 555-559).

THE EXECUTIVE TEAM

How do you put a team together? When I was appointed chief executive in 1989, we were thin in a lot of places. Leadership was good, but times had changed. Most of the executives were beleaguered by the changing complexities of healthcare administration and tired of criticism about financial performance. In retrospect, our problems provided excellent opportunities to recruit new talent for key positions. Almost everyone was subsequently recruited through internal recommendations rather than by search firms.

Factors that spell success or failure in team performance start with a leader who sets the standards for discipline and execution. Other criteria depend on the type of organization: size, composition of services and market forces. Everyone is expected to contribute. Respect is a given. Who you choose to surround you depends on your style and the current exigencies.± Once formed, the executives, about half of whom in our case† were physicians, addressed *issues* that related to their "domains": 1) effective governance; 2) progressive academic excellence; 3) staff recruitment and review; 4) clinical operations; 5) finance-related services; 6) results of tactical plans; 7) compliance; 8) personnel policies, training, and benefits; 9) general operations; 10) marketing and communications. Accurate information must flow freely across their domains. The chief executive needs to be cognizant of the performance profile of each individual executive (strengths, weaknesses and capabilities) in a more critically honest fashion than the executives are likely to perceive themselves.

The best way to make a team work effectively is to assemble talents who have the right fit. Everyone understands the "rules" (expect achievement) and reports only the essentials. We insisted on a good debate about goals and performance. It is naïve to bring together a highly diverse group of people and expect that by calling them a team, they will in fact behave as a team. Professional football teams spend 40 hours per week practicing teamwork for those two hours on game day when the teamwork really counts. Teams and organizations seldom spend two hours per week practicing, and yet they have to function as a team for 40-plus hours per week.[2]

±   The first method for estimating the intelligence of a (leader) is to look at the men he has around him (Machiavelli N. *The Prince*, trans. H.C. Mansfield Jr., University of Chicago Press 1985.)

†   Physicians on the executive committee included the chiefs or directors of staff, information technology, payer contracting, and regional practice. Other professionals were responsible for finance, operations, human resources, marketing and the committee administrator.

Incidentally, don't assemble a large executive management group. In Peter Drucker's words, "Don't forget that Jesus picked only 12 Apostles. If he had picked 60, he couldn't have done it. He had a hard enough time with those 12, always saying to them, 'Don't you understand?'"[3] Finally, don't jump to simple solutions and be careful if everyone readily agrees. As Alfred P. Sloan is reported to have said, "Gentlemen, I take it we are all in complete agreement on the decision here.... Then I propose we postpone further discussion of this matter until our next meeting to give ourselves time to develop disagreement and perhaps gain some understanding of what the decision is all about."[4±]

If the leader has picked a talented group of executives, they are likely to behave as a "team of rivals."[5] Therefore, the leader had better act like Abraham Lincoln. The only behaviors strictly not allowed are loss of credibility and too much "acting out." Harriet Beecher Stowe wrote that President Abraham Lincoln demonstrated his great might less by standing firm than by bending in ways that brought others to his cause. Lincoln's strength, she wrote, "is like the strength not so much of a stone buttress as of a wire cable... swaying to every influence, yielding on this side and on that to popular needs, yet tenaciously and inflexibly bound to carry its great end."[6] In their finest hours Lincoln's successors have all recognized that.

The "trust, but verify" quote generally attributed to Ronald Reagan applies to the chief executive's responsibility for the executive team's performance. Simply put, trust without accountability amounts to blind faith. The chief executive should always insist upon validation of goals and delivery on commitments, even if such action sometimes is subtly resented.

Trust between people does not necessarily mean that they like one another. It means they understand one another.[7] You can even respect those who are risk averse – they just might not be right for the top job. Diversity in talent and personality matters. Homogeneous teams do little to enhance expertise and creative thinking.[8] Give me strong-willed, tough but fair, dedicated and really smart executives, and we will show great results and real progress no matter how onerous the market or the reimbursement. As one of the Cleveland Clinic founders wrote, "What a remarkable record Bunts, Crile, and Lower have had all these years. We have been rivals in everything, yet could differ in opinion about anything and through all the vicissitudes of personal, financial and professional relations, we have been able to think and act as a unit."[9]

In my experience, a culture of loyalty to the institution definitely exists in a good team. Even a good leader can't assure that individual members are loyal to

---

±   Confucius said, "When everyone dislikes something, it should be examined. When everyone likes something, it should be examined." (Analects: 15:28)

each other or even to the leader, but in a great organization, the team is loyal to the mission, vision and credo of the institution that they serve. Quoting de Tocqueville, "The idea that progress comes naturally into each man's mind; the desire to rise swells in every heart at once and all men want to quit their former social position. Ambition becomes a universal feeling."[10] Sound judgment, good management skills and a sense of urgency are found in the best teams in any organization. The role of leadership is to push and drive and build and develop all areas that advance the mission.

A good meeting exercises constructive dialectic tension. Reasoned discussion and debate can be healthy exchanges, if moderated thoughtfully. Most of our solutions or ideas came from or were stimulated by dialogue. Communicate everything you possibly can to your partners. Sam Walton wrote, "The more they know, the more they'll understand. The more they understand, the more they'll care. Once they care, there's no stopping them. If you don't trust your associates to know what's going on, they'll know you really don't consider them partners. Information is power and the gain you get from empowering your associates more than offsets the risk of informing your competitors." [11]

An effective team has a multiplier effect. A poorly performing team breeds competing agendas and turf issues; a high-performing one has organizational coherence and focus. Teams have to master three dimensions of performance. First, they require a common direction, a shared understanding of goals and values. Second, effective group interaction is crucial if teams are to go beyond individual expertise to solve complex problems and if they are to withstand the scrutiny of the rest of the organization. Third, top teams must always be able to renew themselves – to expand their capabilities in response to change.[12] If you have good team leaders, they will attract good players. This is true at the executive level and in each department.

Ideally, all personnel should be aware of the history of the organization and values set forth by its governing bodies. Most people who enter the medical profession want to be part of a hospital or a medical group that gives them the opportunity to help a variety of patients, to work with skilled colleagues, to grow personally and professionally, and, above all, to learn about and participate in medical advancement. Problems arise when the culture is not addressed or when the management is so inflexible that the organization becomes resistant to necessary change.

Twenty years ago an anesthesiologist and division chair with whom I worked throughout my career wrote to me about optimal team characteristics: 1) always have a vision for the future; 2) be challenging and competitive within; 3) engage in constructive criticism but respect and support one another; 4) be timely and responsive to the changing environment; 5) commit to quality in medicine and moreover to the institution that one serves.[13]

An executive group becomes a real team through disciplined action. They shape a common purpose, agree on performance, define a common working approach, develop (through interaction) complementary skills, and hold themselves accountable for the results.[14] The Japanese management concept, *kaizen*,[15] or continuous search for better processes, is founded on disciplined teamwork. The key factors are elimination of waste, environmental discipline and standardization. Quality is prioritized above profit. The culture involves free recognition of problems and cross-functional improvement. Everything can be improved. Inertia is the worst corporate disease.

I remember Ross Perot's observation about the contrasting cultures of his company, EDS, and its buyer, General Motors. "The first EDSer to see a snake kills it. At GM, first thing you do is organize a committee on snakes. Then you bring in a consultant who knows a lot about snakes. Third thing you do is talk about it for a year."[16] A good team can act decisively. Don't become a prisoner of your legal department. Find lawyers who show you how to get things done, not lawyers who tell you why you can't do it. Beware of committee creep. Each committee assignment takes doctors away from their practice. As Thomas Sowell pointed out, "People who enjoy meetings should not be in charge of anything."[17]

The other team "executives" are the *physician-managers* throughout the organization. Their responsibilities multiply each year due to medical progress, compliance and patient demands. A few physicians or managers wilt as their role enlarges. Some are insecure about their position in a large organization or question their "job description." Tell them authority is 20 percent given and 80 percent taken. Occasionally you will see signs of burnout, which may be caused by boredom or inability to work in an academic environment. Victims of this malaise need to know that there is one sure way to escape monotony: that is continual learning, keeping up to date in your field. As a department or division chair, one of the great contributions that a physician executive can make is to instill a sustained enthusiasm for learning. However, if they don't have this drive early in their careers, it is hard to teach later on.

THE NURSING PROFESSION

The Gallup poll honors nursing as the most honest and ethical of all professions. Nurses are a team in and of themselves. Registered nurses are the largest workforce in hospitals. They are the direct caregivers patients see most often and are responsible for the day-to-day implementation of care. The chief nursing officer generally reports to the chief executive,± chief of staff, or the chief operating officer. Whoever the

±   If the organization is a Magnet designated hospital.

nursing director reports to needs to assure the staff that nurses are integrated into the delivery of inpatient and outpatient healthcare, and more important that they have a voice in how it is delivered. Increasing RN staffing is costly but there is a case to be made that you can increase patient satisfaction and safety by doing so. Reducing adverse outcomes may offset the cost.[18] Currently, licensed practical nurses (LPNs) account for a quarter of the workforce.[19] The greater selective use of RNs in preference to LPNs appears to pay for itself.[±]

The most common concern for the nurse executive relates to nurse recruitment and retention.[†] Although the number of nurses has increased about 8 percent from 2000 through 2004, the forecast is for a shortfall over the next decade. There are a number of myths about the nursing shortage.[20] The first is that not enough Americans want to be nurses. Actually, tens of thousands of nursing school applicants are being turned away because U.S. nursing schools lack educational capacity, especially faculty, which is aging. The average age of the RN workforce has increased to 43.7 years and is projected to reach 44.5 years in 2012. RNs in their 50s will be the largest age group in the workforce numbering about 750,000. The demand for RNs is expected to increase at a rate of 2-3 percent per year over the next 20 years, leading to a significant deficit of nursing personnel that will begin around 2015.[§]

As output fails to meet demand, we have fewer young nurses: In 1980 nurses under age 30 constituted 25 percent of the workforce; in 2004 they represented less than 10 percent.[21] Nurses are in short supply around the world. We can't solve our shortage of nurses by recruiting internationally. Currently only about 3 percent of U.S. nurses are not trained in this country. Opportunities for nurses are expanding

---

± A large survey of patients' perception of care based on data from the Hospital Consumer Assessment of Healthcare, Providers and Systems (HCAHPS) indicated moderately high levels of satisfaction. When the satisfaction results were divided into quartiles, the top rating correlated with high nurse staffing levels. However, ratings varied widely across the 40 largest hospital referral regions. (Jha AK, Orav EJ, Zheng J, Epstein AM. *Patients Perception of Hospital Care in the United States.* N Engl J Med 2008: 359 (18); 1921-31).

† There is a 70 percent attrition rate among acute care nurses within three years or less (Healthcare Advisory Board. Reversing the Flight of Talent. Washington, D.C.: The Advisory Board Company, 2000). The estimated cost to replace a medical-surgical nurse is $42,000 and replacement cost for a specialty RN is $64,000. A hospital with 700 nurses and a 14 percent turnover rate had an added annual cost of approximately $3 million taking into account expenses associated with agency and premium labor cost and lost profit margin (Healthcare Advisory Board. *H*Works:Case Study Quantifies Cost of Staff Vacancies.* Washington, D.C.: The Advisory Board Company, September 10, 2001).

§ For detailed projections, see Buerhaus P, Staiger DO, Auerbach DI. *The Future of Nursing Workforce in the United States: Data, Trends and Implications.* Jones and Bartlett Publishers, Boston, MA. 2008.

as outpatient services enlarge and the workforce demands nurse clinicians and nurse practitioners. The need for outpatient nurses will increase, but intensity of hospital care has also increased, with a net effect that more nurses are probably needed in both areas. We require more investment in nurse education and more continuing education for nurses in the practice setting.

The average nurse spends less than a third of his or her time in direct patient care. Data presented by The Healthcare Information and Management Systems Society (HIMSS) show that nurse charting was all on paper in 43 percent of surveyed hospitals, with 30 percent using electronic documentation at a stationary location and 28 percent with mobile devices. Only 20 percent had individual pagers or cell phones.[22] Considering the static RN output, we must explore every possible way of improving nursing efficiency, such as charting through wireless tablets, having the right nurse in the right unit, relying on technicians for operating room assistance, computerizing order entry, and reducing supply problems. These objectives are aimed at reconfiguring the nursing unit so that the nurse has more time for patient interaction and less administrative work. Nurses engage in a lot of "hunting and gathering" activity that wastes time. Targets for improving the efficiency of nursing care include improvements in documentation, medication administration and care coordination.[23] Workflow redesign, electronic charting and leadership training enable greater nurse efficiency and safety in practice. Proactive nurse management and open access to the hospital administration can enhance the role of nursing in hospital practice. Start with supervisors and directors who listen and are advocates. Nurses should be involved in the design of new or modified medical facilities, in the purchase of new electronic applications and in personnel policies.

As hospital leaders, we all rely on operations and finance, but apart from the physician staff, good nursing leadership is the glue that holds it all together. Nurses have to be a continuous institutional priority. Nursing represents 30 percent of a hospital's operating budget. No surprise that finance often looks to nursing when attempting to cut costs, which leads nurse managers to feel that the administration does not adequately prioritize patient care.[24]

If chronic high nurse turnover is a problem in your organization, survey employee satisfaction. Magnet designated facilities are required to collect this information. Another method of addressing high turnover is to conduct exit interviews the moment a nurse resigns. You might be able to prevent the resignation. The information on why there is a desire to separate will be helpful in reducing the number of defections.

Analyze assignments and supervisor abilities and make pay and benefits commensurate with responsibilities. Address mandatory overtime, abusive work environments, unsafe conditions, and poor or nonexistent equipment. Nurses make relatively few medical errors but they encounter an enormous number of problems –

many of these are system-based – in the course of everyday work.[25] The majority of failures arise from the fact that they do not have the supplies, equipment, information, etc. to accomplish a task, or something interfered with the designated task to be performed. In large measure the failure was not the people but the system. Some examples include missing information, missing or broken equipment, inadequate staffing, incorrect supplies or multiple demands on time. Your survey may be distilled into three questions. What does the nurse want to do? What does management want the nurse to do? What does the patient want the nurse to do? The answer to all three is to take care of patients.[±]

At our medical center, we studied a number of solutions aimed at improving nurse retention. These included redeploying the workforce in certain areas where technicians and nurse assistants were able to help the nurse. We offered a retention bonus, child care, tuition subsidy, flexible hours, educational partnerships, differential salaries, temporary staffing, and online teaching. We constantly addressed the nurse/patient ratio and monitored the work hours per patient day. In specialties where nurses were in short supply, we instituted post-retirement work programs, started a patient service associate program and advertised widely. We considered all employment incentives such as part-time work, flextime, temporary work, job sharing, seasonal employment, and on-call shift work. We "marketed" nurses and their activities in many publications. Our idea program elicited many ideas from nurses involved in the process of care and these nurses were recognized individually. The bottom line for nurse retention is listening to the nurses and empowering them to make changes to improve their work environment.

Magnet status is an award given by the American Nurses Credentialing Center to hospitals that meet certain criteria measuring the strength and quality of their nursing. More hospitals apply for Magnet hospital status every year, but only 5 percent of all the hospitals in the United States enjoy Magnet designation. A Magnet status boosts reputation and morale. The program rewards strong professional practice environments, helps recruit and retain nursing staff, draws patients to the facility, helps improve patient outcomes, and indirectly improves hospital finances.[26] If morale is down, there is something wrong within the hospital system: human resources, supervisors or policies. Nurses respond to incentives just as we all do. The most important of these are good working conditions, flexibility in addressing lifestyle issues, the opportunity to provide the best patient care, to be busy and appreciated, to be treated fairly, to work under a good supervisor, and to be rewarded competitively in the market.

±   In an eight-hour shift, a nurse spends about two and a half hours with patients (Tucker AL, Edmondson AC. *Why Hospitals Don't Learn from Failures*. California Management Review, 45 (2), 55-72, 2003).

THE LEADERSHIP FORUM

There is no formula for team management. In our administration the style was to convene the executive group three or four times weekly for approximately two hours to review reports and follow-up and to assure that quarterly goals were met. We had to manage one of the larger non-profit delivery systems in America. Therefore, productivity and budgetary issues were constant topics. Continuous improvement metrics were essential for departments of clinical medicine and were reviewed monthly. In all, 70 controls were reviewed periodically. Too much, you say? Maybe so, but most of the time we knew what was going on.[±] And this is not command-and-control, which doesn't work in any large enterprise. Instead, it is an appreciation of trends and an early warning exercise.

Lonnie Smith, the chief executive and chairman of Intuitive Surgical, Inc., developed a set of rules for effective meeting management:

Before the meeting:
- establish purpose
- define the agenda
- identify participants and roles
- plan desired outcomes

During the meeting:
- review purpose and agenda
- respect the ground rules:
  > keep on time and topic
  > allow no silent disagreement
  > have one conversation at a time
  > focus on the problem or process
  > practice mutual respect
  > insist that everyone participates
- capture the previous discussion
- facilitate the dialogue to achieve desired outcomes
- use prevention and intervention skills
- clarify agreements and decisions

[±]   If I had to do it all over again, I would schedule all important meetings early in the day. George Marshall said, "No one ever had an original idea after three o'clock in the afternoon." (Cited in Atkinson R. *The Day of Battle. The War in Sicily and Italy, 1943-1944*. Henry Holt & Co., New York, 2007).

- summarize group memory
- confirm assignments
- determine the follow-up method and timeline

Meeting guidelines can also be useful in creating focus, discipline, and individual ownership among team members from multiple disciplines who don't typically work together. Dr. Curtis Rimmerman, a cardiologist who led a patient-oriented, world-class service team at the Cleveland Clinic, developed a set of meeting guidelines that have come to be known affectionately as "Rimmerman's Rules." They are: 1) leave rank at the door; 2) no whining; 3) contribute at least one "bright idea" per session; 4) no "sidebar" communications allowed; 5) if you have something to say, say it in the room; 6) assume that each person wants to be present; 7) identify problems and focus on solutions (input – discussion – decision); 8) review the objectives to ensure they are realistic; 9) leave with a sense of accomplishment; 10) expect work outside of the meeting.

The executive team should address two hardwired agenda items: 1) clinical quality, which includes service issues; 2) brainstorming[±] – I believe that the team has to generate a really bright idea every day, an idea that improves the organization or process of care, saves money or improves safety. Motivation is a given, because the tasks at hand should be enough of a stimulant. A leader should not have to motivate the team, but his or her presence and the style of good chairmanship should be inspirational and confirm that people are on a good team.[27] To all this I would add that 1 ½ or 2 hours for a meeting is the maximum. We always tried to limit the executive team meeting agenda to three or four items – often in vain, I admit.

Discontent is the first step in the progress of man or nation.[28] Meeting conflict is inevitable. Personalities may clash when there is lack of understanding, no rules of engagement, a weak leader, personal dissatisfaction, overwork, disorganization,

---

±   Brainstorming: A term coined by the advertising executive Alex Osborn in 1941 to describe a thinking methodology he had developed "by which a group attempts to find a solution for a specific problem by amassing all the ideas spontaneously suggested by its members." Over the years Osborn developed and refined a series of rules for brainstorming meetings. His original rules: 1) Criticism is ruled out. Adverse judgment of ideas must be withheld until later. 2) Freewheeling is welcomed. The wilder the idea, the better; it is easier to tame down than to think up. 3) Quantity is desirable. The greater the number of ideas, the more likelihood of useful ideas. 4) Combination and improvement are sought. In addition to contributing ideas of their own, participants should suggest how the ideas of others can be turned into better ideas or how two or more ideas can be jointed into another idea. (Hurson T. *Think Better: An Innovator's Guide to Productive Thinking*. McGraw-Hill, New York, 2007).

or worse, high output failure. In any debate there can be some minor conflict, but personal conflict between team members is unacceptable. Above all, do not allow turf battles. The unpleasant personal qualities that could lead to chronic conflict are generally screened out when a person is selected to assume an executive position. In the case of incessant disruption, the question is how to handle it. First, I talk privately to combatants. If that conversation doesn't work, I refer you to the following anecdote. I call this the "and you will disappear from the face of the earth" meeting, which happens rarely, but can be used as a last resort.

> Two feuding knights from Yorkshire and Lancashire were ordered before the king when he was just sitting down to dinner. Whose men are you? he asked them. Yours, they replied. And whose men had they raised to fight in their quarrel? Yours, they replied again. "And what authority or commandment had ye, to raise up my men or my people, to fight and slay each other for your quarrel?" Henry demanded, adding that "in this ye are worthy to die." Unable to answer, the two knights humbly begged his pardon. Henry then swore "by the faith that he owed to God and to Saint George" that if they could not resolve their quarrel before he had finished his dish of oysters, "they should be hanged both two." Faced with such a choice, the knights were immediately persuaded to settle their differences, but they were not yet off the hook. The king swore his favorite oath again and told them that if they, or any other lord within or without his realm: whatsoever they were, ever caused any insurrection or death of his subjects again, "they should die, according to the law."[29]

A round table supposedly emphasizes a lack of pecking order, but personally I think this is nonsense. If people are worried about dominance, they're spending too much time thinking about their careers and need to spend more time on exceeding their goals. Also, I don't believe that an administrative group or cabinet has a group personality. It is the role of the person in charge to assure that results occur in the context of the mission and the vision of the organization. Cohesiveness depends on how the meeting is managed. I mentioned previously that our council was akin to the Knesset (or a Viking dinner). However, virtually every meeting stuck to the agenda and, at the end of the day, almost always resulted in progress. An effective team depends on relationships, mutual respect and a collective sense of achievement. Disagreement often produces a better decision. As Senator Patrick Moynihan put it, "Everyone is entitled to his own opinions, but not his own facts."[30]

In forum management, there are two givens: one is trust and the second, respect.± Not everyone has worked with a team or thought about managing to one set of values. I know respect is said to be earned, but if you have recruited wisely, respect is mutual and present from the outset. Healthcare executives have the same interest as any other skilled professional. They want to be part of an environment that is conducive to personal and group success. They want to win; they want to be respected and recognized; they want to grow personally and professionally and have economic security.

There is a story about ensuring trust and it relates to one of the most prominent events on the Lewis and Clark expedition. At the foot of the Rocky Mountains, the party first met the Shoshone tribe. There were a few tense moments before they were welcomed.† Droulliard (the legendary guide) needed no extensive knowledge of the language or signs to inform the chieftain that the strangers desired him and his companions to join them in a friendly smoke. Then a singular event happened. Hardly had Lewis started to extend the pipe toward the chieftain, than he (the chieftain) and his warriors began to take off their moccasins. This act intended to signify that if anyone were to prove unfaithful to whatever they might agree upon in the forthcoming discussion, they would walk barefoot forever afterwards, in summer and winter, for the rest of their lives.[31] Now, that may be frontier lore, but the point should apply to any deal or arrangement in any business. Trust was lost only one time in my administrative career, but I sure would like to see that guy walking around forever barefoot.

MANAGING CHANGE

In healthcare, the changing times mean more complex regulations, more pressure to verify results, more demands from informed patients, potentially more money to support highly targeted investigations, the move toward bundled physician reimbursement.§

The economic pressures of modern healthcare are driving private practice physicians into new business relationships. Many of these relationships relate to

---

±   The five team dysfunctions are: 1) absence of trust; 2) fear of conflict; 3) lack of commitment; 4) avoidance of accountability; 5) inattention to results. (Lencioni P. *The Five Dysfunctions of a Team*. Jossey-Bass, San Francisco, 2002.)

†   The chief turned out to be Cameahwait, Sacagawea's long-lost brother.

§   Medicare would pay a hospital and affiliated physicians a fixed amount to cover costs of providing care during the hospital stay, plus 30 days after discharge. (Hackbarth G, Reischauer R, Mutti A. *Collective Accountability for Medical Care – Toward Bundled Medicare Payments*. N Engl J Med 2008: 359 (1); 3-5)

technology. Between 2000 and 2005 the volume of procedures in Medicare patients increased significantly: knee replacements up 47 percent; arthroscopy, 65 percent; colonoscopy, 40 percent; cardiovascular stress test, 45 percent; computerized tomography, 65 percent; magnetic resonance imaging, 94 percent.[32] The outpatient surgical and imaging sites have proliferated as have partnerships to build them. Most academic medical centers have not entered into this type of joint venture, but depending on reimbursement, that is likely to change.

Joint ventures with physicians for offices, outpatient facilities and informatics are increasing. In many cases your own doctors have become your competition. When a joint venture with those doctors can add value for the community, it may be worthwhile to explore the possibility. Joint ventures, however, are not without shortcoming. Don Williams, former chief executive and chairman of Trammell Crow Company, illustrates their potential drawbacks in a story about Japanese businessmen with whom they were in discussion. The Americans often used the term "joint venture" but their Japanese counterparts did not understand the phrase. After the phrase "joint venture" was translated repeatedly to the Japanese principal, he looked up and exclaimed, "Ah. Now I understand. Joint venture means same bed, different dreams."

Doctors are inherently skeptical of change. So, as the old order inevitably changes, leadership has four options.

1) We can resist change, but this doesn't advance the organization, and the tide of change carries the resisters along anyway. The fates lead the willing and drag the unwilling.

2) The second option: We can whine, which some people think makes you feel better by "getting it out of your system." Actually, it's better to substitute handwringing with activity. As Osler pointed out, "waste of energy, mental distress, nervous worries dog the steps of the man who is anxious about the future."[33] The point is that commitment, hard work, persistence, and innovation have always been responsible for the advances in medicine.

3) The third option: We can panic, which could be fatal. In Hampton Side's book, *The Ghost Soldiers*,[34] he describes a group of 1,600 American prisoners during World War II who were placed in a small cargo hold – way below deck, ill-ventilated, unbearably hot and dangerously life-threatening. The prisoners were gasping for air, passing out, and because they were suffocating, they panicked. Then their captors shut the hatch and

made it even worse. When all seemed lost, a man, not high ranking, stood up and shouted, "We're in this together and if any of us want to live, we're going to have to work together. Calm down. The men in the far corners are suffocating. Take off your shirts and fan the air toward them." The improvement was immediate. He then negotiated for water and brought those who had passed out up to the deck. So, this seemingly nervous, intense, overeager fellow rose to the occasion on that day in a remarkable act of poise and resolve. You fight panic through faith in leadership and faith in each other. Sometimes people rise to greatness at critical times and you can't predict who it will be. That's why leadership development is important.

4) Taking a lesson from that story, the fourth option is what our group practice model of medicine is all about – to pull together… to act as a unit. Real teamwork is unity of purpose and a natural diversity of excellence. Medicine is the single greatest profession that we could ever hope to be in and everyone in management contributes to the greater value we see each year.

The formula for a successful team rests foremost on the understanding that we are in the business of results for clinical medicine, science and education. We move ahead by decisions based on team analysis and discussion. Just as healthy debate is important at the executive level, the same should be true in the departments. In fact, thoughtful disagreement should be encouraged. However, when a decision has been reached, everyone should walk out the door "holding hands." No disagreement, grousing or backbiting afterwards. Period.

Every executive should have time to think, to reflect, to get away. Real accomplishment is the key to mental health. Ariel Sharon wrote about the "mountain of problems" throughout the history of Israel. "I think back when I was a child working with my father on that arid slope of land, walking behind him to plant… exhausted to go on, he would stop for a moment to look backwards, to see how much we had already done. And that would always give me heart for what remained."[35] Accomplishment lifts frustrations. That is one good reason why I always kept a notebook, so that we could look back and see how much we had already done.

Adair[36] believes that certain offices should carry a time warning: Working in this office could damage your time. I read many years ago that the optimal vacation is three weeks: The first week, people don't relax; the second week, they are beginning to rest; and the final week is enjoyment and full recharge. This makes sense, but I confess I never did it. However, if you can get away even for a day or so, just to reflect and rest, it is reinforcing. Solitude is a wonderful thing when one is at peace with oneself and when there is a definite task to be accomplished.[37]

THE KEY EXECUTIVES

The role of leadership and those of the key executives reflect the changes in healthcare and must be shaped to the needs of their specific market. The job descriptions are dynamic. In our institution, not all key executives sat on the administrative council. We respected their time and their responsibilities, which were better served attending to their principal duties. For example, the nursing director, legal counsel, the chief academic officer, and the director of communication met with the administrative group as needed but were not regular members. There are no set rules for this type of forum, which will ultimately reflect the table of organization.

This section describes our executive team functions. My impression of the individual roles and qualifications begins with the *Chief of Staff* (chief medical officer), who operates across the entire academic enterprise. The clinical departments, however organized, ultimately report up to this office. In our organization, so did regional clinical directors. The chief executive must assure that all chairs and chiefs cooperate for progress. There is a fine line between dispute resolution and meddling. It depends on the culture of the institution. If the key executives have a controversy with subordinates, the leadership at the highest level should know the issues and step in before it becomes nuclear. Most of the time all key executives were able to solve problems in their respective domains. The majority of issues involved budget matters and less often personnel.

In dealing with so many constituencies, the chief of staff has to have unshakeable credibility. This office must be respected. Whoever holds it must be fair but firm and uphold all the principles of the medical practice, and where applicable, scientific investigation and education. This is a hard position to fill and to execute.

The chief executive can usually find operation executives and a financial staff, lawyers, department heads and scientists easier than recruiting a great chief of staff. The reason is that the chief of staff has both a leadership and management position and a people's job. The chief of staff is judge, jury, parent, confessor, adjudicator, peacemaker and stand-in for the chief executive, and has to be interactive with outside private practitioners. The chief of staff may chair the council of institutes or divisions. All this requires negotiating skill, patience, toleration, and courage. No waffling. Apart from the chief executive, the chief of staff in a large medical organization is key to good medical relations and academic excellence.

In our model, the *Chief Academic Officer* functioned as the provost. Education and research activities were coordinated through the academic officer, who also had a reporting relationship (a dotted line in the table of organization) to the chief of staff. The chief academic officer generally reports to the chief executive, but communication to the chief of staff is essential and expected.

The role of the *Chief Operating Officer* is variable. Some businesses have divided the responsibilities so that there is in effect no operations post. In our healthcare organization, the chief operating officer had parity with the chief executive, but elsewhere it might depend on the level of operational interest held by the chief executive. An operating officer certainly has to have the same objectives as the chief executive. The functionality of that position depends on the size and scope of the healthcare system. There is no real playbook for the operating officer. It can be a hybrid position, but knowledge about hospital and system administration is important. The operating officer has to keep the engines running throughout the system. The operating and finance officers should coordinate the supply chain management together. Growth, cost and revenue cycle may not be the responsibilities of the operating officer, but he or she must oversee the profitability and free cash flow in the parent hospital and throughout the system hospitals. The operating officer works with the community hospital executives to assure that goals are met. Other responsibilities that are more standard include security, energy, buildings and grounds. The operating officer is the manager who oversees the structural integrity of the system.

The *Chief Financial Officer* is in charge of business intelligence. The financial officer manages the balance sheet, emphasizes the importance of operative performance and directs financial planning. In academic health centers and large hospitals, returns from investment income and philanthropy, expense growth, and uncompensated care are increasingly important markers of income. In addition, we now have increased self-pay collection, revenue cycle complexities and refined coding.

Planning requires financial discipline and assurance about integrity of the numbers. Real-time cost accounting is no longer elusive. As healthcare systems become more complicated, the finance officer is required to communicate effectively, execute the system financial strategy and understand the other executives' responsibilities. What has changed in the chief financial officer's role is that it has become much more strategic and requires more communication compared with even a decade ago. Finance is more involved today in risk management and deal oversight. Investment bankers provide advice regarding managing the balance sheet and executing in the financial markets. They should provide wise counsel in managing bank debt, insurance, commercial paper and private placements. This is one area where I don't believe that investment bankers are mere consultants. Instead they are partners who are involved in financial structure and executions throughout the system.

The objective of *Human Resources* is to leverage the organization's human capital by helping employees to achieve their maximum potential. The director and team are expected to recruit the best available talent,± oversee competitive pay and benefit practices, supervise training and development programs, instill service orientation, and help to create a positive work environment. When human resources executives are under consideration, ensure they have no bias against management, or, conversely, believe that people don't want to work and are lazy. Be sure you are hiring an assertive manager who holds everyone accountable and understands that preventing problems is far easier than solving problems. The responsibility for human resources comprises more than writing fair polices and maintaining good employee relations. The human resources director should also have legal and business expertise and be able to influence strategic planning.

In the best medical organizations, human resources has become less transactional and more consultative. The new human resources is more of a strategic business partner to the individual operating units and less confined to black and white rules. These managers are active participants in the staffing process. Their experience should give them a keen understanding of the business of medicine, the environment and the strategic pressures.

In our business, a brand name is important, but not for premium pricing. Instead, the *Marketing Director* has a unique opportunity to market quality and access. New services, physicians and specialties, and where they are located are informational. The community appreciates information about doctors, scientific breakthroughs, patient testimonies, and education about wellness. There are always great stories about nursing and successful heroics. Use your Web site to advertise and educate from articles, videos, and podcasts.† Place the Net Generation at the center of marketing. Trustees are very helpful in marketing and public relations. They are out in the community and know firsthand about the hospital's image. Ask them what the customers are saying. The organization must learn to think of itself not as producing goods or services but as *buying customers*, doing the things that will make people *want* to do business with it. And the chief executive has the responsibility

---

±   See Appendix V

†   There are ten target "consumer" groups to consider: patients (especially mothers), physicians, payers, government employees, unions, trustees, suppliers, affiliates, researchers and educators. Women are generally more reliable, better informed, have more interest in health services, have more follow-up visits and are more likely to practice preventive medicine.

for creating this environment, this viewpoint, this attitude, this aspiration to set the company's style, its direction, and its goals.[38] The best advice I can offer is to integrate communication, market research and marketing. Otherwise, they will work separately and less efficiently.

If you are hiring a marketing executive, try to find one who has healthcare operational experience. Marketing can aid access by developing dedicated telephone lines and a Web site to handle appointments, executive health, and international queries. Medicine is like a catalogue order business. It's best to have an informed human answer with minimal hold time and prompt follow-up. On your Web site, one call or click takes care of all arrangements. Other facilitators are cancer answer and nurse-on-call lines, and one communication site to arrange hospital transfers instead of having referring doctors queue up for a transfer to individual services.

A good *Director of Communication* will change the organization from a passive reactive instrument for the media into an active, knowledgeable source that the media will respect. The best advice is to develop a constant positive and low-key press presence.[39] Finding a great expert in this field takes some creativity. The best ones have a background in journalism or in a newsroom. This is a tough position to fill. Finding experts in a particular field and asking them for their recommendations is an excellent method for recruiting executives.

There is a difference between public relations and media relations. The former shapes opinions. The latter must excel in talking to the media, becoming an advocate for the media and sometimes using tough love with the media. A communications director has to be scrupulously honest and can't be in awe of or afraid of doctors. The media can see right through someone who is untrustworthy. Get your side of the story out first. Set up really good media training for the doctors. Insist that nothing big appears without the communications director's knowledge.

The extent of *Legal Counsel* depends on the size of the academic organization, the table of organization, system composition and activities extraneous to the core mission. The characteristics of the chief legal counsel have to suit the involvement of the chief executive… "a lawyer that I would want beside me in most negotiations"… a common-sense lawyer… a lawyer we can understand – not too many "whereases"… a lawyer who gives one-hand opinions. The best legal counsel is primarily motivated to serve and promote the enterprise rather than control and restrain it. Too often, legal training leads to narrow thinking that sacrifices real opportunity in favor of risk avoidance. Good healthcare lawyers also need to be good office managers in order to lead their increasing number of legal colleagues. A large hospital or academic medical center can have as many attorneys as a midsize law firm. Chief counsels sometimes are good lawyers but poor managers, and unable to coordinate their group. You also want them to concentrate on their primary role. A good vice counsel can serve as the "managing partner" or administrator and allow the chief counsel to fully exercise his or her talent in other areas.

The above broad overview of the executive team is written only to provide a view of our organization. The chief executive has to select a team with the right skills and chemistry. Follow your instincts. The credo of businessman Karl Eller sums up recruitment admirably, "When you're looking at (personal) characteristics, first comes integrity; second, motivation; third, capacity; fourth, understanding; fifth, knowledge; and last and least, experience. Without integrity, motivation is dangerous. Without motivation, capacity is impotent; without capacity, understanding is limited; without understanding, knowledge is meaningless; without knowledge, experience is blind. Experience is easy to provide and quickly put to good use by people with all other qualities."[40]

If the organization is in disarray, the challenge is to address the issues rather quickly. In each area of executive management, the individual team members require skill in planning, project development and completion, and getting people to work for progress. The role of the leader is to coordinate these activities, elicit ideas, mentor, and above all, support the leadership team.

HOSPITAL VOLUNTEERISM

In our country, volunteering for community services is part of our culture. Volunteerism is the "willingness to help." At the Cleveland Clinic, we started an "ambassador" program in 1992. Now our hospital has approximately 1,200 beds with high occupancy rate, and in 2007 there were 1,700 ambassadors. The program has unique features that deserve commentary.[±] We shall use the term ambassadors and volunteers interchangeably.

Healthcare volunteers are looking for a way to give back something to the community and to the institution that perhaps took care of them. Half of the volunteers are students, either high school students earning community service credits or college students who request experience in healthcare. The other volunteers are senior citizens who have the same motives as their younger counterparts but also see the social benefit as they meet other volunteers and establish friendships. Another volunteer group is comprised of active employees, a third of whom volunteer extra hours for special events. Volunteers generally work four hours once a week.

Our ambassadors have become a major component of service. They provide directions, image, a friendly face, and give ideas about patient satisfaction and

±   For further information, contact Beth Stein, Director, Program Services, at steine@ccf.org.

efficiency back to the organization. The Joint Commission has very specific rules about training requirements, especially in regard to disaster planning, fire safety and infection control. There are five full-time employees in the ambassador program who are responsible for orientation and continuing training for all volunteers.

There is another type of ambassador, not volunteers, but full-time employees, who wear red coats and are stationed in high-traffic areas providing answers and help of every kind. These redcoats are few in number but are, in effect, a type of ambassador. I remember during my tenure, there was a redcoat named Robert who was stationed at the Taussig Cancer Center. This fellow was entertaining, informative and invaluable for many people who were depressed or troubled by their illness. We gave him a top hat to wear. I am convinced he actually saved lives.

There are a growing number of support groups that interact with the volunteers. Some examples are Mended Hearts, volunteers who have had previous orthopedic procedures and counsel patients pre- and post-operatively, and other volunteers for the alcohol and drug rehabilitation area as well as in the subacute or skilled nursing care units.

A pediatric literacy group staffed by volunteers reads to children and gives out books to parents. The volunteers put on a theme party four times a year in the Children's Hospital, which has been highly successful. We have a caring canine pet therapy program that has 41 dogs that visit seven selected nursing units. Volunteer programs may run gift shops, although for variety and profitability those shops should probably be outsourced. We have turned over our gift shops to a noted bookstore that will add literature and gifts for a greatly expanded clientele. Any profit is returned to the volunteer program.

All of the hospitals in our healthcare system have volunteer programs but they are managed autonomously. The leaders of these volunteer programs meet periodically throughout the year to discuss community needs. The annual budget for our ambassador program is $500,000 funded by operations.

Volunteers today are not the candy stripers of old. They are a legion of bright and compassionate men and women, young and old, who help patients and personnel and add immeasurably to the value of healthcare.

MISTAKES

Mistakes and failures are inevitable. "My own success was attended by quite a few failures along the way," said Kemmons Wilson, "but I refuse to make the biggest mistake of all: worrying too much about making mistakes."[41] Most catastrophes or major crises are unanticipated. Success is almost always credited to policy, diplomacy or operations while failure is blamed on intelligence[42] (meaning knowledge, not IQ).

In healthcare, this results from a failure to understand the profession and the market. A disciplined, experienced executive team will minimize the error rate.

I always ask myself three questions before making a decision: 1) Do I really understand the issue at hand and could I explain it to my colleagues?; 2) Will there be any unintended consequences?; 3) What will happen if we don't decide now? As James Thurber wrote in the *New Yorker* many years ago, "It is better to ask some of the questions than to know all the answers."[43] It's said that Japanese businesspeople, once they have all the facts, will ask *why* five times before making a decision. Personally, I took notes at team meetings as the discussion proceeded – to summarize the pros and cons and also to review as the decision was followed up. The group is inspired and encouraged by successful decisions probably more than any other factor. Inaction demoralizes people far more than failure.

However, failures should not be confused with mistakes. Mistakes produce little new or useful information and, therefore, are without value. Thomke[44] has four rules for successful management. 1) organize for rapid management; 2) fail early and often; 3) avoid mistakes; and 4) anticipate and exploit early information combining new and old technologies. Fewer errors occur when governance is engaged and where attention to detail is the hallmark of leadership. Mistakes usually relate to errors in clinical systems, projected growth and contracting. Oversight and fiscal policies are often slack. I learned a long time ago that the best surgeons don't forget their mistakes. Repetition of error does not constitute experience.

Problems at the healthcare system level are generally attributed to poor clinical quality and lack of operational and financial communication. Everyone thought they were paying attention, but we still misjudged the early impact of the initial Balanced Budget Act. Mistakes in the growth category relate to building or acquiring before financial planning. Bad contracts result from inept negotiations, failure to obtain clinical input regarding volume and pricing, acquiescence to low per diem contracts or capitation, or no bargaining leverage. Failure in the oversight area indicates diffuse attention, no discipline, change resistance or simply bad judgment.[±] Finally, fiscal mistakes may relate to high-risk deals, poor planning, too much debt, no fund development, or continued declining profit for all the reasons above. (If you want to learn about a classic compilation of mistakes and failure, read *The Fall of the House of AHERF: The Allegheny Bankruptcy*.[45]

An inherent weakness in many large academic centers is the slow development of new physician leaders and especially physician executives. Hospitals tend to have

---

±　I have not failed ten thousand times. I have successfully found ten thousand ways that will not work. (Thomas Edison)

pretty thin bench strength. Great doctors and great scientists don't necessarily want to be key executives. They often aspire to be department or division or institute chairs, but to sit in the mahogany row offices is not very interesting. They want to be real doctors and investigators, not professional administrators.

All organizations make mistakes in recruitment, but very few people, especially managers, need to be terminated. Firing large numbers of people who were originally hired for key positions – or repeated periodic purges or layoffs – are an indication of unstable management. When I read about massive layoffs, I have to wonder what all those people were doing there in the first place. Certainly, disagreement is not grounds for dismissal. The best way for a group to be smart is for each person in it to think and act as independently as possible.[46]

Communication is the hardest to teach. Directives, even in the digital age, often don't reach intended personnel or are distorted along the way. When considering a decision, the mind gives disproportionate weight to the first information it receives.[47] We tend to subconsciously decide what to do before figuring out why we want to do it. Most of us are overconfident about our judgment, which can lead to bad decisions. One of the examples of poor management style is the supervisor or manager who says, "Look at what they are doing to us now" or, "I don't agree with this change but I have to do it." Even worse are managers who rigidly maintain the status quo because they have no creative ability to develop or advance the department. Many administrators in medicine are afraid to speak out or hide behind the clinical department head or are intimidated by all physicians. Many hospitals have changed administrative reporting for clinical departments to a central administrative command that bypasses the clinical department heads.

Department managers, being in the middle, are subject to a different set of pressures, shortcomings, and temptations from those above and below them. Too many manage reactively. They fail to understand their role in management and how their actions affect performance up and down the process stream. Many have reached a dead end in their careers. Having moved up from labor to management, they're now "stuck," not having the education or training to move higher. Because they may not have the high-level contacts that are needed to have clout, they lose the respect of employees. Where supervisor turnover is high, workers feel they can outwait – and outwit – any boss. Powerless managers create a monotonous work environment, where performance measures are strictly based on rules devoid of change.[48] A good executive empowers subordinates and gives them security to act without fear. Tell them you prefer smart mistakes, but errors are inevitable – don't hide from them. Learn and don't repeat if possible.± Prevention is always better than cure. Or as

±   Avoid making the wrong mistakes. (Yogi Berra)

Warren Buffett says facetiously, "Failing conventionally is the route to go; as a group, lemmings may have a rotten image, but no individual lemming has ever received bad press."[49] For most chief executives, only one thing is worse than making a huge strategic mistake: being the only person in the industry to make it.

The sense of responsibility is often the most difficult to imbue because it is more than the outcome of patient care. Responsibility also applies to the management of cost, thoughtful consideration about the process of care, and scrupulous attention to the needs of the patient. The best executives and managers are impatient about finishing the tasks at hand. I love impatient people. However, they are not the best negotiators.

CONSULTANTS

Identify an issue or problem, form a committee, set up an office, hire a consultant and table the decision. This is what happens in many businesses. I kept a lid on consultant spending because the yield was low… probably more so in healthcare than other businesses. We don't manufacture an array of products or manage global divisions. Pricing is less of an issue and we don't have "distribution" problems outside the supply chain. The data amassed by the consultant comes mainly from the client and may even be erroneous. Their recommendations generally don't include methods of implementation.[±] There is an adage: If you're not part of the solution, there's good money to be made in prolonging the problems. Worse, the consultant knows what the chief executive requires justification for and produces conclusions accordingly. Having said that, we had some great consultants during my tenure, and in widely disparate areas: acquisitions, billing, and service. In each case the advice was transformational. In healthcare, consultants are useful in finance, including preparation for bond rating, automation in the revenue cycle, expansion of the delivery system (acquisitions and site development), and service, which includes ongoing personnel education. Consultants are especially valuable when they can stimulate strategic thinking.

± "In my long life, I have never seen a management consultant's report that didn't end with the same advice: 'This problem needs management consulting services.' Widespread incentive-caused bias requires that one should often distrust or take with a grain of salt, the advice of one's professional advisor, even if he is an engineer. The general antidotes here are: 1) especially fear professional advice when it is especially good for the advisor; 2) learn and use the basic elements of your advisor's trade as you deal with your advisor; and 3) double check, disbelieve, or replace much of what you're told, to the degree that it seems appropriate after objective thought." (*Poor Charlie's Almanack: The Wit and Wisdom of Charles T. Munger*, Ed., Kaufman PD. The Donning Company Publishers 3rd Edition 2008)

Hiring consultants± should not be a knee-jerk response to every problem. The majority of them know less about your business than your team does and may not understand the local market. An organization generally calls for help in highly technical areas, for service improvement or sometimes when you are just stumped. What you hope for is fresh ideas. Too often, what you get is an analysis of the problem based on interviews of your own personnel, which you could have done yourself. Good recommendations generally coincide with your own opinion from the outset. What you don't get, unless consultants become embedded (at high cost), is implementation.

We contracted with three exceptional consultants over the course of 15 years: 1) a healthcare consultant hired to interview a hospital system that we wanted to acquire. The consultant informed us that the administrators and some trustees of the target system were leaning away from us and toward our chief competitor – we changed our approach and won the competition; 2) a technology consultant was hired to manage our charge master updates – we ended up outsourcing the charge master maintenance to them; 3) a service consultant, Quint Studer, who facilitated the inception of a world-class service program that greatly added to quality assurance and reputation.

Some successful executives rely heavily on consultants. God bless them. I would caution against excessive use of consultants because of the overall low yield of exceptional results and the cumulative high cost. The biggest downside is reliance on paid consultants to do what you could easily do yourself. Dependence on consultants spreads throughout an organization, and soon management, even leaders, stop thinking – at great expense.

There are a lot of potential advisors within a large medical complex: experienced physician managers, trustees, personal business acquaintances and, best of all, your own team. The question is: Do I really need help in these areas going forward or am I just hiring somebody to justify what I intended to do all along? If you have the courage of your convictions and have discussed the issue widely, you can save a lot of money by not hiring outside experts. If consultants are needed, one or more of these three results should occur: 1) the organization should realize added revenue of ten times the advisor's fee after two years; 2) the organization should gain a competitive position; 3) the organization should be transformed to fit a new competitive market.[50]

Mark Shapiro, general manager and vice president of the Cleveland Indians, believes that "an organization differentiates itself by focusing on team building even

---

±   I have not considered outside law firms, investment managers or lobbyists as consultants. They are an integral part of most large hospital systems. The same applies to salary and benefit consultants, which were essential for a group practice and large workforce.

more than acquiring individual talent."[51] Remember, teams and teamwork are not the same thing. A strong performance ethic, disciplined action and integration across operational boundaries are essential in building a real team. The best teams generally are comprised of a small number of people who have complementary skills and shared purposes and hold themselves individually and mutually accountable for all actions and results. Skill is more important than personality. A good leader shares leadership and develops an almost symbiotic relationship among team members. The purpose of the team at the top is identical to the purpose of the company.[52]

CHAPTER 9

INNOVATION

And it ought to be remembered that there is nothing more diffi-cult to take in hand, more perilous to conduct, or more uncertain in its success, than to take the lead in the introduction of a new order of things. Because the innovator has for enemies all those who have done well under the old conditions, and lukewarm defend-ers in those who may do well under the new. This coolness arises partly from fear of the opponents, who have the laws on their side, and partly from the incredulity of men, who do not readily believe in new things until they have had a long experience of them. Thus it happens that whenever those who are hostile have the oppor-tunity to attack, they do it like partisans, whilst the others defend lukewarmly....

— Niccolo Machiavelli
The Prince, 1515
W.K. Marriott (translated 1908)

Invention and innovation are not the same. Invention is pure knowledge based on new science or technology that is protectable. Innovation is invention that produces economic value. There may be a considerable time lag between the two.[1,2] Many inventions and innovations are modified substantially over time.[3] Innovation means new ideas or research that leads to new methods, products, technology, scientific endeavors or services, which are then brought to the market or become standard practice. Innovation involves bringing the idea into existence.[4] Innovation does not depend on invention but generally involves many interactions and feedbacks in knowledge creation.[5] Innovation has become the core driver of growth, performance and valuation.[6] An innovation requires an idea and an investment in it. As the 2002 World Economic Forum Global Competitiveness Report concludes, "Innovation has become, perhaps, the most important source of competitive advantage in advanced economies."[7]

There are about 300 academic health centers and large teaching hospitals in the U.S. that have the capability to develop new drugs, devices or services that are commercially viable or in some way add new value. All of the 5,000 hospitals in the U.S. are filled with creative people, who, under the proper conditions, can think and talk about ways to improve patient care – if only someone will listen. We don't sell products, but the products that we use have a measurable impact on efficiency. Look for ideas that improve patient processing, case management, safety, accounting, or other measures that might improve the results. Define the innovation that meets the organizational strategic objectives: innovations that improve healthcare and conserve resources; innovations that increase patient and personnel satisfaction. There should be a direct link between strategic priorities and ideation.[8]

Innovations may be categorized as transformational, substantial and incremental.[9] *Transformational* innovation turns the field upside down, the way the pacemaker or magnetic resonance imaging transformed cardiology and radiology. The term disruptive innovation[10,11] is defined as technology that introduces a significantly lower cost or easier-to-use product into an existing category. Clayton Christensen points out that disruption often doesn't involve big technological breakthroughs; instead, it involves mastering the intricate art of simple solutions to improve convenience, accessibility or affordability. Disruption allows a whole new population of consumers to afford and use a product or service that was historically limited to people with a lot of money or special skills. *Substantial* innovation is defined as the second generation of transformational invention, such as coronary artery stenting, which followed balloon angioplasty. Most innovation in healthcare is of the third type, *incremental,* which involves process more than products. This is the least extreme (and disruptive) type of innovation and occurs widely in healthcare because technology and processes are already in place and ripe for new ideas. Foster and Kaplan call incremental innovations the red blood cells of the economy.[12] Incremental innovation may not create wealth directly; however, even small innovations can improve efficiency and signal important change in process. The opportunities are staggering. Wherever you find waiting lines, congestion, inefficiency, duplication, and processing dissatisfactions – there is the opportunity for innovation. Incremental innovation is the signature of continuity. The innovation may not catch on immediately, but when it does, it creates a new dimension of performance and occurs mostly through collaboration.[13] Innovation is now part of continuous improvement.

HEALTHCARE INNOVATION

Traditionally, the mission of academic medicine was seen as a three-legged stool supported by science, education and patient care. Today, this mission might be more accurately visualized as a 3-dimensional pyramid with innovation as the base. Innovation is a core part of healthcare, finding application in: 1) plans for new services; 2) the creation of new products, especially devices and pharmaceuticals; 3) improved safety, outcome and service; and 4) greater operating efficiencies. In a receptive culture, ideas are easy to generate. Ideas, however, can't stand alone on their own merits. The rate of adoption is the hard part.

Procedure technology, genomics and pharmaceutical blockbusters are all potential disruptors. Less obvious opportunities have included: retail clinics staffed by nurse practitioners; nighthawk radiology; supply delivery robots; radiofrequency asset tracking; robotically assisted surgery; and simulation software for medical education. Outside the hospital there are less expensive modular systems for telehealth and monitoring, which include remote video consultation to correctional institutions, nursing homes, emergency departments, and psychiatric facilities.[14] Technology improves faster than people's lives change.

Herzlinger believes that innovation is still difficult because healthcare is so fragmented and change resistant with so many forces repelling new ideas.[15] Our human nature is such that busy managers resist the responsibility of generating or even accepting new ways of doing things and are even less likely to champion an idea through to implementation. A resistant attitude is pervasive in many industries. The old saw *it won't work* or *we tried it before* is an excuse not to think about making healthcare more efficient and safe. Although progress is shown through same-day admissions for elective procedures, improved transmission of laboratory and radiology results, attention to quality indicators, electronic billing and capacity management, hospitals tend to operate the same way as they have for decades. They are hierarchical systems.

A culture that stimulates idea generation has to be driven by medical and scientific leadership. If an academic medical center, or any hospital for that matter, expects to stay on the leading edge, the leadership should make innovation the highest priority for safety, for greater efficiency, and to promote market differentiation. Ideas are opportunities. To meet the challenge of eliciting innovations, an organization has to be able to assess its abilities and disabilities beyond the personnel level. Three factors affect an organization's capacity to absorb innovation: its resources, its processes, and its values.[16] When a culture of decentralized innovation is established, it becomes possible to implement a really great new idea that has practical application. Everybody has the opportunity to make a difference, but the leadership team has to encourage idea generation and then bring those ideas to fruition. An innovation pipeline depends on the number of people involved.

Although a great deal of incremental innovation relates to operational process, safety is even more important. All medical organizations should embrace the Institute for Healthcare Improvement, which was created to save 100,000 lives by preventing avoidable hospital deaths.[17] The founder, Dr. Donald Berwick, believes that it is not the workforce but the governance and senior leadership of the hospital that is responsible for improvements in care. The frontline workers are ready, willing and able but they need guidance to practice more effectively. Their methodology involves checklists. Would you get on an airplane where the pilot said that he didn't use checklists because he had plenty of experience?[±][†]

In their program, there are six evidence-based practices that add to safety:

- permit any staff to call a rapid-response team for patients in decline
- use aspirin and beta blockers early in treatment of myocardial infarction
- have a protocol to prevent sepsis from central venous catheters
- post hand washing protocols to reduce surgical infections
- record prescribed drugs accurately
- develop protocols to prevent ventilator-associated pneumonia

In each of these practices, there is a list or a bundle of checks that assure compliance. It's not quite as simple as it seems, but it has been proven to be lifesaving.

Inefficiency in the U.S. health system is as pernicious as it is pervasive. The remedy is innovation. Consistent hospital innovation requires three elements: 1) the right culture and an environment that fosters new ideas; 2) a skilled workforce with knowledge and experience who understand the importance of thinking about their jobs and the surrounding environment; and 3) managerial promotion and support. These are the critical conditions for successful innovation in healthcare.

±   See also Haynes AB, et. al. *A Surgical Safety Checklist to Reduce Morbidity and Mortality in a Global Population.* (N Engl J Med 2009: 360 (5); 491-9) They report favorable results after implementation of a surgical (non-cardiac) checklist.

†   John J. Nance wrote a good book about "the ultimate flight plan and barrierless communication" titled *Why Hospitals Should Fly.* Bozeman, MT: Second River Healthcare Press, 2008.

For healthcare leadership, the diplomacy of communicating change is essential to motivation.[18] Innovation has resulted in many improvements, but huge problems in patient logistics, supplies and patient accounts still exist. Components of the revenue cycle are poorly automated and not well integrated. Billing is problematic because payment is complex. Cost accounting is slow and generally estimated by a formula. Improvements have been made in discharge planning, but it's still hard to get patients out early in the day. Non-critically ill patients languish between tests and procedures and may wait unnecessarily long in the hospital in order to get scheduled for a procedure. Drucker observes "that any of these incongruities [in any field] is a *symptom* of an opportunity to innovate."[19]

Today, there's no excuse for insularity. We live in a global marketplace of ideas, where opportunities to share ideas and new practices abound. Personnel should be recognized for innovations that improve safety and efficiency. As Geoffrey Moore advises, "put yourself in service to an attractive target market to work on a solution to a seemingly intractable problem."[20] Mass collaboration fits very well into healthcare, especially in the service of innovation. The Web exposes us to breakthroughs happening across the industrial environment.

Wikis[±] bring the collective intelligence of the world to bear on projects of all kinds. The Web becomes a participatory platform. Many operational problems can be prioritized, qualified and sent out for commentary, particularly for the development of customer solutions.[21] Corporations manufacturing pharmaceuticals, consumer products, chemicals and polymers contract with, for example, InnoCentive or 9-Sigma, which post research and development challenges worldwide. The problem is posted anonymously. Solutions are submitted confidentially. Monetary awards are provided for top solutions. As companies learn to use these tools, they will develop managerial innovations – smarter and faster ways for individuals and teams to create value through interactions – that will be difficult for their rivals to replicate. Companies in sectors like healthcare and banking are already moving in this direction.[22] The Agency for Healthcare Research and Quality (AHRQ) launched a new Web site called the Health Care Innovations Exchange (http//www.innovations. ahrq.gov) that is designed to support healthcare professionals in sharing and adopting innovations that improve the delivery of healthcare to patients.[23] It is another way of "operationalizing innovation."[24]

[±] *Wiki* is the Hawaiian word for "quick" with *wiki wiki* meaning "super quick." (Lih A. *The Wikipedia Revolution. How a Bunch of Nobodies Created the World's Greatest Encyclopedia.* New York: Hyperion, 2009).

BROAD AREAS OF PROCESS IMPROVEMENT

Innovation is part of continuous improvement. The huge opportunities listed below pertain to efficiency, accuracy, education for the betterment of the workforce and for informed consumerism. The list could easily double or triple in length but these are some of the immediate priorities.

1) database integration$^{\pm}$
2) wireless tablets for nurse record management
3) quality metrics online
4) automated inventory utilization and charge capture
5) staffing for weekend procedures/outpatient visits
6) improved physician productivity
   - appointment coordination
   - practice management module
   - patient financial services combined with the electronic medical record
   - selected use of nurse practitioners
7) communication of ideas across departments, institutes and systems
8) staff education on leadership and management
9) health improvement programs (wellness)
   - staff (personnel)
   - newsletter on health for patients
10) Medicare and Medicaid patient education to better navigate the healthcare system

Integration of the electronic health record (also called patient or medical record) heads the list of priorities. Wireless tablets for nurses' recordkeeping are less disruptive of the nurse-patient relationship than carts with computers. Automation along the supply chain has been discussed earlier (chapter 7). Hospital utilization has many inefficiencies, but the reduced elective clinical activity on weekends could be remedied. Many staff would welcome weekend shifts for procedures if the hospital capacity permits. A modification of workflow and workforce also depends on the market supply of skilled personnel.

Physician productivity is a sticky subject today because doctors want to work fewer hours in clinics. Nonetheless, patient appointments can be made more efficiently by online access. Chart the trends in no-show and cancelled visits. Access

---

$\pm$ An electronic medical record means integration of outpatient and inpatient records, ordering capabilities, and research applications. Integration depends on a single patient identification number across the healthcare system.

can be improved by better confirmation of appointments and efforts to keep schedules totally booked. Practice management modules are available for ambulatory electronic patient records including outpatient billing directly from the electronic record.

Leadership training is catching on, but nurses still get short shrift in areas of service, efficiency, communication, and best practices. It's difficult to staff good in-house programs. There are excellent companies that specialize in medical staff education. This is one area that outsourcing may pay big dividends. I recall a trip to Wal-Mart in Bentonville, Arkansas. As part of the visit, we attended a sales/marketing course for advanced leadership. A contracted education group was very effective and later on we hired them for leadership seminars. For advanced leadership courses, most large hospitals will outsource this capability.

The challenge is to communicate the best ideas, especially best practices, across the system. That we still don't do effectively. There are plenty of great innovations that don't reach the community hospitals or vice versa. Many of these ideas relate to patient information. Provide help desks for Medicare and Medicaid patients to aid them in navigating the complex healthcare system. At the same time, provide information about health improvement and show them how to access more information, yours and health information available on the Internet and in most libraries.

OVERCOMING RESISTANCE

Idea killers. These are phrases for thoughtless idea rejection. They're used by people who are too unmotivated to give useful criticism or direction, who fail to ask idea-provoking response questions, or who dismiss others not believed to have the potential for good ideas. Phrases like, "It's not in our budget" or, "We don't have time" are half-truths. All budgets and schedules can be changed for a really good idea.[25] Here are some excuses and I'll bet you have heard each of them at one time or another.

- We tried that already.
- We've never done that before.
- We don't do it that way here.
- That never works.
- Not in our budget.
- Not an interesting problem.
- We don't have time.
- Executives will never go for it.
- It's out of our scope.
- People won't like it.

- It won't make enough money.
- How stupid are you?
- You're smarter with your mouth shut.
  A complete list of idea killers is at
  http://www.scottberkun.com/blog/?p=492.

In hospitals, the barriers to new ideas are usually 1) fear of risk; 2) budget constraints; 3) apathy or the excuse of no time; 4) no one will listen; 5) new ideas not solicited or recognized; 6) internal politics that crush creative thought; and 7) incompetent managers.

Another real barrier to innovation is described by IDEO's chief executive, Tim Brown, who believes that, "If you don't have a process for choosing projects, starting projects, and ending projects, you will never get very good at innovation. Projects need some form – you call them something; you run them in a certain way; you fund them in a certain way.... The biggest barrier to innovation is needing to know the answer before you get started. This often manifests itself as a desire to have proof that your idea's worthwhile before you actually start the project: 'Show me the business proof that this is going to be a good idea.'"[26]

The challenge for any enterprise is to get people to think about their jobs and about the organization. Personnel want to express themselves, to be heard, to improve the processes around them, to be successful, and to be recognized. Unit managers or supervisors are the gatekeepers for new ideas. They must encourage personnel to think about their jobs and how they relate to the process of care. There are a lot of reasons to think while on the job: You see room for improvement, for personal knowledge, to learn new skills, to create something, and relieve frustration.[27] Your biggest concerns are the ABCs of failure: Arrogance, Bureaucracy and Complacency."[28]

THE INNOVATION PROCESS IN HOSPITALS

Hospitals are challenged in many ways. Innovation has to be turned into competitive advantage. At the same time, a medical center has to create a system of discovery so that the environment stimulates a continuous process of innovation. Every organization has to have a purpose. Innovation without purpose is flat and satisfies only commercial needs. With purpose, innovation can not only help you understand customers, technology and the competition, it can bring out the latent sense of discovery, altruism and heroism of your personnel.[29] The secret is to see beyond the existing market dynamics.

The diffusion of new ideas is the process by which innovation is communicated among members of a healthcare system. New ideas help us escape from old, often inefficient practices.[30] The best ideas come from people who are knowledgeable about their work and how their jobs affect others. Ideas create compound interest, boosting performance, adding knowledge, improving the work environment and creating a system of discovery. There has to be communication and organization built into the process of innovation. As Confucius said, "...Never innovate randomly."[31]

Ideally, a self-perpetuating process works like this:

FIGURE 9.1

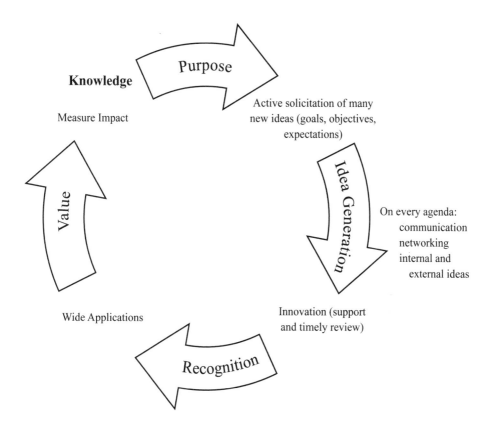

Generally, innovation requires baseline knowledge. There are many smart, skilled people among hospital personnel who are doing the minimum amount of labor they need to do to get by. They do their jobs and go home without giving much thought to their roles in the overall patient care episode, or how their roles influence patient flow before or after the patient enters their "space." These people can be affected by incremental innovations that relate to efficiency, patient convenience, or quality, which includes service and safety. Start by asking, "Why are we doing these activities (in the process)?" Eliminate the pseudo work.[±] Solicit ideas constantly. Try to engage everyone. A large pipeline of ideas depends on the number of people involved. Bring innovation up at meetings and not in a perfunctory way. For success, ideas need support, recognition and discipline.

In a recent interview, Nicholas Carr discussed the right and wrong way to be creative.[32] "Creative people are great, but creativity tends to be a messy process. There are going to be areas of your business where that's okay, and there are going to be areas where the last thing you want is messiness. In those areas, you should value and reward competent people who can do routine tasks very, very well." Having a reliable core of steady people is just as important as having brilliant, breakthrough thinkers. Discipline and creativity can coexist. Creativity is just connecting things. When you ask creative people how they did something, they feel guilty because they didn't really do it; they just saw something. It seemed obvious to them after awhile. That's because they were able to connect experiences they've had and transform them into new ideas. And the reason they were able to do that was that they've had more experiences or had thought more about their experiences than other people.[33] Scientists and educators are more likely to be the breakthrough guys, while the rest of us tend to be incrementalists. What we all have in common is a need to begin with the problem at hand.

Innovation should add value for the patient. Value equals benefits plus convenience divided by cost. To determine the value of an idea or innovation, apply the acronym NABC[34] Need – Is the market crying out for your product or service? Approach – Does it have a unique advantage or approach? Benefits – What are the benefits to the patient? Competition – How does it compare to what else is out there? Freidman writes that the world is flat.[35] Carlson and Wilmot take this further by saying that the world is not just flat, it has been reduced to the size of a dot. Information and capital move around the world at the speed of light. Location does not matter for many knowledge-intensive activities.

The business of medicine can always learn from the business of business. The 3M Corporation is consistently ranked among the world's most innovative companies. How has it remained so inventive? One engineer at 3M cites the company's seven pillars of innovation: 1) commitment to innovation from the CEO on down; 2) a tradition of hiring the best people and encouraging them to innovate; 3) a broad base of technology where one innovation may lead to other ideas or technologies; 4) communication up and down the organization about generation of ideas;

[±]   Pseudo work is that paid activity (or indeed, inactivity), the performance of which has no effect whatever on the scheme of things and of which the main purpose is the provision of employment, the advancement and the consumption of resources. (Kirwan L. *Political Correctness and the Surgeon*. Jackson, MS: AuthorHouse UK Ltd., 2008).

5) recognition and reward; 6) measuring the effects of innovation; 7) always thinking about customers and their needs.[36]

Japanese companies have a slightly different approach to knowledge creation that emphasizes:[37]

- absence of overplanning
- brevity of paperwork
- acceptance of mistakes as normal
- regular crossing of boundaries
- encouragement of initiative-taking
- flow of ideas from below
- minimum interference from above
- inability of top to kill an idea
- maintenance of a small and flat organization structure

Regardless of the approach, staff members are inspired when they see the positive impact of a great idea being implemented in their area. Being able to do more for patients lifts their spirits and gives them greater satisfaction in their work. "Ideas are like rabbits. You get a couple and learn how to handle them, and pretty soon you have a dozen."[±]

THE IDEA PROGRAM

"Why do so many men never amount to anything?" Edison asked. "Because they don't think…. The man who doesn't make up his mind to cultivate the habit of thinking misses the greatest pleasure in life. He not only misses the greatest pleasure, but he cannot make the most of himself. All progress, all success, springs from thinking."[38] One of the reasons we went into healthcare and related fields is to make a real difference. Not only do we have the opportunity to render compassionate care and gain experience, but we have the opportunity to help reinvent healthcare. That is really making a difference.

The Cleveland Clinic has a long history of innovation and invention. The key drivers are a broad base in science, a large teaching experience and high patient volumes across all specialties leading to great clinical experience, and a generous capital base. From this tradition, we created an idea program that mobilized everyone

---

±   Fensch T. *Conversations with John Steinbeck (Literary Conversation Series),* University Press of Mississippi, 1998, p. 43

in the institution to think about new ways to improve processes and services. Personnel were challenged to submit ideas that added value to patient care, boosted performance, created knowledge, improved the work environment and established a system of discovery. The best ideas were expected to be shared across the system. Some may believe that management should create time for reflection, but there is plenty of time for ideation during work hours if the staff will think about better processes as they go about their work. Time needs to be carved out for dialogue about ideas at all group meetings.

Our idea program was very similar to the one that was used by Toyota, which reported 20 years ago that it elicited 30 suggestions per employee, or two million suggestions per year. It has been reported that 85 percent of these suggestions are adopted.[39] We encouraged idea generation by emphasizing that there are no bad ideas... none too small or too big. We couldn't implement all of them because of scope, duplication, priorities, or fiscal constraint, but everyone who submitted ideas received a personal response, and approximately a third of their recommendations were implemented. We funded ideas from the discretionary budget; however, in retrospect, an innovation fund would have been easier to manage. The process was designed as follows: Personnel submitted ideas in a number of designated categories by using the in-house computer network; these ideas were promptly reviewed by individuals who were familiar with the area about which the idea was being submitted; the accepted ideas were followed in order to assure they were being implemented correctly. It is interesting to note the background of the personnel who submitted suggestions. Of the 46,000 ideas that were processed up to December 2007, administrative personnel accounted for 41 percent; clinical staff, 27 percent; nurses, 15 percent; operations personnel, 5 percent; environmental and food services, 4 percent; research staff, 4 percent; and physicians, 4 percent. Create an online review of implemented ideas, where they originated and their measured impact.

Anyone undertaking such an ideas program would do well to avoid monetary awards, with their potential to incite jealousy, or worse, vindictive behavior.[±] Instead, reward by public recognition, bestowing awards and even job promotions. Ideas precede resources, but discretionary funding for implementation should be allocated without delay. An inflexible budgeting process is the best way to strangle innovation and kill the incentive to submit ideas. In our experience, the most valuable ideas addressed clinical process, patient safety and operations. Nurses and administrative personnel submitted good ideas most frequently and physicians least

---

±   Envy is the most destructive social passion – more so than hatred. Hatred is visible and universally recognized as evil. Envy seldom operates under its own name. It chooses a lovelier name to hide behind and prefers to do its work invisibly. (Novak M. *Business as a Calling. Work and the Examined Life.* The Free Press, New York, 1996, p. 90.)

frequently. Information Technology was often slowest to respond because ideas in that category require complex change. In most large hospitals, IT can barely keep up with maintenance, let alone begin new programs or applications.

The ideas that were implemented ran the gamut of needs. They included a mentoring program to guide employees through the stages of their careers, lunchtime classes in foreign languages, an Intranet database for employee wellness, and a hotline to housekeeping to report environmental emergencies. Early patient care ideas included a special discharge lounge for patients waiting for transportation, patient call-back programs, clearer signage, a new guide for all admitted patients, portable alert devices for families waiting for patient information, and a transfer office that facilitates all outside transfers (recently implemented and highly successful).

Not all of the smart people work for you.[40] Ideas can be solicited or amplified by studying other organizations. One of the axioms at Cisco Corporation is that most innovations don't originate in their company. Sam Walton used to say that every important thing he did he copied from someone else.[41] Benchmarking gives perspective, new ideas, solutions, and an even greater incentive to excel. It has always amazed me that operational and financial supervisors frequently don't know anything about results, efficiencies or organization at the hospital down the street or in any one of the nation's leading hospitals. Does the administration know what personnel are saying and doing? How are their issues addressed? Get off your position and visit them.

The medical process is so redundant and filled with paper records that it often is difficult to determine what activities waste personnel time; what wastes money; what frustrates people in their jobs because of what they are not getting done while they are wasting their time with "busy" work. What do the patients really gripe about most? An innovation program can motivate people to identify what is needed to accomplish work with less effort. Am I wasting time and energy trying to find the tools to do my job? If so, why? Emphasize tools more than rules. Every little positive change may not be a home run, but ideas that result in practical changes represent incremental innovation. Improved communication by itself is an innovation. Start with solving the problem of unproductive meetings. A meeting without action items is a social event.[42] Every important meeting should focus on quality and leave time for ideas.

A great many ideas in healthcare come from patients themselves. They know the flaws in the system. Take your own poll. Where do patients and their families see a need for improvement? In addition to food and cleanliness, what else appears disorganized? Chances are, timely response to nurse call lights and cryptic billing are high on their lists. The point is that ideas come from many sources, but leaders and managers have to keep their idea receptors on at all times. Innovation is based on knowledge and experience, discussion with colleagues, observation from walking around – or are you tuned out? Nicholas Murray Butler, former president of Columbia University, said that there are three kinds of people – "those who make things happen, those who watch things happen and those who have no idea of what is happening."[43] As the leader, which are you?

Remember that you are working in healthcare to make a contribution to the safety and welfare of all patients. Design new process around patients' needs. Being innovative is one way you advance personally and professionally. Failure to innovate locks us into yesterday's medicine. Acknowledged innovation and quality (results) add to the reputation of the medical organization. Don't try to innovate for the future; innovate for the present.[44]

BIOTECHNOLOGY BUSINESSES

"What is distinctive about the capitalist economy is the original discovery that the primary cause of economic development is mind," notes political philosopher Michael Novak.[45] For a city to thrive, it needs to create or nurture new industries. In the early 20th century, Cleveland had built its agglomeration on access to natural resources, low-cost labor, and metallurgy. Later on, in other cities, modern industries were built on education and science often made possible by the presence of university and government laboratories. Cleveland did not develop a concentration of specialists able to connect inventors and entrepreneurs with investors. A lack of emphasis on public education and university-based research compared to other regions in the country also contributed to Cleveland's decline. The majority of modern inventions occurred where technology became science-based and connected to universities. In retrospect, Ohio was irresponsible for failing to support investment in regional economies that emphasized science and education. Entrepreneurialism is attracted by educational excellence, university research activity and a unified community voice and vision, all of which attract industry.

Industries mature. When they do, innovations that make people want more of their products slow down. If the new and growing industries go elsewhere, a region's growth slows down. As industries age, their costs rise and a region becomes less competitive. Lower-cost regions get the new plants. Now, with modern transportation and telecommunications, most regions have to fiercely compete on a global scale. Like it or not, that is the reality, and it won't go away.[46]

Austin, Texas, is a good case study of a public-private partnership driving economic development. Almost a quarter-century ago, Austin decided to be a leader in science and technology. Granted it had a few things going for it: Austin is the state capital; the University of Texas is located there; one-third of the population has the equivalent to a bachelor's degree; and per capita book sales are among the highest in the nation. The business community, the university and the city spoke in one voice. The first part of their plan was the partnership between government, business and the university. The city and county government gave incentives to businesses that sought to expand or relocate. These included favorable utility rates, tax abatement, innovative bonding authority, a research park, agreements not to annex (therefore, not to tax), a plan to expedite permits and approvals, and promotion of entrepreneurialism in the local technology incubator. It's not too late for cities to sponsor biotechnical development, but risk capital and discretionary federal or research funding support will be required. Today a supportive business environment includes skilled workforce training.

For many cities, biotechnology offers more opportunities than any other new business. In biotechnology, the science *is* the business.[47] For biotechnical development, regions and municipalities need first to engage universities with active leadership. University research provides intensive networking across sectors and with industry. To stimulate biotechnology many academic medical centers have invested in an office of technology transfer, the purpose of which is first to attract ideas or inventions from internal or regional sources and, from them, to develop commercial applications. The goal of such an office is to keep innovation within the organization so that the staff doesn't take their ideas (and royalties) for development elsewhere. Technology transfer in academic institutions is defined as the transfer of university (or hospital) research, inventions and intellectual property to industry for commercialization. It is the migration of academic discoveries to useful application in the development of marketable products or processes.[48] Technology transfer is essentially the commercialization of discoveries and innovations. Henry Ford said, "There are three questions: Is it needed? Is it practicable? Is it commercial?"[49]

Passage of the Bayh-Dole Act in 1980 intended to facilitate industrial application of university research by allowing universities to protect and license inventions from federally funded programs (previously, the government owned the intellectual property). Thereafter, technology transfer programs proliferated. Two hundred research institutions maintain offices dedicated to technology transfer. Invention disclosures at universities have increased nearly 300 percent; patents received have improved by 275 percent, and licenses and options executed with private industry have grown more than 500 percent to around 5,000 annually. Licensing income received by universities has surpassed $1 billion annually.[50] The increase in university patents has outpaced the overall growth in patenting.[51]

Abraham Lincoln famously remarked that the patent system was intended to "add the fuel of interest to the fire of genius," and Lincoln himself received a patent.[±52] The university generally retains the patent for a given invention and licenses it for a fee to one or more commercial enterprises. Profits derived from licensing the patent are required by law to be shared with the inventor. This association between academia and industry provides a new avenue to profits for researchers and institutions alike. The academic scientist, lured by the promise of royalties, becomes an entrepreneur, and universities become more like big businesses. They fully understand that "the cause of wealth is invention, detection and enterprise."[53]

The healthcare and related software industries invest more in innovation than other industries – about 11 percent annually. Pharmaceutical companies and device manufacturers lead the list. However, the major innovation sectors in healthcare are increasingly dynamic.[54] Leading universities have capitalized on the expanding federal research budget and opportunities to work with industry. Research and development may be consolidated into dedicated science parks to attract industry and bolster a culture of innovation. A science park composed of related research facilities stimulates flow of knowledge and fosters an environment for the creative growth of innovation-based companies by providing them with high-quality space.[55] A science park attracts money for science from many sources.

Gary Pisano of Harvard Business School points out that much of the debate about activities in the business of university science focuses on the impact of patents, which is the wrong issue.[56] It is not so much a matter of whether universities gain intellectual property, but how they choose to use those patents and the extent to which they make the knowledge in those patents widely available. How is science linked to these institutions and businesses? What influences the sector's capacity to manage risk, achieve integration and facilitate learning? What changes may be beneficial for the region?

The number of patents that were granted per medical school faculty increased significantly from 1981 through 2000. Although most patenting activity was carried out by faculty members in clinical departments, their rate of patent applications was low relative to that of the science faculty. Patents granted to faculty members of medical schools accounted for an increasing share of all academic patents (from 29 percent in 1976 to 53 percent in 2003). There is a strong correlation between recent scientific productivity, as measured by receipt of NIH grants, and involvement in patenting. A university or academic medical center with more resources is likely to generate more patents.[57]

±   Patent No. 6469. A device to lift boats over shoals, which was never manufactured. Lincoln is the only U.S. president to hold a patent.

TECHNOLOGY TRANSFER GUIDELINES

An office of technology transfer has a twofold challenge: 1) how to fund new technology when patents alone do not provide profit, and 2) how to manage conflict of interest. Today, an office of technology transfer operates under less autonomy than in the past. A conflict of interest exists when an individual or organization is in a position in which professional judgment concerning a primary interest tends to be unduly influenced by a secondary interest, namely financial gain. It is a situation in which a personal interest conflicts with a demand of duty, in which regard for one duty tends to lead to disregard of another, or in which one duty tends to interfere with the proper exercise of judgment.[58]

The medical and research staff should understand that disclosure of all industrial ties is mandatory. Consulting agreements with individual faculty members that include payment or ownership of intellectual property created must be reviewed in its entirety before approval. Payments from manufacturers to clinicians for using any type of product are strictly forbidden. The American Association of Medical Colleges has recommended that conflicted individuals should not participate in human subject research involving the company or whichever of its products is causing the potential conflict.[59] In a recent survey of academic medical centers, only a third of respondents had issued a conflict of interest policy.[60]

The Cleveland Clinic now requires that all industry relationships are submitted for approval. Physicians and scientists must disclose these relationships. The new Web site (www.clevelandclinic.org) posts all of the industry ties to Clinic physicians, researchers and their families. The staff is required to report when the relationships change materially and must update the disclosure annually. By accessing the site, patients can ascertain whether their doctor is affiliated with a specific company. These initiatives are widely heralded as a step towards a potential national database that would disclose all physician-industry relationships.

Institutional oversight for technology transfer should flow through an advisory committee (some of whom should be trustees of the organization) and then to a designated office within the institution. In large research organizations, the independent advisors can report directly to the dean of research, chief executive officer or the provost. The audit function and procedure are increasingly important with respect to institutional policy, the administration of intellectual property, licensing agreements and the process of evaluating inventions. Therefore, the financing of inventions and tracking expenses are key audit responsibilities. The press, legislators and regulators all agree that the hospitals' greatest responsibility is to the welfare of the patient and that this responsibility must prevail over competing interests of financial gain, reputation, building, innovation, economic development and the demands of entrepreneurs.[61]

Kassirer, who has written extensively on conflict of interest, concludes:

> Most physicians think of a career in medicine as a calling, and practice the principle they agreed to when they joined the profession, namely to "come for the benefit of the sick, remaining free of all intentional injustice [and] of all mischief." Nonetheless, as we have seen, the line between true professionalism and overt exploitation can be indistinct: collaborating with industry can benefit patient care, but at the same time it can bias physicians' actions. Though an individual's motives may be difficult for an outsider to fathom, in their heart of hearts doctors usually know the real rationale for their actions. In the final analysis, each person must search his own conscience and decide whether or not to make financial arrangements that might compromise them. At issue is whether the public can trust us not only to be at their side, but on their side. Our collective actions will determine what our profession is to become, and I believe that most people are eager to attain the highest standards. Most people become physicians out of noble intentions. But as John Stuart Mill said, "The capacity for the nobler feelings is in most natures a very tender plant, easily killed, not only by hostile influences, but by mere want of sustenance." The profession is under siege by big business, and I do not perceive a vigorous effort to rescue it. [62]

We have reached a point where larger medical organizations should publish standards of conduct. The document should include your position on mission, integrity, care standards and conflict disclosures.[±]

INNOVATION FACTS

The top five university biotechnology transfer and commercialization centers are the Massachusetts Institute of Technology, the University of California System, the California Institute of Technology, Stanford University, and the University of Florida.[63] For these centers, research earns a high rate of return, with every dollar

---

±   Audrey Andrews, Chief Compliance Officer at Tenet Healthcare, has written *Standards of Conduct* for the company. The paper is available through audrey.andrews@tenethealth.com. This publication will give you ideas for your own standards and it applies to for-profit and non-profit hospitals.

invested in the office of technology returning more than six dollars in licensing income. According to the Milken Institute in 2008, Massachusetts leads the nation as the top state in technology and science.[±] Massachusetts just passed a $1 billion life sciences bill to invest high-tech infrastructure in research and development over the next 10 years.

The success of the technology office depends on the size of the academic enterprise. The larger the research base, the larger the portfolio of new technologies made available to license. More years of experience in technology transfer generally mean greater knowledge and know-how of the staff. Better institutional oversight and policies are required for institutions that are aggressive in eliciting and pursuing inventions.[64] The monetization mind-set increasingly influences licensing and disclosure policies in ways that may inhibit the broad flow of critical scientific information. Under the influence of the profit motive, these policies function more to increase university licensing revenues and equity returns than to contribute to the scientific commons.[65]

Obviously, not every invention will turn out to have economic value. One of the strongest predictors of technology transfer success is the diversity of research. The majority of healthcare institutions lose money on technology transfer because the expenses exceed the return from commercial development. A recent survey of technology transfer offices found that only 12 percent of technology that is licensed is ready for commercialization.[66] One question often not addressed is whether the region around the institution will benefit from the technology transfer.

Leaders give lip service to the idea that the world is moving faster and we need to innovate. However, when one asks people in the organization to describe their innovation system, they don't know because they don't have one.[67] As Kanter observes, innovation gets rediscovered as a growth enabler every half-dozen years or so.[68] Frequently, the first wave of enthusiasm is followed by mediocre execution and anemic results. Innovation projects are then "quietly disbanded" in cost-cutting drives. Don't confuse one-time efficiencies with sustained cost improvement. The current call for innovation cannot be allowed to suffer this fate. Medicine can no longer afford it. Continuous innovation is no longer a fad. It is a way of life, and for the academic center, insurance for survival. Healthcare reform must create strong incentives for medical, scientific and managerial innovation. "Innovation... is the only true, long-term solution for high-quality, affordable healthcare."[69]

[±] The Milken Institute State Technology and Science Index, June 2008, provides details on ranking and state funding trends nationwide. (http://www.milkeninstitute.org/newsroom).

HEALTHCARE DELIVERY

Often the same people who want a more humanistic, person-oriented medicine also want a commodity medicine – without realizing that there is an inherent contradiction between the two views. If the patient is a person, so too is the doctor. Only persons can take care of persons as persons – recognizing all the things that make each of us somewhat different and, consequently, introducing the differences into our care when we are sick.

But if every appendectomy is considered to be the same as every other – like a mass-produced table – and every office visit and hospital consultation are the same, where does the concept of the doctor as a person fit in with that? The forces necessary to keep every medical service identical and cheap discourage the intense personal involvement by the physician in the patient's care that is required in order to lift medicine above the merely technical.

Human concern, clinical judgment, knowledge born of experience, time spent in listening, understanding a patient's need, and other personal acts of medicine cannot be considered in third-party regulations, fixed-fee schedules or even as topics of medical care research, because they cannot be measured. So the rewards go to technical services, tests, procedures, numbers of visits, operations – things that can be measured. Not surprisingly, in medicine, as elsewhere, people tend to go where the rewards are. When medical care is to be a social commodity evenly distributed at low cost, whose size and shape are to be determined by primarily economic or management forces, then something has to be last – and that will be humanism.

— Eric J. Cassell
"The Commodity View of Medicine"
The Wall Street Journal, April 30, 1979

Patients want access and affordability. They want competence, compassion and continuity, and they want choice. In short, they want quality medical care.[1] Medical organizations strive to deliver these features in a comprehensive healthcare system. The old way to manage by scent-marking your territory or building fences around the academic center is officially over. Those who continue to manage this way are not going to make it. Today you have to think about system building through virtual networks, mergers, and acquisitions. The Cleveland Clinic system is comprised of a central academic medical center surrounded by regional clinics and affiliated community hospitals. The parent academic foundation controls the alliance, which is structured as a merger of assets. The academic center serves as the hub for the decentralized management of community-based facilities. The hospitals are managed with relative autonomy; however, productivity and service are overseen for quality, operational efficiencies, and continuous cost management. The greatest challenge in system integration is to build clinical integration. Coordination of health services and clinical processes are key factors in value for patients and personnel for which the system has assumed responsibility.

BUILDING A HEALTH SYSTEM

The goals, purpose and moral duty of a healthcare system are to measurably improve healthcare in the community served. In other words, if an academic center doesn't plan to invest time and money into the community hospital, it should not acquire it. Some hospitals and clinics will be only nominally viable, but those facilities are often important to an underserved community, and nearly all can be improved. Unless the area is grossly over-bedded, the "fix it and sell it" approach may even devalue the community. Respect the Japanese business approach. "We believe if you have a family, you can't just eliminate certain members of that family because profits are down."[2] To be successful, you have to give more than you take. Likewise, communities, doctors and hospitals have to put their faith in the academic center partnership.

To create or expand a healthcare delivery system, the academic medical center must first understand the local markets, namely the socioeconomic variables, demographics, payer mix and the origin of hospital and outpatient referrals. A fair and equal partnership is realized when you are able to improve the community hospital and its outpatient clinics. There is no set formula or manual. The objectives are first to provide clear standards for quality in clinical medicine and service. Second, you have the never-ending responsibility to selectively upgrade facilities and equipment. Third, the continuous recruitment of good physicians is a high priority. Fourth, education is an increasingly broad responsibility for public programs and wellness. Fifth, continuing medical education for physicians further benefits the community. Sixth, markets differ but key specialties may serve both the main campus and selected community hospitals. Above all, a healthcare system has to be more than a coalition of hospitals; it has to be a union of people.

If expansion is in your plans, be sure that the new alliances can add value to the system by improving healthcare in the community served. Don't buy hospitals just to match the competition's acquisitions. Too often medical centers react stupidly to competitors' plans. It has to make sense. In our zeal for expansion, we should all be reminded of Drucker's admonition: "I will tell you a secret: Dealmaking beats working. Dealmaking is exciting and fun, and working is grubby. Running anything is primarily an enormous amount of grubby detail work, and very little excitement, so dealmaking is kind of romantic, sexy. That's why you have deals that make no sense."[3]

We followed a particular philosophy in the broader community. We did not buy anything we didn't need or like. We executed well and quickly. We followed a complementary, not a combative, approach in these communities. In managing different community hospitals we always gave more than we received. We worked to reduce our hospital cost to be comparable to that of the community hospitals. Each year, we critically analyzed the individual performance of our specialties at home and in the community. We would not, under any circumstances, compromise our academic mission. We based every decision on what was best for the patient, irrespective of location.

Before taking responsibility for another healthcare facility, ask yourself these questions: Do you have enough working capital? Are you able to recruit skilled personnel from the community? Can you improve current relationships with physicians? Can you manage from a distance? Where could the large size of a new system break down? You need to have this information for business integration and staff relations. If the community hospital under consideration is well staffed and well managed, the task is easier. Unfortunately, that's not always the case. When the academic organization plans to locate a branch, whether it's a clinic, hospital or even a unified campus at a distant site, the most important question to answer is whether you can effectively duplicate your reputation.

If you hope to reproduce your standards offsite, you need to carefully evaluate and possibly recruit additional experienced medical and administrative staff. Before plunging into a new affiliation, ask yourself: Where are the synergies? The objectives of synergy are to increase competitiveness and cash flow. Can governance issues be settled? Where will new referrals come from? What is the estimated time to added profitability? How will the acquisition affect current staff? Are there competitive advantages in the new location? What is our early, best use of resources? In the global healthcare economy, you may have the opportunity to create an international alliance. At that time, you should find out if government concessions are available and if you can manage in a new and different culture.

The strategy to build a healthcare delivery system comprised of multiple hospitals and clinics is foremost to add healthcare value throughout the region. A less discussed reason: If you don't hunt, you will be hunted. An academic-based healthcare delivery system may wish to remove the economic threat of community hospitals consolidating or being sold to for-profit or to other not-for-profit entities. On the offense side, a well-managed academic-community partnership can improve the community hospital and add both value to patient care and job security for personnel. Strategies for improvement might include clinical realignment of services, strengthening existing services, enlarging the primary care base and operational consolidations that favor scalable benefits. These strategies must create added business value, defined as increases in competitiveness and resulting cash flows beyond what the two companies are expected to accomplish independently.[4] Designing a system is not unlike developing a manufacturing strategy. There are three potential areas of focus: the product (advances in medicine), new markets (distant referrals), and customer development (informed patients). Don't lose sight of the fact that the "product" is healthcare and the ultimate beneficiary of any acquisition must be the patient.

Heed Paul Ellwood's observation from his 1988 Shattuck lecture.[5]

> The intricate machinery of our health care system can no longer grasp the threads of experience. The mischief that began long before the health care crises of the 1970s is progressively disabling the vast machinery of medicine. Too often, payers, physicians, and health care executives do not share common insights into the life of the patient. We acknowledge that our common interest is the patient, but we represent that interest from such divergent, even conflicting, viewpoints that everyone loses perspective. As a result, the health care system has become an organism guided by misguided choices; it is unstable, confused, and desperately in need of a central nervous system that can help it cope with the complexities of modern medicine. The problem is our inability to measure and understand the effect of the choices of patients, payers, and physicians on the patient's aspirations for a better quality of life. The result is that we

have uninformed patients, skeptical payers, frustrated physicians, and besieged health care executives.

Twenty years later, we appear to be doing slightly better. If you can create an aligned, integrated system focused on efficient high-quality patient care, your system will have addressed many of his concerns.

People generally want to stay in their communities for most of their healthcare and will use a good local hospital. But there's no point in acquiring community hospitals if the expansion of services doesn't add up to more value than the individual entities. An organization has added value only when the network of customers, suppliers, and complementers in which it operates is better off with it than without it. Then the organization delivers something that is unique and valuable in the marketplace.[6]

We expanded our geographic presence by acquiring eight hospitals in the Cleveland area. Our success resulted from collaboration rather than competition. The new hospital system required good relations with the practicing physicians attending those hospitals. To avoid their resentment, we insisted that the majority of patients seen in the regional clinics were referred to community specialists – and not to the academic center. Exceptions would include high-risk tertiary cases or when the patient requested an appointment at the academic center. Our situation was more challenging because we operated 14 family health centers, most of which preceded the hospital system. The primary care physicians in our satellite clinics were hired in a staff model and their practices operated within the academic medical center organization. It was to our advantage that many community doctors were facing increased costs in practice. We attracted new physicians because we were able to: 1) recruit them into a staff model for primary care; 2) build new outpatient offices for them; 3) hire hospitalists for their support; 4) provide medical liability coverage; 5) include an ambulatory patient record linked to a hospital data repository; 6) give them additional revenue-generating opportunities.

When large institutions, academic or otherwise, buy physician practices, a large part of the sale often is based on the sellers' practice assets and liabilities. Physician-owned facilities or groups frequently lack audited financial statements. Their valuation is generally based upon hard assets, accounts receivable or other forms of working capital and goodwill. We took a different approach. We determined who were the best private physicians in each market. We avoided mediocrity and were willing to pay for excellence. As a tax-exempt organization, we decided not to calculate fair market value to avoid violating private inurement. Instead, we recruited physicians into a staff model based on an estimate of their productivity, reputation and years of practice. In certain instances, we had to pay the tail of malpractice premiums, but we bought no hard assets or receivables. My advice is to not acquire physicians' prior assets or take responsibility for their liabilities.

All doctors, especially primary care doctors, need support. Above all, newly recruited doctors trust the intentions of the academic medical center to make their practices and the facilities better than before. Physicians are increasingly aligning with health systems for reasons of economics, namely, the costs and hassles of practice and medical liability. Other factors include the looming prospect of bundled reimbursement, the potential for a more efficient practice model, further education opportunities and security. The longstanding tradition of primary care doctors working alone in community clinics is less practical or even economically viable. Primary care is the clinical core of the healthcare system and the gateway to prompt convenient service, long-term person-focused care, comprehensive care for most health needs, and coordination of referrals.[7] Community imaging, laboratory medicine and outpatient surgery have changed market dynamics and fueled the demand for one-stop shopping. Your community hospital can be the ideal site for added primary care services. A lot of support is already built in. The physicians who still have hospital practices appreciate the opportunity... and under the right conditions, better offices.

The value of primary care physicians for community health is more evident each year. States with more primary care physicians per capita have lower per capita Medicare costs and higher-quality care in contrast to states with more specialists per capita, which are reported to have lower-quality care and higher per capita Medicare expenditures.[8] Solutions to reverse the shortage of primary care doctors are now a priority in healthcare reform.[9]

BARRIERS TO SYSTEMIZATION

Only the best quality hospitals should be targeted for merger. It would be interesting to find hospitals in the community that are "beloved, bloated and bleeding,"[10] but that is generally too good to be true. Opportunity doesn't come wrapped perfectly. The reality is that most community hospitals seeking affiliation face imminent problems or see bad times ahead. Too many community hospitals are rife with turf issues, beset by rumors and have poor physician-administration compatibility. The incentives for physicians in everyday practice are, sorry to say, often largely economic.

Community physicians have an inherent mistrust of the academic center.[±] For them, the merger spells competition and a personal economic threat. New hospital management may be seen as one more tree poked in their cage. Physicians are already leaving practice prematurely, dissatisfied with reimbursement and regulatory aspects of office management. They see the intrusion of an academic center bringing superfluous rules, forced meetings, more policies, the likelihood of local administrative change, unrealistic productivity demands, mandatory referrals downtown, all of which could reduce their personal income.

To maintain good relations, don't try to force clinical protocols or evidence-based medicine on community doctors too quickly after a merger. Regina Herzlinger warns, "These systems could be wonderful if medicine were a powerful science with a clear understanding of what causes and cures illnesses and disabilities, but currently it's more art than science. Dictating protocols to doctors is as meaningless as forcing artists to paint by numbers."[11] Peer influence from good clinical data is a far more effective method of management. Of all merger factors, physician relationships are the most important. Show them, "Partners are not servants, but neither are they rivals."[12]

There are essentially three types of relationships: parasitic, commensal and mutual. Mutuality should be the goal. The fears of community physicians will be assuaged if the academic leadership delivers on promise, listens attentively, communicates consistently and allows relatively independent management. Unfulfilled promises are a prescription for failure. Doctors do care about a career of contribution. They prefer to be associated with a name brand and a culture that they can respect. Professional opportunity in the market they serve is important, but so is the type of practice, expertise of colleagues, performance of the hospital(s) and the lifestyle afforded by practice. Overall, private physicians are under great strain from cost of practice and decline in real reimbursement. Consequently, they seek additional sources of income. Good relations do not necessarily mean that physicians will be enthusiastic about participating in hospital administrative activities.[13] Some will; involve them. Some resist; leave them alone.

Acquisitions may go according to plan, but not to timetable. Time is one of the biggest obstacles to systemization. It takes time to fix things and organize for changing practice. One of the first priorities is to manage disparate information technologies. Matters of governance are sure to strain negotiations and delay your merger. You'll need to occupy the intersection of community relations, medical

±   Trust is the mutual confidence that no party to an exchange will exploit another's vulnerabilities. (Sabel CF. *Studied Trust: Building New Forms of Cooperation in a Volatile Economy.* Human Relations 1993: 46 (9); 1133-70).

governance, and the academic medical center. Once you've merged you'll need to dissolve or modify community hospital boards or risk an ongoing we-they situation. This can be accomplished by appointing selected community trustees to the academic hospital board. Or you could change the community hospital board of trustees to an advisory board. A third approach would be to consolidate all the community hospitals to form one community hospital board. If none of the above is possible, you should be present at their board meetings.

The best advice I can give is to learn the local market and study the operations of the hospital and its clinical performance before making any changes. First find and improve gaps in the community delivery systems. Recapitalization of the hospitals is essential. You could also build primary care offices at the hospital or surgeon offices in or near the ambulatory surgery center. Develop centers of excellence, e.g., orthopedic and spine centers, bariatrics, or diabetology. Improve imaging and ambulatory surgery, which may suffer from poor equipment or management. Consider remodeling or building new obstetric facilities and women's health centers. Give more attention to post-acute care where it is needed. Encourage an attitude of interdependence rather than independence among providers.

When an academic institution acquires a community hospital, integration of the business functions is one of the highest priorities. Communication with the private practice physicians should be informative and frequent. It is said that when it comes to change, physicians are less adaptive organisms; instead, they are resistant strains. All sorts of rumors need to be addressed and most of them relate to perceived economic threats. No, we are not mandating that you refer patients downtown or to our doctors in the community. No, we have no plans to salarize physicians. No, we are not going to cut personnel in your hospital. We will, however, try to make procedure schedules more efficient, save money by integrating operational, financial and legal systems, and put some cash into the hospital facilities and equipment. With respect to the latter, here is the preliminary plan – for example, radiologic facilities are worn, surgical suites need to be renovated or expanded, outpatient offices refurbished, and so on. The academic center should make medical practice easier by helping the physician in scheduling, precertification, managed care contracting, documentation, and more efficient hospital service. This creates like-minded colleagues.

There are "forces of darkness" within all organizations. Academic physicians are often reluctant to collaborate with community physicians. They may engage in a dialogue of condescension. Your academicians cannot be allowed to discriminate or display a sense of superiority. This is one area where the leadership of the academic center has to be forceful. Some academic physicians fear competition from the community and, of course, the community physicians are likewise uneasy. The affiliated community hospitals and their respective staff are part of the "academic" family, not second-class providers. Referral patterns in the community are based on trust, communication and outcomes. There are no fundamentally incompatible partners. The good doctors will cooperate. As coach Herman Edwards put it, "They will play for the name on the side of the helmet, not just the name on the back of the jersey."[14]

There are a number of competitive issues among doctors that exist with or without a system of clinics and hospitals. Doctors are aggressively competing with hospitals by owning ambulatory centers and specialty hospitals. The motivation for hospitals to pursue joint ventures with physicians on outpatient facilities is that 50 percent is better than nothing. Remember that hospital-physician joint ventures are under close scrutiny and are subject to economic risk for both parties. "[Our caution] makes our relationship with doctors more fractious."[15]

To make matters worse, emergency department on-call interest has waned significantly because of the perceived higher risk of malpractice litigation, low or no reimbursements for treating uninsured patients and unpredictable hours that affect daytime practice. Reluctantly hospitals have to pay specialists extra for these services. In the past decade, hospitalists' ranks have exploded – there are approximately 20,000 hospitalists today, or about the same number as neurologists or gastroenterologists.[16] Hospitalists may have improved safety, but some believe they have contributed to the ongoing disintegration between hospitals and outside physicians. It depends on the physicians' attitude – most want in-hospital support.

The supply of physicians per capita has historically and cross-sectionally correlated with the gross domestic product per capita.[17] Despite increased demand for their services, physician productivity is projected to decline owing in part to more trained women physicians working fewer hours and physicians as a whole seeking more balanced lifestyles. A number of reports have suggested that a low supply of physicians may be associated with higher mortality rates; however, it has been shown that once supply is even modestly greater, patients derive little further benefit.[18] Workforce planning models show a weak link between patient outcomes and physicians per capita with the exception of the primary care physician supply.

As noted earlier, the regional population tends to do better when systems emphasize primary care.[19] In building a primary care network, take advantage of the economic downturn. Many good generalists have retired early; some have lost money in their pension plans and want to return to practice. An economic downturn or any long recession provides splendid opportunities for staff enrichment, or to put it more simply, recruitment of really good doctors, other skilled personnel and executives. Hard times look gloomy, but it is a very good time to upgrade the talent base.

Community hospitals need to anticipate the transformation in the delivery of care. They are likely to survive in the local community if they can adjust to: more regionalization of quaternary care; an increase in minimally invasive procedures and the majority of elective surgery being conducted in outpatient specialty facilities, some with extended stay; more high-tech imaging outside the hospital; and group practice consolidation. These trends are likely to affect the volume of certain medical services and result in a shift of services within systems.

INCREMENTAL INTEGRATION

Leaders at the academic medical center have to answer any questions community physicians may have about intended changes. Clint Eastwood's preacher in *Pale Rider* puts the matter elegantly. When a town businessman tells the preacher that a group of independent gold miners refused to move off their land to make way for his company and are "standing in the way of progress," the preacher asks: "Yours or theirs?" When first talking about change and progress, be prepared for the question, yours or theirs?

In post-merger discussions with community physicians, we held fast to the principle that healthcare is a public benefit, not solely an opportunity to create wealth. We realized change through education and planning, not mandates. Our only firm expectation was adherence to quality guidelines. Four principles – standardization, simplification, clinical relevance, and accountability – will improve performance and address physician needs. Physicians quite sensibly want to reduce their administrative burden and the time spent on administrative tasks. Outlying doctors don't want to trek to your main campus for meetings, especially not in the middle of the day. Make it easier for them to practice good medicine. Cut the red tape. Listen to the doctors. They know the problems, many of which have existed for years. But they can't repair these inefficiencies alone. That's your job. If you can standardize, simplify and make realistic mutual decisions, the physicians will be more willing to be held publicly accountable for their performance. Measure performance in terms of practices they can control. Review procedures and accepted indications, outlier rates, and basic quality metrics. Does the nursing service perform consistently well around the clock? Surgeons understandably want efficient scheduling. Good doctors want a good practice as much as you do. Are their wishes utopian? If you consider physician requests carefully, you'll see that most have practical ideas.

As integration proceeds, it is important to protect new ideas and new programs from the bureaucracy of the existing structure. As we developed the community clinics (family health centers), we were able to progress rapidly, because these new entities were immune from the need to please every constituency inside the parent organization. Building out the system is a never-ending effort and, as previously emphasized, it depends on "experimentation." A new system is a wonderful laboratory for patient service and delivery ideas, such as using medical assistants in some areas instead of nurses, trying different evening and weekend hours depending on the market and group visits for patients with similar conditions. The point is that a new system has to be an incubator. It must be protected from the bureaucracy and entrenchment that always fears a new venture will somehow diminish their own prosperity. This is where leadership comes in – by providing a culture that seeks new opportunities, sometimes fails along the way, but succeeds in the long run. There are always uncertainties and risks. Don't be afraid to take a calculated risk. Constancy of purpose and great persistence underlie the long-term success of the new system.

SYSTEM MANAGEMENT

Discovery is fun; colonizing is work. Consolidation may produce economies of scale in a number of clinical and operational areas, but nothing is guaranteed. Manage where the action is. In the experience of The Advisory Board, the biggest cost reduction opportunities are achieved within the first year after a merger. Each area of potential consolidation should show opportunities for a decrease in infrastructure cost. An academic center may reposition or expand services like obstetrics, pediatrics, rehabilitation and psychiatry into the community. Look to administration, not the clinical departments, for most of the savings. Most clinical costs are variable, not fixed. According to The Advisory Board, 87 percent of cost savings come from nonclinical areas.[20] On the clinical side, less morbidity (after treatment) saves money.

The ambulatory electronic record for community clinics is much easier to install and maintain compared with the more complicated in-hospital record. An ambulatory electronic record with a practice management component and a data integrator, a hub that is linked to the hospital repository, is an important priority. Our community clinics became paperless in 2002. According to a recent healthcare industry report, fewer than 10 percent of doctors communicate with their patients online. Many fear that confidentiality can be compromised, that they will be deluged by patient e-mail that adds hours of uncompensated work to their already busy schedules, and that patients will send e-mails about urgent matters that the doctor will not see on time.[21] The big challenge is to develop a data interchange with physicians in the community.

Health information exchanges (HIEs) share patient data electronically across disparate sites of care. The exchange involves integration of data between hospital and outpatient electronic medical records and all outside laboratory and radiology entities. This sharing of clinical data among all providers, regardless of affiliation, can improve care coordination and reduce duplication of services. HIEs were introduced in 2004 to facilitate the development of a national health information network.[±] Providers have been slow to adopt because of concerns about loss of competitive advantage, cost, and misuse of data. The ultimate objective is to have an HIE through a single interface. The advantages of a regional data exchange could affect public health, a broad base of research, clinical quality, pay-for-performance, and payer communication.[22]

Can hospitals incent staff to be more efficient by enhancing coordination and collaboration? Gain sharing engages physicians in targeted cost-reduction initiatives by rewarding them with a percentage of cost savings. The goal of this is to reduce unnecessary costs related to purchase and use of physician preference items. It has its advocates, but I agree with Donald Palmisano, a past AMA president, surgeon and attorney, who said, "First off, a physician has an ethical and fiduciary responsibility to do what's in the best interests of the patient. I think it's insulting to think that giving me an additional amount of money will make me do what I'm supposed to do."[23] Given the complexity of what is being asked, it would be difficult to reward physicians fairly. In addition to responsibility for outcomes, credentialing for hospital practice should entail responsibility for cost and good service, which includes communicating effectively to the patient and to colleagues. If those criteria for credentialing and privileges are not met after counseling, privileges should be suspended. The effectiveness of hospital leadership is reflected in how well individual physicians understand the goals of the organization and how well they relate individually and collectively.

How do you get private practice physicians to refer to your community hospital? Leadership plays a big role. Doctors are attracted to a hospital with a good reputation, one that is financially healthy and has a good consultant staff. Physicians will look for a consistently high standard of care, including a good physical plant and high patient satisfaction. Admitting physicians will pay attention to their patients' impression of service, especially those perennial targets of complaints like cleanliness, waiting time, and food. One study of patients' comments found that more than half were negative about room conditions, and a third were negative about hospital discharge.[24] Interestingly, patients are more critical of their physical surrounding than of their care. Patients' number one priority is how quickly and effectively personnel respond to their concerns and complaints.

±   Forty-two HIEs were operational at the state and local level in 2008 – up from 32 in 2007 – and 36 were in implementation phases. (*Health Information Exchange Efforts Lower Healthcare Costs, Survey Finds*. The Advisory Board Company. Daily Briefing, September 12, 2008).

Community doctors will not tolerate heavy-handedness, intimidation or silly rules. Make it easy for community hospitals to enjoy collaboration with the academic center. In other words, add value for the patient and provider; don't detract from programs that are already in place. Wherever possible, stress the advantages of physician alignment with the hospital. Never talk down to community physicians who can be fiercely independent, street-smart, and sometimes as good or better in the care of patients as their counterparts on the academic staff. In our merger experience, we began by interviewing the leading physicians in each hospital to find out how we could help them in their practices. Most physicians want to grow their practices, and for proceduralists this means workflow efficiency. In operating room management, we offered them extended hours, fast-track scheduling blocks, variable staff scheduling, and faster room turnover time. Optimal scheduling creates capacity for extra cases. The physician's office location and proximity to the hospital are important as well as access to a well-run emergency department. Surgeons have relatively simple requests such as a preferred time slot; a consistent operating room team; a good and reliable floor assignment; competent anesthesia. Academic center executives can win the trust of the community hospital by attending community hospital meetings.

Community physicians should provide regular input at their administrative meetings and, if possible, a physician executive from the academic center should facilitate the discussion. Sorry to repeat this, but all physicians must understand that they are in charge of quality, performance and cost. In addition to transparency about finance and operations, the community hospital staff can benefit from seminars and discussion about prevention of medical liability. Good information about hospital outcomes should include national and regional benchmarks.

In our setting a local hospital operational council with physician input worked reasonably well. The parent organization must address deficiencies brought up by community physicians and sort out the cause or where the ineffectual management lies. Patient financial services should be attended to first because most frequently the community hospital is not working the accounts satisfactorily. Service improvement and capacity management are other important areas of investigation. Communicate with non-physician personnel through a nurses' council, wellness newsletter, and by giving personnel input into service and marketing plans. Advertise success at the local hospital and especially celebrate the accomplishments of the local administration.

Approximately 25 to 50 percent of the operating expense of a company can be attributed to not doing it right the first time. The same applies to medicine. It is estimated that companies could boost profits 100 percent by holding onto 5 percent more of their customers.[25] Put yourself in the patient's shoes. How would you like to waste half a day seeing one doctor and then have to come back for more tests and then back again to see another doctor and so on? Why don't clinics try to coordinate all appointments and tests at one visit—at least meet the specialist on the same day? When we lose patient loyalty, we lose an asset.

CONSUMERISM

The patient is becoming a more knowledgeable purchaser of healthcare services. The obvious reasons relate first to price sensitivity because payment out of pocket is increasing. A second factor is an awareness about variations in quality. As more information is available about hospital outcomes and service, the informed consumer will survey reports on clinical quality, cost and even recommendations (and complaints) from personal experiences.

Patients still trust their physician's judgment, and see healthcare largely in terms of their personal relationship with their doctor. Even when admitted to the hospital, they focus on the doctor more than the organization. This is changing fast. Patients will learn to look for organizational markers of quality care from online public reporting, patient satisfaction surveys, ranked hospital reputation, and signs of perverse incentives to over- or undertreat.

A recent poll conducted by McKinsey reveals how patients choose hospitals.[26] (Figure 10.1) The reasons for hospital admission based on source and requests are shown below.

FIGURE 10.1

Factors influencing patients' choice of hospitals

Have you ever requested a specific hospital from your physician?
% of patients

Would you request a hospital if it were distinctive for patient experience, all other things being equal?
% of patients

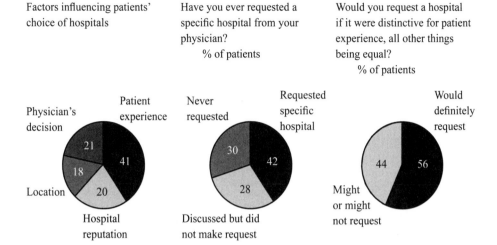

*For commercially insured patients, excludes those patients (39% of total surveyed) who can go to only one facility in community given current health coverage or severity of condition.

Source: 2007 McKinsey survey of >2,000 US patients with commercial insurance or Medicaid and >100 physicians.

According to this survey, patients have become much more independent about their choice of hospitals. The graph on the left shows that physicians' influence about where to hospitalize is waning. More than half of patients did not seek the treating physician's advice about a specific hospital. Even today, nearly half of the patients may request a specific hospital known for treating their particular ailment. In an emergency, the options are limited. In a small community, the options may be even fewer. Patients tend to go where they are referred because they trust the judgment of their personal doctor; however, consumers are getting choosier because of the available information including individual physician profiles on the Internet.[27] As consumers learn to shop for healthcare, the concept of value becomes the leading driver of consumer choice.[28] One of the best new publications available to surgical patients is a book titled *I Need an Operation... Now What? The Patients' Guide to a Safe and Successful Outcome* published by the American College of Surgeons.[29±] This informative publication shows the patient how to "size up" the doctor, what to ask the surgeon, and how to assure good follow-up. All surgeons should read it too.

Finally, nearly everyone is waking up to the concept of wellness. Seventy percent of all healthcare costs in the United States are attributed to preventable risks and unhealthy choices (Wellness Councils of America and the Center for HealthCare Economics). The estimated savings in healthcare gained by participation in health promotion programs is significant. Forty percent of healthcare costs are related to three lifestyle choices: tobacco use, physical inactivity, and unhealthy food.[†] Weight reduction and active lifestyle are strongly correlated with lower total healthcare charges.

At the forefront of employee wellness, Dr. Toby Cosgrove, the Cleveland Clinic chief executive, has instituted in-house and external wellness initiatives. Realizing that the majority of diseases are preventable, he has changed certain practices. These include not hiring smokers, serving healthy foods in the cafeteria and vending machines, and workforce education about obesity and management of chronic illness. The Cleveland Clinic has also started a disease reversal program[§] supervised by wellness expert Dr. Michael Roizen. This includes disease-specific group therapies for exercise, stress management and nutrition education. The group therapy sessions are classified as visits and approved by Medicare and other carriers.

We don't categorize health-related absenteeism; instead we lump it into "paid time off." Even worse, businesses don't measure health-related presenteeism. Attention to wellness will help us better understand the reasons for time away and reduced performance. Wellness does more than improve health and reduce employee healthcare costs. As people learn about a healthy lifestyle, they become *informed consumers*. Disease prevention and health promotion by medical personnel depends

---

±   CMS has produced an excellent brochure, titled *Planning for Your Discharge: A Checklist for Patients and Caregivers,* preparing patients to leave a hospital, nursing home, or other healthcare setting. (CMS Pub. No. 11376 September 2008.)

   Another good book for patients, written by Davis Liu of the Permanente Medical Group, is titled *Stay Healthy, Live Longer, Spend Wisely: Making Intelligent Choices in America's Health System.* Dr. Liu combines recommendations for doctors and guidelines for patients who enter the doctor-patient relationship. He shows patients how to make every office visit count and to make sure that the diagnostic testing, treatments and future evaluations are clearly understood. It's a really good book for patients and it wouldn't hurt doctors to read it too.

†   Surprisingly, 67 percent of American adults are overweight or obese; 60 percent don't exercise and more than 20 percent continue to smoke. (www.welcoa.org/freeersources/pdf/whyandhow/chapter1.pdf).

§   For more information about Lifestyle180, a program that addresses nutrition, exercise and stress management, email lifestyle190@ccf.org.

on leadership, good communication, economic incentives and case management. Today, wellness is fast becoming part of quality assurance. As in any business, success is measured by employee satisfaction and a reduction in medical claims.

There are challenges for the provider in this new era. The majority of hospitals are unprepared for inquiries about accurate estimates of out-of-pocket costs. Often times, financial counseling is poor or absent and "patient-friendly" billing is more like friendly fire. Patients are increasingly dissatisfied about payer benefit obfuscation. With the consumerism tidal wave, patients will demand better access to parking, surrounding hotels, and a well-maintained facility. Consumerism complements the quality movement and the provider should be ready for it.

QUALITY

"Physicians can no longer retreat into their practices and laboratories and wait for it (quality) to blow over. Conversely, reacting with angry indignation will only aid those who wish to gain control of the profession because it will ignore the existing problems. The very nature of medicine as a profession is at stake."[30] Quality assurance is not a guest relations program; it's about leadership: purpose, worthwhile work, and making a difference.[31]

We know that quality is the efficient and effective application of medical care.[±] Universally, quality means conforming to standards and it includes setting the standards. Although quality costs money, spending alone does not necessarily improve quality. Not all data gathering is cost effective. But doing a thing right the first time is free.[†] Quality depends on yourself, your specialty and the internal environment. Quality is the conscience of the medical organization.

The emphasis on quality is to make your health system the best place to work and care for patients so that we enlarge the value of healthcare for patients and staff. Service expert Quint Studer has developed what he calls the "five pillars of excellence": people, service, quality, finance and growth.[32] Studer has shown the link between employee satisfaction, patient satisfaction and business performance. We used his pillars as the basis of measurement in our service award program. However,

---

±   High-quality care means effective, well-coordinated, safe, patient-centered and timely care. (Schoen C, Davis K, How SK, Schoenbaum SC. *U.S. Health System Performance: A National Scorecard*. Health Affairs 2006: 25 (6); ww457-w475).

†   Phillip Crosby, in his industry classic, *Quality Is Free,* credits ITT CEO Geneen for the concept that "Quality is not only right, it is free. And, it is not only free, it is the most profitable product line we have." What costs money is all the actions that involve not doing things right the first time. While we are not an industry in terms of a quantifiable product and cannot establish industrial quality control programs, we must plan for a more quantifiable assessment of results in every field. (Crosby PB. *Quality Is Free*. Denver, CO: Mentor Books, 1979, p. 131).

we added a foundation beneath the pillars. That base is *innovation*. A great effort was placed on change, ideas, how to do things better (see chapter 9). We constantly emphasized the importance of innovation. We taught managers not to be afraid to make decisions and to learn from all mistakes.

Each of the five pillars and their base has an economic impact. For example, attention to quality, clinical service, and employee satisfaction enabled us to decrease nursing turnover from 13.5 to 11. 4 percent, a 15 percent improvement that reduced nursing cost. We formed a Quality Institute to measure, assess and improve quality throughout the system, and the effort earned two Codman Awards. Attention to service is one of the most important roles in management. It stimulates ideas, rewards performance, increases personnel satisfaction, and is appreciated by patients.

Surprisingly, past polls of hospital executives reveal that their priorities include finance, operations systems, physician issues, and expansion – but rarely customer satisfaction and employee retention. World-class service begins by making customer satisfaction and employee retention top priorities. It means improving communication between ourselves and our patients. It means quantifying performance and cross-organizational improvement. It means better education of patients, personnel and executives. It means setting priorities and goals and refining accountability to give a sense of ownership.

Fred Smith, founder of Federal Express, says, "We discovered a long time ago that customer satisfaction really begins with employee satisfaction."[33] Inspired by the Disney Corporation, hospitals are focusing on the "guest" experience. You can revitalize a service-excellence initiative by shifting your analysis from what kind of service your caregivers are providing, to what kind of experience your patients are having.[34] In effect, Toyota did the same thing calling for "customer first" in everything. Together, these companies make the exceptional customer experience every person's job, every day.

This pyramid signifies our approach to quality.

FIGURE 10.2

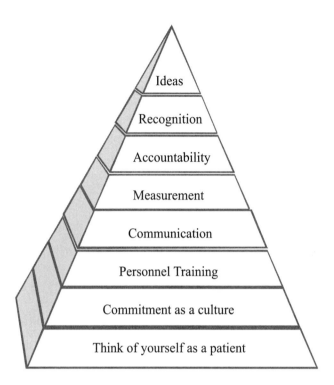

The base reminds all the staff to think of themselves as patients. Each step up the pyramid is another component of quality. Our commitment to patient care and superior service defines our culture. How well we train our staff about policies and communication assures this commitment. Our outcome metrics, accountability, and recognition of great performance are all part of clinical quality. Hospital personnel throughout a medical organization know how to improve the process, but they often are not heard. Innovation can occur anywhere in the organization and it's contagious.

Quality in healthcare is vulnerable to the sins of overuse, underuse and misuse. The hospital defends against errors by hiring skilled, dedicated and knowledgeable personnel. Not only are policies and protocols in place but communication and teaching about those policies are in effect. If the organization has a punitive culture, you will never find the source of the problems. A bureaucratic culture will celebrate a near miss, but a high reliability organization reacts to a near miss as if it were an adverse event.[35]

The Institute of Medicine concludes that the problems with medical mistakes are not principally caused by individual human error but rather by faulty systems, processes, and conditions that lead people to make mistakes or fail to prevent them.[36]

Medical errors may be portrayed by lining up slices of Swiss cheese. This metaphor represents the defensive layers between a potential hazard or error and the resulting complication.

FIGURE 10.3

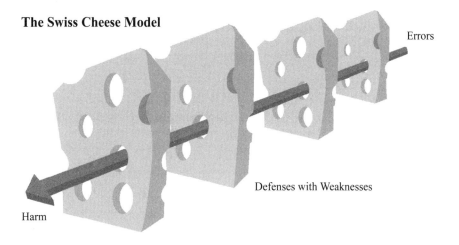

The Swiss Cheese Model

Errors

Defenses with Weaknesses

Harm

Reason J. Managing the Risks of Organizational Accidents (Ashgate, 1997).

The slices are the barriers to error and the holes are the gaps in protocols or policies or untrained personnel. Ideally, there are no holes in the defensive layers. Unfortunately, human and system lapses break down the defense. When active failure or latent conditions, such as poor design, supervision, manufacturing defects, training shortfalls, etc., produce holes in the defense, an accident trajectory may occur because the holes are lined up and the hazard passes through. No single error necessarily caused the event. Yet, there are many opportunities for individuals to intervene and prevent harm.[37] A pathological or bureaucratic culture does not encourage ideas about prevention. Neither commitment nor competence will suffice unless the organization is aware of the dangers that threaten operations. The repetition of error does not constitute experience.

Quality experts have produced an array of improvement methods, all of which have valuable components. They include CQI (continued quality improvement), which incorporates plan, do, check and act; idealized design (brainstorming about processes, culture and facilities); lean thinking (the Toyota Lean approach of 10 management principles and many tools to improve quality and efficiency). There also is Six Sigma, which attempts to assure defect-free service. For example, three defects in a million would equate to 99.9997 percent of defect-free products or services. Statistical tracking of complications for quality improvement is an indicator of quality assurance. You should be aware of Six Sigma protocol and apply it to new measures that could include prescription errors, patient falls, certain infections, "never" events, vaccinations, and counseling about tobacco cessation. Start small and add to the list. Make sure that morbidity is specific, measurable, and timely. Six Sigma is one good way to reduce variations.

Vanderbilt University has 300 metrics that are online and accessible to every employee.[38] These metrics are reported in a full-day session on a quarterly basis so that processes may be modified to obtain a better outcome. The doctors appreciate having data that is current, reliable, and presented in a comparative context. (It's hard to define a "defect" where performance spans initial service all the way to long-term outcome.) But all this data is meaningless without a well-supported plan to use the data to improve results. The federal government's HCAHPS initiative should stimulate hospitals to further improve. HCAHPS is a standardized survey for measuring patient satisfaction during the hospital experience. It is currently composed of 27 questions that entail communication with doctors and nurses, responsiveness of staff, cleanliness and quietness, pain control, communication about medicines and discharge information. Nothing like data to show where you stand in the community.[39]

Leadership must assure that the organization engages in a continual self-appraisal process. Ideally, all hospitals should have a permanent organizational entity for assessing quality, a routine system for gathering risk-adjusted data, benchmarks against which quality is assessed, a means of assuring that the data is accurate and representative, a policy of sharing this data with patients and other hospitals, and methods for instituting corrective action. The goal is to become a "high reliability" organization.[±]

We are finally getting around to Donabedian's observation from 20 years ago:

> ...at the grassroots, where people, awash in the alphabet soup of acronymic healthcare providers, are beginning to murmur their

---

±   High Reliability Organization. (*Becoming a High Reliability Organization: Operational Advice for Hospital Leaders.* AHRQ Publication No. 08-0022, April 2008). See also LaPorte TR, reference 35 in this chapter.

discontent; in the boardrooms of corporations where those who buy healthcare by the carload are wondering what precisely their dollars have bought; in the labyrinthine folds of governments, where politicians and bureaucrats, their wetted fingers to the wind, have felt the chill of public opprobrium; and in the rarefied reaches of academe, whose denizens, exquisitely attuned to the ebb and flow of grants, see new, rich pastures before them. It is an awakening to wonder at, a return to sanity we must applaud. I celebrate our rededication to quality in healthcare.[40]

As you review your approach to healthcare quality, remember that it's not enough to "inspect" quality; you have to build it into your system permanently.

PATIENT SATISFACTION

Patient satisfaction can be addressed by improving access, reducing waiting time for appointments, and eliminating the long process of hospital admission. The Center for Learning at the Cleveland Clinic reminds the quality service classes about the parallels between inpatients and those who go to jail. Remember, you are thinking of yourself as a patient. How would you like to:

- have your clothes taken away
- enter a bleak environment
- be assigned a number and known by that number
- turn over your valuables
- have a stranger as a roommate
- see family on a limited basis
- live according to the institution's schedule
- have very few choices/little control
- have virtually no privacy
- eat food that may be distasteful

Given that most of the above applies to the majority of patients in most hospitals, this would be a good time to revisit the basics. Let's start with physician etiquette, which is often sorely lacking in the mechanistic approach to patient care today.[41] Here is a modified protocol that doctors might consider when visiting a hospitalized patient.

- Coat and tie or clean white coat; no scrubs.
- Ask permission to enter the room; wait for an answer.
- Introduce yourself, showing ID badge.
- Shake hands (wear glove if needed).
- Sit down. Stand only if appropriate.
- Briefly explain your role on the team.
- Preserve dignity.
- Address patients by their formal last name, not first name.

This list can be easily modified, but it goes a long way towards improving patient satisfaction and a return to professionalism. We should be cognizant about patients' concern for privacy and their sensitivity to inconveniences. Patients are aware of the general ambience, especially cleanliness and the attitude of nurses. Most of all, they want a treatment plan that they can understand... and trust.

In-house satisfaction surveys are imperfect – compiling your own scores is akin to cheating at golf. You may look good but you don't learn anything. Satisfaction scores don't mean anything unless they translate into future loyalty. Satisfaction studies are often poorly conceived and conducted because they measure the wrong activity or the wrong customers, are easy to manipulate and encourage organizations and their employees to invest time and money unproductively. Interview the "failures" and make failure analysis an ongoing program.[42] High patient satisfaction scores are not relevant unless they are compiled during high patient activity. A low volume operation tends to have higher scores. Don't forget to survey personnel satisfaction. If the personnel are pleased, the patients are even more pleased.

Access needs continuous attention. If you want to find out about the barriers to scheduling and admission, hire a mystery shopper or be one yourself. Call in for an appointment and see what kind of a reception you get. After you are sufficiently surprised, change the attitude of those who schedule, remove the restrictions, and emphasize on-time appointments.

Patients and their families expect a perfect result today, and what's more, they want to be part of an efficient process that includes consistent exemplary service. Patients want to understand the diagnosis, the intended treatment, and the probabilities for "cure."[43] Most of all, patients want someone to listen, give sound advice, and attend to their follow-up. Dr. Richard Farmer, who for many years chaired the Cleveland Clinic Division of Medicine, believed in four maxims that should apply to patients at every medical center: you shouldn't have to be physician-referred, be rich or famous, pay exorbitant fees, or be inconvenienced.

In any business, management must understand foremost that your brand is a statement of trust between you and the customer. In healthcare, a respected brand signifies experience. As Reichheld[44] has observed, a lot of people who receive healthcare are influential, not necessarily rich, but invariably intelligent, usually educated, often activists civically, in church and at work or politically. In short, they're connected – and have a wide range of family and friends. These influential people will form lasting impressions of clinical services and will communicate through their connections with surprising strength and breadth. People seek their advice. They are recognized to be informed consumers. You want them to seek out your hospital and have a satisfactory experience there.

Satisfied customers will often tell other people about your "company" and many of those who are told will become your customers. Therefore, the best opportunity for increasing sales is through satisfying your present customer base and cultivating new customers. Superior service will bring in customers, keep them, and multiply the value of their accounts. The cost of a lost customer is five times the annual value of that account. It takes five times as much time, effort and money to attract a new customer as it does to keep a current one.[45]

Hospital executives often don't understand that most complaints never reach the chief of staff or the chief executive's office. It's in human nature that people complain in different ways. Therefore, it is the role of the ombudsmen or the department head or the individual doctor to listen and follow up with corrective action and to make amends. The worst "diseases" among healthcare personnel are arrogance and ignorance. This is another example where prevention is the best medicine. A patient can be a great source of innovation. The best advertisement is a satisfied patient.

THE PRACTICE OF MEDICINE

Basically, patients want doctors they can trust. They want to know what is involved in follow-up, especially how to communicate with the lead physician. When your patient asks, "What are my chances, doc?" he surely doesn't mean in Houston or Cleveland or someplace else a thousand miles away. He means where you are, and more importantly, where he is. You owe it to him to tell him. You owe it to yourself to know (the answer).[46] Sorry if that seems like too big an order, but that is the standard to which we must all manage. Administration, personnel and physicians must work together to decrease both annoyance and wasted time in the process of care. The healthcare team would do well to remember these patient management "rules."

Think of yourself as a patient.
There are no trivial questions.
Improve by finding problems in the system and fixing it.
Talk to patients about their experience – learn from it.

Don't hire anybody that doesn't like people.
Train personnel to meet the new standards.
Monitor patient satisfaction metrics from independent surveyors.

Modified from Robert Kay, M.D.,
former Chief of Staff, Cleveland Clinic

If you are a patient, how do you pick a good doctor? Obviously, you want the physician to be well educated, communicative, compassionate and considerate. You want him or her to have common sense and, above all, to carefully listen to what you are saying. It is reasonable to want the doctor to return your calls, be available and have an on-time office. When the physician is unresponsive in thought or action, the patient should seek another physician. Even under the strictest HMO guidelines, a patient has the right to request another primary physician.

Physicians who spread an array of choices in front of the patient and say, "Go ahead and choose; it's your life," are, in my opinion, shirking their duty.[47] The physician should review the alternatives and describe the options, but the physician has to take the responsibility and not shift it to the shoulders of the patient. An informed patient balances the "asymmetry." A good doctor wants to do the same thing. It's also acceptable for the physician to admit that he doesn't know the best treatment. If that's the case, he should give an informed opinion and help the patient seek a second opinion. That is part of quality and service.

Interactions with patients should start with the consideration that patients and their families really don't want to be in the hospital. Each has different circumstances – emotional, social, and those related to the severity of illness. Basically, patients want a smooth, effortless process. They want prompt response to their needs, no waiting, or other frustration. To them, communication has to be understandable, the surroundings pleasant and the staff capable and caring. Patients need to have answers to basic questions. What is wrong with me? Why do I have this problem? What *should* be done, not what *could* be done?

> When I'm sick, I want a doctor who will treat me and not an average. I want a doctor who will recognize the various ways in which I differ... in my particular demographic, clinical and other pertinent attributes. I want a doctor to recognize that the average obtained is a mixture of different results and different kinds of people. The doctor should then sort out those treatments and apply... the treatment... most suitable to me.[48]

People value process as much as substance. Kaiser Permanente trains thousands of physicians through their "four habits" model: 1) foster rapport and communication about process; 2) elicit the patient's perspective; 3) show empathy; 4) deliver diagnosis based on the original concern and explain, summarize and review the next steps.[49]

One way to find a good doctor is to interview a physician, a nurse or someone who has been severely ill and under the care of physicians. They know where the good doctors and hospitals are. They have experience and won't mind at all if you ask their advice. The patient has responsibilities in this relationship as well. The patient must be open with the physician about primary complaints, as well as other medical issues, even if they are embarrassing. If the patient feels uncomfortable about a course of action recommended by the physician, discuss the need for a second opinion. If the doctor is upset, that is a sure sign that you need another opinion and probably a new doctor. As a friend of mine advises, "Find me a doctor who can handle a lot of worry."[±]

On the other side, noncompliance is a major source of unexpected outcomes of care. Tell patients to give their health more attention. You can be the richest man in the world and the most successful man alive, but if you lose your good health, you will be a very unhappy man.[50] The hallmarks of the physician-patient relationship are openness and honesty in both directions, protected by confidentiality. This can occur only in an atmosphere of mutual respect, without which the relationship will fail.

What do doctors want? Efficient, clean facilities; an office location that benefits access and their personal logistics; a good ambulatory electronic record; competent colleagues and personnel wherever they practice. That is not too much to ask. Doctors are just like everyone else. They need appreciation. Ronald Reagan used to tell a story about a teenager who worked all day filling sandbags and building barricades to prevent a flood. A television reporter saw him working there cold and tired at night. The reporter asked, "Do you live here?" "No." Then why was he doing this? The teenager said, "I guess it's the first time I ever felt needed." That answer, says Reagan, "tells us something so true about ourselves that it should be printed on a billboard."[51] When a large number of internists were interviewed about their profession, they talked about the miracles and the lessons, sharing their own lives and their patients' lives, witnessing profound experiences and receiving acknowledgment for a job well done. These factors gave them a deeper appreciation of what it means to be a human being and a doctor, and how their caring actions and not just technical ability are important to their patients.[52] *Medicine is a mix of science and soul.*[53]

[±]   Dr. Roger Mee, former Chair, Department of Congenital Heart Surgery, Children's Hospital, Cleveland Clinic.

John Steinbeck wrote, "There is no other story, a man, after he has brushed off all the dust and chips of his life, will have left only the hard, clean questions: Was it good or was it evil? Have I done well or ill?"[54] As physicians, we are privileged to share the most profound moments of people's lives. As surgeon George Crile, Jr., wrote, "No physician, sleepless and worried about a patient, can return to the hospital in the midnight hours without feeling the importance of this faith. The dim corridor is silent; the doors are closed. At the end of the corridor in the glow of the desk lamp, the nurse watches over those who sleep or lie lonely and awake behind the closed white doors. No physician entering the hospital in these quiet hours can help feeling that the medical institution of which he is a part is in essence religious, that is built on trust. No physician can fail to be proud that he is part of his patients' fate."[55]

People facing death, young or old, do not think about what accolades they have earned or what social functions they have attended, what positions they have held, or even how much wealth they have accumulated. At the end, what is on their minds is who they loved and who loved them, who respected them, their family and friends; that circle is everything and is a good measure of one's life and whether or not one has made a difference.[±]

±   From Bernadine Healy

THE HIGH NOTE

These are my feelings at the present juncture, what I put before you in all sincerity and knowing that you will share many of them and that you will not resent the expression of any.

— Winston Churchill
Quoted in Jenkins R. *Churchill: A Biography*
Farrar Straus and Giroux, New York, 2001

These lessons and experiences serve to reacquaint the reader with the role of leadership in healthcare. The best leadership in all professions requires knowledge, common sense, and decision effectiveness, along with other characteristics described earlier.

Although the leader has to judge the performance of the executive team, leaders must appraise themselves more critically. No one ever accused me of being an extrovert, but there are times when you must be visible throughout the healthcare system – and not only in times of trouble. By interacting with staff, you will be amazed by their perceptions and needs that have not been addressed. This is where progress, or lack thereof, becomes evident. This is part of growing into the job.

What you were in your previous life as a physician or scientist or educator or all three, you are "no longer in the before." You are in a new and much larger role with far greater responsibilities and human interactions. It's okay to tread lightly when you're trying to get a grip on a very special field, but pretty soon everyone expects results. Directing one of these big medical organizations is not still life. There is a lot of activity whizzing around in the local environment, most of which the leadership team and managers can deal with. But you as chief executive should know the issues and their resolution. If you have inherited or recruited talent, they will deal with it effectively. If you have a lousy team, it's your fault, not theirs.

The big picture includes the changes and opportunities in clinical medicine, science, medical education, and fiscal policy that affect everything from quality to payment. You have to keep your eye on all the aforementioned and at the same time on market conditions and national issues. If you devote your energy solely to the inside or only to external matters, you will be in for surprises. Remember, a leader can be excused for mistakes, even short-term failures, but not for surprises.

Team leadership starts at the top but it has to reach far into the ranks to achieve long-standing success. Performance leadership depends on being an effective learner and listener and not repeating mistakes. Along the way many people will offer advice, none of which should be dismissed without careful thought. This is where common sense comes in. Don't be preoccupied with turning the medical organization into a real business. There are business practices that hospitals should emulate, but don't compromise humanism.

The economy, health policies and the regional market are all important factors. However, the single greatest factor between success and average or worse performance is the acquisition and retention of *talent*. The most successful chief executives have attracted clinical and scientific excellence across the organization.

The role of leadership is to concentrate on finding and funding opportunities at reasonable risk. And the chief executive is the responsible risk manager. It's not enough to protect the mission. You must advance it and you don't have to turn the organization upside down to show progress. In my experience, improved results are found in a series of small steps that lead to a large net effect. However you reach your goal, you will reach it faster if you insist on follow-up for all the tactical plans. Discipline in follow-up relies on leadership emphasizing a culture of responsibility and accountability.

Although we were ahead by having a staff model of salaried physicians and scientists, numerous inefficiencies still exist in all medical organizations. A focus on best practices and process innovation will reduce these inefficiencies and their attendant cost structure. Don't think you're too big to learn from other medical organizations. They should be part of your best practices survey. Most really good medical organizations will open their doors and show their approach to operations and finance, and even their design and performance in regional practice.

My final piece of advice covers six areas. *First,* never be afraid to remind people of the nobility of our calling, improving the health and lives of the people we are privileged to serve. Budgets and revenue are designed to achieve that vision, not the other way around. Celebrating the successes of your staff in providing extraordinary care reinforces the core values in healthcare and brings out enthusiasm and pride. *Second*, the inevitable move towards government-dominated healthcare should stimulate hospital leadership to focus on the payment/cost ratio. The challenge is to integrate operations, finance and clinical systems to gain full payment at or close to provision of service. Concentrate on better organization of data. *Third*, if you are in academic leadership, protect the research and education budgets, because they are less able to withstand indiscriminate cuts. *Fourth*, the organization will distinguish itself through exceptional outcomes and service. The leadership team at the top has to be inspirational and engaged to assure that leaders throughout the organization are managing proactively. This is why investment in leadership and holding everyone accountable for individual and collective performance is the new culture for medical organizations. Research may add a valuable aura but it can't drive referrals. Research and education are not immune to this process and their metrics are equally important as those of clinical medicine. *Fifth*, medical leadership and human resources have to find and retain the best and the most educable talent. The key to progress and endurance is to have the best staff at every level. *Sixth,* prepare for more flexibility in your business model, which will depend on your awareness of impending changes. The earliest signs of change are the transfer of more economic risk to the patient, the specter of unionism, the fragmentation of inpatient and outpatient care, and the emphasis on wellness. There is an old footballer axiom that warns, if you don't prepare, prepare to fail. There are no stepwise prescriptions, but you'll find that good ideas are everywhere if your receptors are on. In healthcare everyone is "busy," and we don't solicit ideas nearly as well as we should – ideas about better ways to practice with less redundancy and without compromising safety. In this world at this time, to win you have to be an innovator. And it is not only about efficiency. It also involves finding new sources of revenue.

Above all, don't mind the critics. The only way to avoid criticism is to do nothing, say nothing and be nothing. Most of it is not to your face, and if it is helpful, your true friends will advise you accordingly. Most of the criticism comes from those who are uninformed or from those who do nothing and wait for things to get better. It's like art critics or book reviewers who tell the reader what they would have done differently if they had done the work, which they hadn't.

When the organization shows real progress, the leadership team will achieve the personal satisfaction of knowing that they have enriched the people around them. If a genie could grant healthcare leaders one wish, I suggest that we try to take this advice offered many years ago.[±]

[±]   Modified from Christian D. Larson, *Optimists Creed,* 1912, Your Forces and How to Use Them.

Be so strong that nothing can disturb your peace of mind. Talk health, happiness and prosperity to every person you meet. Make all your friends feel there is something in them. Look at the sunny side of everything. Think only the best, work only for the best and expect only the best. Be as enthusiastic about the success of others as you are about your own. Forget the mistakes of the past and press on to the greater achievements of the future. Give everyone a smile. Spend so much time improving yourself that you have no time left to criticize others. Be too big for worry and too noble for anger.

Today, more than ever, medical leadership extends beyond the hospitals. A great medical center can renew communities by improving population health through wellness programs and coordinated patient care. The insight and experience of a great staff will overcome these challenges. And, they will look to leadership for wisdom and fortitude.

Reforming the health insurance industry will not be an easy task. To make health insurance more affordable and offer a wider choice of plans, these areas of reform should be considered.

1) Create an insurance market so that people can find benefits that suit them anywhere nationwide.[±] Consumers should have a wide choice of plans to meet their needs and tax relief to encourage health insurance coverage. The goal is to have access to more affordable insurance.

2) Allow interstate plan comparisons and purchasing so that individuals and groups can avoid some of the onerous state mandates that add significantly to the premium. Legislate insurance portability whether it is employer- or individual-based. Policies should be carried anywhere in the country and used anywhere. (A typical worker changes jobs ten times by the time he or she is 42 years old.) (Emanuel E., Wyden, R. A New Federal-State Partnership in Health Care, Real Power for States. JAMA 2008: 300(16); 1931-38)

3) Prevent cherry picking in the individual insurance market. Ensure guaranteed issue of insurance policies, but risk adjust so that every indemnity company has a similar distribution of risk. Risk adjustment can be accomplished by age alone or by accounting for additional risk factors, such as smoking. Some would advocate an added premium for smokers. Preexisting conditions should be known at the time of purchase to assess risk for the insurer. If the insurance company has taken on younger or healthier patients, it should pay some "tax" that covers the high-risk selection in other companies.

4) Standardize catastrophic coverage and establish risk pools at the state and/ or regional level to moderate individual health plan exposure.

5) Agree to contractual terms within the provider contract, which will ultimately increase the efficiency and lower the operational costs of the relationship. This will include prompt payment terms, immediate denial explanation and effective customer service.

6) Encourage and support physicians, particularly independent community practitioners, in the adoption of the electronic medical record. Currently only a minority of independent physicians have adopted EMRs. The EMR can improve quality and efficiency by reducing duplication, preventing

---

±   Because state mandates, disease prevalence and practice patterns vary widely, a regional approach to interstate health insurance purchasing would likely precede nationwide access.

medical errors, and improving communication between physicians, patients and health plans.

7) Provide consumers with actionable information about coverage and cost. Insurers need to provide clearly stated information about what they pay for a given condition and what they don't pay for, including plan co-payments and deductibles. All insurers should post understandable terms for each purchase option.

8) Provide consumers with information about outcomes and other value metrics. According to the Wennberg/Dartmouth Atlas data, there is enormous variation in the cost and quality of similar healthcare services. It is time that insurers and providers collaborate to publish quality and outcomes data. Having accurate cost and quality information available will allow referring physicians and consumers to choose the most appropriate and efficient providers.

9) Standardize benefits covered in HSA plans.

10) Encourage responsibility for personal health improvement by actively supporting workplace and community wellness programs, publishing wellness information and offering economic benefits for wellness and prevention services. This will allow consumers to gain a healthier lifestyle that has shown to lower the probability of future illness and possibly to avoid later expensive treatment.

ELECTRONIC PATIENT RECORDS AND FINANCIAL SERVICES

Consumer-directed healthcare (in various forms) is increasing in enrollment. Regardless of plan type, higher co-payments and deductibles raise administrative costs. Currently, hospital revenue cycle management is bloated, poorly coordinated, and frequently inaccurate. Components of the revenue cycle are not efficiently coordinated because charge is not entered in real time. The prospect of a 24-hour claim is elusive for inpatient transactions. To accelerate payments, improvement will require faster and more accurate claims and billing. Patient financial services-medical record integration can significantly lower cost, improve payment, and accelerate adoption of the electronic patient record. See pages 238-239 for detailed information.

Payer aligns with bank to facilitate these patient benefits

- smart (affinity) card issued, which automatically completes all registration activities including patient access to medical record
- smart card serves as debit or branded credit card for healthcare services
- patient may choose card as identifier-only or tie to HSA-type accounts
- web-based access to medical/claim information
- no membership fee
- card = facilitated access

Healthcare System and Logo

1234 5678 9101 1122

Member Name

Exp Date

credit card logo

credit or debit
insurance benefits
current medications
allergies
record of surgery
vaccinations
employer information

Card controls

- access to selected physicians – pricing disclosed
- unique patient identifier
- eligibility (benefit info)
- medical record access
- pharmacy benefits
- co-payments/deductibles (when bank card is used)
- discount for prompt payment
- credit limit
  ↓
  → secure pin

Electronic medical record converts provided services into real-time charge using

- practice management system
  registration, verification,
  authorization
  scheduling
  coding events
  claim and bill
- EMR includes
  computerized order entry
  real-time quality data
  ambulatory record interface
  ↓ Claims transmitted to
  → payer by electronic data
  interchange (switch)

Virtual clearinghouse

- retained by employer or payer
- financial transactions
  payer portal
  confirm eligibility, pharmacy
  and plan design
  electronic claims transactions
  real-time adjudication of
  claims
  bank card authorization
  discount authorization
  maintain benefit plan data
  send to bank for distribution
- call center – problem resolution
- reports to member, payer and provider
- produce 1099 forms for provider
  ↓

Provider paid through bank

- immediate payment
- eliminates point-of-service collection by providers
- guaranteed payment of out-of-pocket (co-payment/deductibles) for qualified cardmember

Advantages

To the patient:
- facilitates personal health account
- provider rates known up-front
- discount for prompt payment
- immediate claim status
- plan benefit information
- up-front knowledge of financial responsibilities
- identifier card flexible – banking optional
- access personal health record
- eligibility review/updates/ beneficiary and dependent changes
- e-mail communication with provider
- wide range of financial services available
- stop-loss, catastrophic care built in
- receives on-line healthcare information for prevention/ wellness

To the provider:
- outsource most of revenue cycle management – less paper and cost
- eliminate point-of-service cash collection
- accelerated payment → cash flow
- exclusive health system contract
- guaranteed collection
- devote more resources to quality, including service and operations
- added patient loyalty

To the payer:
- outsource claims and transactions (eliminate claims systems)
- significantly reduce back-office process
- eliminate provider and patient hassle
- retain contracting
- sell non-covered services insurance

To the purchaser:
- more responsibility to employee
- eliminate third party administrator
- decrease health plan cost
- more incentive to promote CDHP

To the bank (credit card):
- outsource transaction processing
- receive percentage of all transactions
- provide account balances
- interest on debt
- loans for co-payment/deductibles
- facilitate sale of non-covered products
- reward programs
- financial planning

Cleveland Clinic Market Penetration 1994

The yellow shade shows the highest referral areas. In 1944, the presystem referrals were local and modest. Ten years later, the referral market grew consonant with the family health center expansions. Today, the patient visits to the family health centers are equivalent to the patient visits on the main campus. Nearly half of the physicians in this regional practice are now specialists.

The top frame shows the market penetration in 1994. The bottom frame shows the growth in market penetration ten years later in 2003.

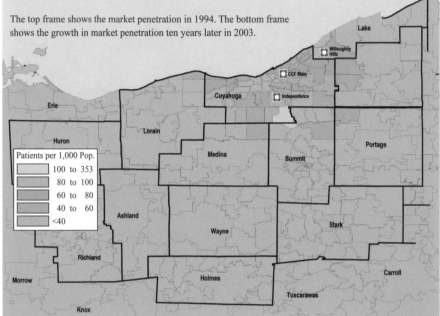

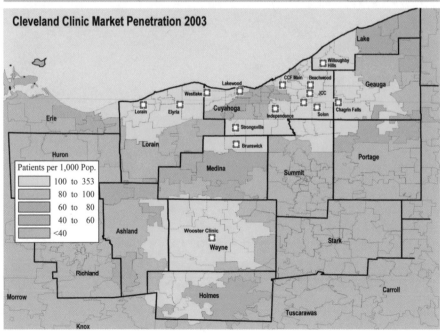

The Losers' Ten Commandments (John R. Graham, Graham Communications, marketing and sales consulting, Quincy, Massachusetts):

1) Always have an excuse. Develop a series of phrases and rehearse them regularly so you will always have one ready when you need it. Examples: My car wouldn't start. Our prices are too high. The alarm clock didn't go off. I didn't have time. The customer made a mistake. I can't get through to him on the phone. The computer fouled up. The economy is bad, etc. Never be speechless when it comes to making excuses for yourself.

2) Be sure to blend into the pack. Losers know that it is important to be invisible. Vanilla is their favorite flavor. Never call attention to yourself. Look, act, and work the way you really are – mediocre.

3) Keep your eye on the competition. Think and breathe the competition. Know all about them, their weaknesses, their opportunities, their problems and their needs. Never think about your customers.

4) Avoid taking risks at all costs. Risk taking is extremely dangerous. You may either fail or succeed. Either one will put you in great jeopardy. Risk takers lead the pack by always wanting to test themselves. They are never satisfied with their performance. They want to do better. They welcome risks as opportunities. Such thinking makes you shudder.

5) Never let yourself become enthusiastic. If you do, you will want to do more. Become more deeply involved in your work and place your company, coworkers, and customers ahead of yourself.

6) Always put yourself first. Before you agree to anything, ask yourself, "What's in it for me?" If something requires extra time and effort, it could lead to more sales, increased productivity and higher profits for your company. By putting yourself first, you will avoid all these problems.

7) If something goes wrong, blame someone. This is very important. Taking responsibility causes difficulties, so make sure you always have someone in mind to blame when a problem arises. Taking responsibility only makes you more valuable. You might even be viewed as a leader.

8) Spend a lot of time second-guessing the boss. This is your real job. A top priority. By never showing initiative, you are guaranteed a permanent position – at the bottom of the ladder.

9) Never learn anything new. Knowledge is dangerous. It means you will become a problem solver. If this happens, customers will view you as

essential to their success and your company will give you regular promotions.

10) If all else fails, say, "I don't know." The less you know, the better off you are. Whenever you are asked a question, just say, "I don't know." You will quickly become exactly what you are. Useless. By the way, it is easy to become a winner. All you have to do is go to work and break these ten commandments.

A P P E N D I X   V

An enormous amount of money is wasted on new hires who leave within the first few months. The organization has to evaluate character, capacity, energy and experience during the initial interview and later after 90 days on the job. A new method of personnel evaluation has been developed and named after Dr. Virginia Apgar, the first woman to be named a full professor at Columbia University College of Physicians and Surgeons in 1949. In 1953, she devised a rating system on a scale of 0-10 for newborns. It was the first standardized method for evaluating a newborn's transition to life outside the womb. The system is credited worldwide for reducing infant mortality. This "rating" has been cleverly adapted to employee evaluation.

Below is a sample tool for a 0-2 rating system at interview and later at 90 days. This method is practical and easily modified to fit healthcare.[±]

Character	
	Will not bend or wink at truth – will describe the situation as it is
	Has the confidence to speak up if they disagree
	Answers questions consistently regardless of audience
	Shares praise & accepts responsibility
	The person is passionate/engaged
	Contributes personally and appreciates the contributions of others

Capacity	
	Demonstrated ability to actively understand problems
	Demonstrated ability to discern patterns
	Can come up to speed without excessive handholding or structure
	Street smart, not just book smart

Energy	
	Desire & urgency to contribute in any way they can, including small things to start
	Trust that they will deliver on directives and/or tasks without constant follow-up
	Will not be a bystander

Experience	
	Acts decisively based on prior knowledge, from here or elsewhere
	Comes with different ideas, contacts and approaches that apply to new situations
	Changes the feel of the group for the better by bringing new perspectives

±   Intuitive Surgical, Inc. 1266 Kifer Road, Sunnyvale, CA 94086

ACKNOWLEDGMENTS

The author acknowledges the valuable input from the following friends and colleagues: Gene Altus, Jim Bennett, Eugene Blackstone, M.D., Jim Blazar, David Bronson, M.D., John Clough, M.D., John Costin, M.D., Fred DeGrandis, Al Dobson, Michael Feuer, Bernadine Healy, M.D., Norman Hertzer, M.D., Robert Ivancic, Ray Leach, Frank Lordeman, Roger Mee, M.D., Michael McMillan, Michael O'Boyle, Peter Osenar, Robert Replogle, M.D., Stanley Sieniawski, Mark Smith, M.D., William W. Stead, M.D., Michael Tanner, Angela Wonson, Claire Zangerle.

As the manuscript proceeded, these experts provided excellent suggestions and healthy criticism. Some were interviewed only; others reviewed sections or chapters, and a few read the entire book. If this book has any merit, I credit the sound advice I have received from their knowledge and experience.

The inestimable collaboration of Ms. Kathy Vaughn with assistance from Pat Cogan brought the collection of manuscripts to book form. They checked facts and verified all references. They are wise beyond their technical skills, and I always listened to their counsel. Finally, my profound gratitude is reserved for the Cleveland Public Library, one of the very best libraries in America. Their abundant resources and their inter-library loan services aided my efficiency and research significantly.

R E F E R E N C E S

INTRODUCTION
1) Drucker P: Managing the Non-Profit Organization. HarperCollins Publishers, New York, 1990.
2) Polanyi M. Personal Knowledge—Towards a Post-Critical Philosophy, Chicago University of Chicago Press (1956).

CHAPTER 1: LEADERSHIP
1) Adair J. Not Bosses But Leaders: How to Lead the Way to Success. Talbot Adair Press, London, 1987, p. 145
2) Gardner JW. Attributes and Context. (Leadership Papers 6). Leadership Studies Program. Washington, D.C.: Independent Sector, 1987, p. 15.
3) Black B. On the Edge of Common Sense: Differences Seem Subtle, But Are Substantial. Amarillo.com, Amarillo Global News, August 20, 2005.
4) Zaleznik A. Managers and Leaders: Are They Different? Harvard Business Review 2004: 82 (1); 74-81.
5) Raynor ME. The Strategy Paradox. Why Committing to Success Leads to Failure [and What to Do About it]. Currency Books, New York, 2007.
6) Etzioni A, Dual Leadership in Complex Organizations, American Sociological Review 30:4, October 1965, pp. 688-698.
7) Cited in Janove J. A 3,500-Year-Old Lesson in Delegating. HR Magazine 2005, p. 110.
8) Fraser GM. Quartered Safe Out Here. HarperCollins 1995.
9) Fraser GM. Ibid.
10) Cawthorne N. Military Commanders. The 100 Greatest Throughout History. Enchanted Lion Books, 2004, p. 189.
11) Slim W. Field Marshall, Viscount. Defeat into Victory: Battling Japan in Burma and India. 1942-1945. New York: Cooper Square Press, 2000.
12) Russo JE. and Schoemaker PJH. Decision Traps: The Ten Barriers To Brilliant Decision-Making & How To Overcome Them. Doubleday 1989.
13) Slim W. Ibid.
14) Slim W. Sheffield Lecture. Cited in Adair J. Effective Strategic Leadership. Pan McMillan, London, 2003, p. 194.
15) Slim W. Field-Marshall, Viscount. A Soldier Looks At Business. An address before The Empire Club of Canada. 22, April 1963.
16) Chapman TW. Management Learning Experiences of CEOs. Xlibris Corporation 2008.
17) Moore G. Interview in Strategy and Leadership. 35, Number 5, 2007.
18) Houghton JR. Chapter Two. Corporate Transformation and Senior Leadership. IN: Hambrick DC, Nadeler DA, Tushman ML. Navigating Change. Now CEOs, Top Teams, and Boards Steer Transformation. Harvard Business School Press, Boston, MA, 1998, p. 37.
19) Luntz F. Words That Work – It's Not What You Say, It's What People Hear. Hyperion, 2007.
20) Cited in Ambrose SE: Personal Reflections of an Historian to America. Simon & Schuster, New York, 2002, p. 98.
21) Morris B. Tearing Up the Jack Welch Playbook. Fortune Magazine, July 11, 2006.
22) Slater R. Jack Welch and The GE Way. McGraw Hill, 1999, p. 117.
23) Hesiod 700 B.C. Hesiod: Work and Days. Translated by Richard Lattimore. Ann Arbor Books, 1959, p. 95.
24) Collins J. Level 5 Leadership: The Triumph of Humility and Fierce Resolve. Harvard Business Review 2005: 82 (7/8); 136-46.

25) Kanter RM., Power Failure in Management Circuits. Harvard Business Review, July-August 1979, Harvard Business School Publishing 2000.
26) Cited in Benson JH. So You Want to Be a Leader?: Advice and Counsel to Young Leaders. Trafford Publishing 2007.
27) Walpole H. Fortitude. New York: Modern Library; 1913.
28) Cited in Ward Connerly's 2001 Commencement Address "Warriors of Freedom," Hillsdale College, May 12, 2001.
29) Slywotzky A. The Art of Profitability. Warner Books, Inc., New York, N.Y. 2002, p. 167.
30) Famous words of Trajan when he delivered the sword to the governors of the provinces, as the emblem of their authority. IN: Preface. Diary of Thomas Burton, esq., Vol 1:July 1653-April 1657 (1828). URL: http://www.british-history.ac.uk/report.asp?compid=36719.
31) Adair J. Effective Leadership, Gower Publishing, Ltd., 1993, p. 103.
32) Calloway DW. The Promise and Paradoxes of Leadership. Directors & Board, Winter 1985, Vol. 9 (2); 12-16.
33) Lagnado L. Poison Pill: Elite Medical Schools Seemed Perfect Mates, Except to the Doctors. Wall Street Journal, Mar 21, 1997; Sect. A1.
34) Attributed to Henry Cisneros
35) Firestone H. Cited in Poor Charlie's Almanack. The Wit and Wisdom of Charles T. Munger. 3rd Ed., Edited by Peter D. Kaufman. Donning Company Publishers, 2008, page 70.
36) Ross SJ. Cited in Cohen R. New York Times, December 21, 1992.
37) Atkinson R. An Army at Dawn. The War in North Africa, 1942-1943. Henry Holt & Co., NY, 2002, p. 485.
38) Address by Henry Kissinger. 106th Landon Lecture, Kansas State University, Manhattan, Kansas, April 29, 1996.
39) Coughlin T. Personal Communication.
40) Told to him by Dwight Morrow. IN: Monnet, J. Memoirs. Doubleday, 1978.
41) Firestone HS. What I Have Learned About Men. IN: Krass P. Book of Business Wisdom. John Wiley & Sons, Inc., NY, 1997.
42) Ambrose SE. To America. Personal Reflections of a Historian. Simon and Schuster, 2002.
43) Gerald Buckberg, M.D., personal communication.
44) Deutsch CG. Building the Global Bank. An Interview with Jamie Dimon. The McKinsey Quarterly, 12/18/06.
45) Miller LM. Barbarians to Bureaucrats. Corporate Life Cycle Strategies. Clarkson N. Potter Inc., New York, 1989, p. 180.
46) Welch J, Welch S. Being a Leader, It's a Whole New Mindset. Business Week, January 30, 2006
47) Barondess JA. On Mentoring. J R Soc Med, 1997; 90:347-9.
48) Wright S. Examining What Residents Look For in Their Role Models; Acad Med, 1996; 71(3):290-2.
49) Jenkins R. Churchill: A Biography. Farrar Straus and Giroux, NY, 2001,p. 455.
50) Dohn DF. Mentoring: A Neurosurgical Odyssey. Cleveland Clinic Distinguished Alumnus Lecturer, 2001 Neuroscience Days, May 29, 2001.
51) Salacuse JA. The Art of Advice. How to Give It and How to Take It. Times Books, New York, 1994.
52) Letter from Lincoln to W.T. Sherman. Cited in Memoirs of General W. T. Sherman written by himself, Vol. II, D. Appleton & Co., New York, 1875.
53) Blackmun HA. Remarks at the Commencement Exercise of Mayo Medical School. Mayo Clinic Proc 1980: 55; 573-578.
54) U.S. Supreme Court Justice Antonin Scalia, commencement address, College of William and Mary, 1996.
55) Costin J. Personal communication.
56) Cited in Charlton J. The Military Quotation Book. St. Martin's Press, New York, 2002, p. 83.
57) Gardner JW. The Role of the Leader. Health Care Forum Journal, May-June 1990, pp. 31-34.

58) Russo JE, Schoemaker PJH. Decision Traps: The Ten Barriers To Brilliant Decision-Making & How to Overcome Them. Doubleday 1989.

59) Sarkozy N. Speech to the French-American Foundation, Washington, D.C., September 12, 2006.

60) Gardner JW. On Leadership. New York: Free Press, 1990.

61) Lansberg I. The Tests of a Prince. Harvard Business Review, September 2007, p. 99-100.

62) Finkelstein S. Why Smart Executives Fail: And What You Can Learn from their Mistakes. Penguin Books, 2003.

63) Maister D. True Professionalism. The Free Press, New York, 1997, p. 71.

64) Quoted by Jim Calhoun, head basketball coach, University of Connecticut, in an interview with Charlie Rose, December 27, 2007.

CHAPTER 2: THE PHYSICIAN CHIEF EXECUTIVE

1) Loop FD. Presidential Address. The First Living and the Last Dying. J Thorac Cardiovasc Surg 1998: 116; 683-88.

2) Lorsch JW, Kurana R. Changing Leaders. The Board's Role in CEO Succession and Why They Often Pick the Wrong Leaders. BusinessWeek.com, October 25, 2007.

3) Russell B. Power. A New Social Analysis. Routledge: New York, 2004, p. 13.

4) Jennett B. High-Technology Medicine: Benefits and Burdens. Oxford, Oxford University Press, 1986.

5) Jenkins R. Churchill: A Biography. Farrar Straus and Giroux, NY, 2001, p. 536.

6) Bennett WJ. America: The Last Best Hope, Volume 1 From the Age of Discovery to a World at War, Nelson Current 2006.

7) French President Nicholas Sarkozy. Cited in Reza Y. L'aube Le Soir Ou La Nuit ("Dawn Evening or Night"). Editions Flammarion, 2007.

8) Reischauer E. My Life Between Japan and America. HarperCollins, New York, 1986.

9) Gardner JW. On Leadership. The Free Press, 1990.

10) Bennis W. and Nanus B. Leaders. New York: Harper and Row, 1965.

11) Acheson D. Quoted in Wall Street Journal, September 8, 1977.

12) Adair J. Effective Motivation, Pan McMillan, London, 1996.

13) Menninger WW. Adaptation and Morale. Predictable Responses to Life Changes. Bulletin of the Menninger Clinic 1988: 52: 198-210.

14) Drucker PF. Management: Tasks, Responsibilities, Practices. Harper & Row, New York, 1973.

15) Franklin B. Poor Richard's Almanack: Being the Choicest Morsels of Wisdom, Written During the Years of the Almanack's Publication. Peter Pauper Press, Inc., 1986, p. 38.

16) Ury W. Getting Past No: Negotiating Your Way From Confrontation to Cooperation. Bantam Books, New York, 1993.

17) Bruck C. The Big Hitter. The New Yorker, December 8, 1997, p. 82.

18) Mitchell G. Making Peace, New York: Knopf, 1999, p. 13.

19) Anders G. The Best Acquisitions Start With The CEO Who Charms Sellers. Wall Street Journal, August 21, 2006.

20) Huxtable AL. Frank Lloyd Wright. Penguin Group, 2004, p. 41.

21) Alstadt DM. Human Knowledge, the Legalistic Mentality, and National Survival. Presented to the Federation of Societies for Coatings Technology; Oct 29, 1975; Los Angeles.

22) Dohn DF. Mentoring: A Neurosurgical Odyssey. Cleveland Clinic Distinguished Alumnus Lecturer, 2001 Neuroscience Days, Cleveland Clinic, May 29, 2001.

23) Podhoretz N. World War IV. The Long Struggle Against Islamo Facism. Doubleday, 2007.

24) Attributed to Eugene Stead IN: Rubin ER. Leadership Amid Change: The Challenge of Academic Health Centers. IN: Eastwood G. Mission Management. A New Synthesis, Vol. 2, Association of Academic Health Centers. 1998 p. 67-84.

25) James Willerson, statement given in public presentations and motivational speeches over the years.

26) Donne J. Devotions. Chapter VI: Meditation.

27) Waldroop J, Butler T. Managing Away Bad Habits. Harvard Business Review 2000; Sept-Oct.; 89-98.

28) Ramsay D. The History of the American Revolution. Volume 1, 1749-1815, edited by Lester H. Cohen (originally published 1789), Liberty Fund. Rev. ed, 1990.

29) Grant US. Personal Memoirs. Penguin, New York, 1999, p. 381.

30) Steve Nash, professional basketball player, interviewed by Charlie Rose, August 27, 2007.

31) Twain M. Pudd'nhead Wilson's Calendar. The Tragedy of Pudd'nhead Wilson, Chapter 16, 1894.

32) Krauthamer C. The Hounding of Doctors Has Just Begun. The Seattle Times. May 31, 1993.

33) Delbecq AL, Gill SL. Justice as a Prelude to Teamwork. Healthcare Management Review 1985: 10; 45-52.

34) Blackstone E. Personal communication.

35) Peters JP, Tseng S. Managing Strategic Change in Hospitals. Chicago: American Hospital Publishing, 1983, pp. 63-69.

36) Collins F. Language of God. Free Press, A Division of Simon & Schuster, Inc., New York, NY 10020, 2006 , pp. 214-217.

37) Gardner K, ed. The Excellent Board. Practical Solutions for Health Care Trustees and CEOs, American Hospital Association, 2003. (Ingram J and Kenney RM: Spinoffs: How to Build Just the Right Board. Directors and Board, 3rd quarter, 2006.)

38) WSHA Governing Board Orientation Manual, Second Edition, September 2000. www.wsha.org.

39) Gardner K, ed. The Excellent Board II. New, Practical Solutions for Health Care Trustees and CEOs. Health Forum, Inc., Chicago, IL, 2008.

40) Bowen WG. The Board Book. W.W. Norton and Company, New York, 2008.

41) Governance in Nonprofit Community Health Systems. Prybil L and others. College of Public Health, University of Iowa. A Report in Three Phases, 2007-08.

42) Wiehl J. Roles and Responsibilities of Nonprofit Health Care Board Members in the Post-Enron Era. J of Legal Medicine, Vol. 25, 2004.

43) Smith JE. Grant. Simon and Schuster, 2001, p. 288.

44) Charan R. Boards That Deliver. John Wiley & Sons, Inc., San Francisco, 2005.

45) Leap T. Keys to Spotting a Flawed CEO – Before It's Too Late. Wall Street Journal, December 1, 2007.

46) Boardrooms in 2003: Directors Speak Out. Board Alert, New York, NY, pp. 8-23.

47) Carver J. Boards That Make A Difference: A New Design for Leadership in Nonprofit and Public Organizations. Jossey-Bass, 1991.

48) Garman AN, Tyler JL. CEO Succession Planning in Freestanding U.S. Hospitals: Final Report. Prepared for the American College of Healthcare Executives, October 27, 2004.

49) 10 Best Practices for Measuring the Effectiveness of Non-Profit Health Care Boards. Bulletin of the National Center for Health Care Leadership, Educational and Advertorial Supplement to Modern Heathcare, December 2006, p. 9-20.

50) Peregine MW. New Guidance to Governing Board on Compliance Plan Oversight. Corporate Governance Task Force, Executive Summary, January 2007, American Health Lawyers Association.

51) Steiner JE. Understanding Compliance Legal Standards as a Key Element in a Compliance Program. On the Front Lines CCH Health Care Compliance Letter, April 1, 2008.

52) An Integrated Approach to Corporate Compliance. A Resource for Health Care Organization Board of Directors. United States Department of Health and Human Services, Office of the Inspector General and the American Health Lawyers' Association, July 1, 2004.

53) Case Western Reserve University Regulations (Amended 2005), Article I Trustees.

54) Quoted in the *Sunday Times,* London, November 15, 1992.

55) Mitroff II, Anagnos G. Managing Crises Before They Happen. What Every Executive and Manager Needs to Know About Crisis Management. Amacom, American Management Association, New York, 2001.

56) Luecke R. Crisis Management. Master the Skills to Prevent Disasters. Harvard Business Essentials. Harvard School Press, Boston, MA, 2004.

57) Dezenhall E, Weber J. Damage Control. Why Everything you Know About Crisis Management is Wrong. Penguin Group, New York, 2007.

58) Pfeffer J, Sutton RI. Hard Facts. Dangerous Half-Truths And Total Nonsense Profiting From Evidence-Based Management. Harvard Business School Press, Boston, MA, 2006.

59) Attributed to William Rees Mogg. IN: Gardner H. Leading Minds. The Anatomy of Leadership. Basic Books, 1996, p. 244.

60) Guttridge LF. Mutiny: A History of Naval Insurrection. Shepperton, UK: Ian Allen, 1992, p. 73.

61) Burns,JM. Transforming Leadership. Atlantic Monthly Press, 2003.

62) Neil Cavuto interview with Rupert Murdoch; Rupert Murdoch on Super Bowl Ratings, News Corp's Earnings and Presidential Race. Tuesday, February 5, 2008.

63) Cited in Brownstein R. The Second Civil War: How Extreme Partisanship has Paralyzed Washington and Polarized America. The Penguin Press, New York, 2007.

64) Feuer M. Strong Caveat to New Management. Smart Business. September 2008.

65) Lacey R. Ford: The Men and the Machine. Little Brown & Co., 1986, p. 274.

66) Ruark R. Something of Value. Doubleday. 1955.

67) Kerr C. The Uses of the University. Harvard University Press. 1963.

68) Thatcher M. Interview for Press Association (10th anniversary as Prime Minister). May 3, 1989.

69) Sevareid E. This Reporter, Two-Part Edward R. Murrow Portrait, August 2, 1988 on PBS.

70) Advice from Donald Regan to Wm. P. Lauder. Lauder WP. The Best Advice I Ever Got. Harvard Business Review, May 2008, p. 21.

71) Wooden J, Jamison S. Wooden: A Lifetime of Observations and Reflections On and Off the Court. Contemporary Books, Chicago, Ill., 1997, p. 94.

72) Jenkins R. Churchill. A Biography. Farrar Straus and Giroux, 2001, p. 612.

73) Clough JD. To Act As A Unit. The Story of The Cleveland Clinic, Third Edition, Cleveland Clinic Foundation, Cleveland, OH, 1996.

CHAPTER 3: THE ACADEMIC MEDICAL CENTER

1) Murray C: Human Accomplishment. The Pursuit of Excellence in the Arts and Sciences, 800 B.C. to 1950 HarperCollins Publishers, New York, NY 2003, p. 207.

2) George Crile, Sr., M.D.. The Clinic Foundation. Speech at the official opening of the Cleveland Clinic, February 26, 1921; Cleveland Clinic Archives.

3) Dubos RJ. Louis Pasteur, Free Lance of Science. Boston: Little, Brown & Company, 1950, p. 85.

4) Groopman J. How Doctors Think. Houghton Mifflin 2007.

5) William E. Lower, M.D. The Importance of a Patient. First known printed version in Notice to Interns, Fellows and Staff of the Medical Division, April 6, 1967.

6) Darwin C. Introduction. IN: From So Simple a Beginning. The Four Great Books of Charles Darwin (Voyage of the H.M.S. Beagle), Edward O. Wilson, ed., W.W. Norton, 2005.

7) Stevens RA, Rosenberg CE, Burns LR. History and Health Policy in the United States. Rutgers University Press, 2006.

8) Science, The Endless Frontier. A Report to the President by Vannevar Bush, Director of the Office of Scientific Research and Development. July 1945.

9) Darwin C. The Life and Letters of Charles Darwin: Including an Autobiographical Chapter. Edited by his son Francis Darwin. In two volumes. Vol. 1, New York, NY; London: D. Appleton and Co., 1911, pp. 85-86 [available online at http://landsat.ohiolink.edu/EBooks//OSU/LifeDarwin1.51463657.pdf; accessed June 12, 2008].

10) Drucker PF. Managing in the Next Society. St. Martins Press, New York, 2002.

11) Cited in Wheeler, H.B. Shattuck Lecture-Healing and Heroism. N Eng J of Med 322:1540-48, 1990.

12) Cited in Manning PR, DeBakey L. Medicine: Preserving the Passion. New York, Springer –Verlag; 1987.

13) Joubert J. Pensées, 1842.

14) Jolly P. Medical School Tuition and Young Physicians' Indebtedness. Health Affairs 2005; 24: 527-535.

15) Morrison G. Mortgaging our Future – The Cost of Medical Education. N Engl J Med 2005: 352; 117-119.

16) Cooke M, Irby DM, Sullivan W, Ludmerer KM. American Medical Education 100 years After the Flexner Report. N Engl J Med 2006: 355; 1339-44.

17) Osler W. Counsels and Ideals from the Writings of William Osler. Boston: Houghton Mifflin, 1905, p. 129.

18) Spence J. The Need for Understanding the Individual as Part of the Training and Function of Doctors and Nurses. [Speech delivered at a conference on mental health held in March 1949]. In: The Purpose and Practice of Medicine: Selections from the Writings of Sir James Spence. London: Oxford University Press; 1960, p 273-4.

19) Report to the American Medical Association's Judicial Council, June 1930. IN: Lasagna L. The Doctors' Dilemma. Harper & Brothers: New York, 1962.

20) Mayo, M.D., W. The Medical Profession and the Public. Presented at the opening of the Cleveland Clinic, February 26, 1921. JAMA 76;921-25, 1921.

21) Presented at the opening of the Cleveland Clinic, February 26,1921.

22) Condensed excerpt from speech by George W. Crile, M.D., at the opening of the Cleveland Clinic, February 1921; quotation edited by William E. Lower, M.D. in the program for the Clinic's 25th anniversary ceremony, February 24-25, 1946).

23) Kovner AR. Improving the Effectiveness of Hospital Governing Boards. Frontiers of Health Services Management 1985: 2 (1); 4-33.

24) Bunts AT, Crile, Jr. G, (eds). To Act as A Unit. The Story of the Cleveland Clinic. Published by The Cleveland Clinic, 1971, page xii.

25) Wyngaarden JB. The Clinical Investigator as an Endangered Species. N Engl J Med. 1979; 301:1254-1259.

26) Nathan DG, Wilson JD. Clinical Research and the NIH—A Report Card. N Engl J Med. 2003;349:1860-1865.

27) Rosenberg L. Medicine: Physician-Scientists—Endangered and Essential. Science, 1999; 283:331-332.

28) Ley TJ, Rosenberg LE: The Physician-Scientist Career Pipeline in 2005. Build It, and They Will Come. JAMA 2005: 294: 1342-1351.

29) Neilson EG: The Role of Medical School Admission Committees in the Decline of Physician-Scientists. J Clin Invest 2003; 111: 765-767.

30) Wang S. Cleveland Clinic's Medical School to Offer Tuition-Free Education: Move Seeks to Spur Students' Interest in Academic Careers. Wall Street Journal, May 15, 2008, p. D3.

31) Feuer M. The Dreaded Annual Performance Review. Not a Time for Retribution But a Roadmap for the Future. Smart Business Magazine and SBN Online, May 2006.

32) al-Sihhah FT, 'anh_ M. Moses Maimonides' Two Treatises on the Regimen of Health. Translated from the Arabic and edited in accordance with the Hebrew and Latin versions by Bar-Sela A, Hoff HE, Faris E. Trans Amer Philosophical Soc 1964: 54 (4); 3-50; p. 21.

33) Ludmerer KM. Chapter Sixteen. Internal Malaise. Time to Heal. American Medical Education from the Turn of the Century to the Era of Managed Care. Oxford University Press 1999, p. 331.

34) Goldsmith J. Hospitals and Physicians: Not a Pretty Picture. Health Affairs 2007: 26 (1); w72-w75.

35) Reinhardt U. The Economics of For-Profit and Not-For-Profit Hospitals. Health Affairs 2000; 19 (6); 178-186.

36) Fleishman JL. The Foundation. A Great American Secret. How Private Wealth is Changing the World. Public Affairs, New York, 2007, p. 16.

37) Strome S. Big Gifts, Tax Breaks, and a Debate on Charity. New York Times, September 6, 2007.

38) Cited in Johnson P. A History of the American People. HarperCollins Publishers, 1998, p. 555.

39) Attributed to Yogi Berra in Novak M: Business as a Calling. Work in the Examined Life. The Free Press, New York, NY, 1996.

40) The Modest Visionary. Time Magazine, May 23, 1960

41) Haderlein J. Can You Bank on Philanthropy? Health Care Financial Management. May 2006, 102-105.

42) DeMaria AN. Philanthropy and Medicine. JACC 2006: 48; 1725-26.

43) Milligan S. Puckoon. London:Blond; 1963; Chapter 6, p. 69. .

44) Envisioning the Future of Academic Health Centers. Final Report of the Commonwealth Fund Task Force on Academic Health Centers 2003.

45) Healy B. Medicine, the Art. U.S. News & World Report, July 15, 2007.

CHAPTER 4: HEALTHCARE TRENDS, POLICIES AND PROPOSED REFORMS

1) Emmott B. 20:21 Vision. Twentieth-Century Lessons for the Twenty-First Century. Farrar, Straus and Giroux, New York, 2003.

2) Stevens R. In Sickness and in Wealth: American Hospitals in the Twentieth Century. The Johns Hopkins University Press, Baltimore, MD, 1999, p. 365.

3) Peterson PG. Will America Grow Up Before It Grows Old? Random House, New York 1996, p. 82.

4) Caudon D. Price of Seniors' Care to Soar as Boomers Age. USA Today, February 14, 2008.

5) Walker DM. America at a Crossroad. Vital Speeches of the Day 2006: 72 (26): 258.

6) Henry WA. In Defense of Elitism. Chapter One. The Vital Lie. Anchor Books Doubleday, NY, 1995, p. 12.

7) Brook Y. The Right Vision of Health Care. Forbes, January 2008.

8) Newhouse JP. An Iconoclastic View of Cost Containment. Health Affairs 1993: 12 (Supp 1): 152-171.

9) Emanuel EJ, Fuchs, VR. The Perfect Storm of Overutilization. JAMA 2008: 299 (23): 2789-2791.

10) Peterson PG. Running on Empty. How the Democratic and Republic Parties are Bankrupting our Future and What Americans Can Do About It. Farrar, Straus and Giroux, New York, 2004, p. 115.

11) Morgan PC. Chapter 1: Health Care Spending: Past Trends and Projections. Congressional Research Services, The Library of Congress, Washington, DC., 2004.

12) Poisal JA, Truffer C, Smith S, et al. Health Spending Projections Through 2016: Modest Changes Obscure Part D's Impact. Health Affairs 2007: 26 (2); w242-w253.

13) Orszag PR, Ellis P. The Challenge of Rising Health Care Costs. A View from the Congressional Budget Office. N Engl J Med 2007: 357; 1793-95.

14) Lubitz J, Beebe J, Baker C. Longevity and Medicare Expenditures. N Eng J Med 1995: 332; 999-1003.

15) Pear R. States Differ Widely in Spending on Health Care, Study Finds. New York Times, September 18, 2007.

16) Hall RE, Jones CI. The Value of Life and the Rise in Health Spending. Quarterly Journal of Economics 2007: Feb. (1); 39-72.

17) Cutler DM, McClellan M. Is Technology Change in Medicine Worth It? Health Affairs 2001: 20 (5); 11-29.

18) Murphy KM, Topel RH. Measuring the Gains from Medical Research. An Economic Approach. The University of Chicago Press, Chicago, IL, 2003, p. 4.

19) Marmot MG. Status Syndrome. The Challenge of Medicine. JAMA 2006: 295 (11); 1304-06.

20) White C. Why Did Medicare Spending Growth Slow Down? Health Affairs 2008: 27 (3); 793-802.

21) Eugene McCarthy. *Time* Magazine, February 12, 1979.

22) Averch H, Johnson L. Behavior of the Firm under Regulatory Constraint. American Economic Review 1962: 52; 1052-69.

23) Wattenberg BJ. The Good News is the Bad News is Wrong. AEI Press, Washington, D.C., 1995, p 174.

24) Drucker P, Dyson E, Handy C, Saffo P, Senge PM. Looking Ahead: Implications of the Present. Harvard Business Review 1997: 75 (15); 18-32.

25) He W, Sengupta M, Velkoff VA, DeBarros KA. U.S. Census Bureau, Current Populations Reports, P23-209, 65+ in the United States: 2005. U.S. Government Printing Office, Washington, D.C., 2005.

26) Spillman BC, Lubitz J. The Effect of Longevity on Spending for Acute and Long-Term Care. N Engl J Med. 2000: 342(19); 1409-1415.

27) Minkler M, Fuller-Thompson E, Guralnik JM. Gradient of Disability Across Socioeconomic Spectrum in the United States. N Engl J Med 2006: 355 (7); 695-703.

28) DeRose K, Escarce J, Lurie N. Immigrants and Health Care: Sources of Vulnerability. Health Affairs 2007: 26 (5); 1258-68.

29) Mohanty SA, Woolhandler S, Himmelstein DU, Pati S, Carrasquillo O, Bor DH. Health Care Expenditures of Immigrants in the United States: A Nationally Representative Analysis. Am J Public Health 2005: 95; 1431-8.

30) Goldman DP, Smith JP, Sood N. Immigrants and the Cost of Medical Care. Health Affairs 2006: 25 (6); 1700-11.

31) The Commonwealth Fund Commission on a High Performance Health System. Framework for a High Performance Health System for the United States. New York. August 2006.

32) Mankiw NG. Beyond Those Health Care Numbers. New York Times, November 4, 2007.

33) Thorpe KE, et al. The Impact of Obesity on Rising Medical Spending. Health Affairs 2004: 23; w480–w486 (published online 20 October 2004; 10.1377/hlthaff.w4.480.

34) Weissman JS. The Trouble with Uncompensated Hospital Care. N Engl J Med 2005: 352 (12); 1171-73.

35) Dobson A, DaVanzo J, Sen N. The Cost-Shift Payment 'Hydraulic': Foundation, History, and Implications. Health Affairs 2006: 25 (1); 22-33.

36) Iglehart JK. Improving Tomorrow's Health Care with Today's Tools: A Conversation with Larry C. Glasscock. Health Affairs 2006: 26 (1); w13-w21 (web exclusive).

37) Gold M. Commercial Health Insurance: Smart or Simply Lucky? Health Affairs 2006: 25 (6); 1490-93.

38) Geyman JP. Health Care in America: Can Our Ailing System Be Healed? Butterworth Heinmann, Boston, MA, 2001, p. 256.

39) Lawrence D. Bridging the Quality Chasm IN: Building a Better Delivery System. A New Engineering/Health Care Partnership. National Academy of Engineering, Institute of Medicine, National Academies Press, Washington, D.C., 2005, p. 100.

40) Sox HC. Leaving (Internal) Medicine. Ann Int Med 2006: 144; 57-58.

41) Bodenheimer T. Primary Care—Will It Survive? N Eng J Med 2006: 355 (9); 861-64.

42) Lynge DC, Larson EH, Thompson MJ, Rosenblatt RA, Hart LG. A Longitudinal Analysis of the General Surgery Workforce in the United States 1981-2005. Arch of Surg 2008: 143; 345-350.

43) Cannon MF, Tanner MD. Healthy Competition: What's Holding Back Health Care and How to Free It. Cato Institute, Washington, DC, 2005, pp. 91-92.

44) Anderson G, Frogner B, Reinhardt U. Health Spending in OECD Countries in 2004: An Update. Health Affairs 2007: 26 (5): 1481-89.

45) Reinhardt U, Hussey PS, Anderson GF. U.S. Health Care Spending in an International Context. Health Affairs 2004: 23; 11-12.

46) Donahue TJ. The State of American Business. U.S. Chamber of Commerce, 2007.

47) McKinsey Global Institute. Accounting for the Cost of Health Care in the United States. January 2007, p. 11.

48) Mandel M. What's Really Propping Up the Economy. Business Week, September 25, 2006.

49) American College of Physicians, Achieving a High Performance Health Care System with Universal Access: What the United States Can Learn from Other Countries. Ann Inter Med 2008; 148; 55-75.

50) Goodson JD. Unintended Consequences of Resource-Based Relative Value Scale Reimbursement. JAMA 2007: 298 (19); 2308-2310.

51) Phillips RL, Dodoo M, Jaén CR, Green LA. COGME's 16th Report to Congress: Too Many Physicians Could Be Worse Than Wasted. Ann Family Med 2005: 3 (3); 268-70.

52) Iglehart JK. Grassroots Activism and the Pursuit of an Expanded Physician Supply. Health Policy Report. N Engl J Med 2008: 358 (16): 1741-49.

53) Iglehart JK, Ibid.

54) Kane CK. Physician Marketplace Report, 2001. American Medical Association, Chicago, IL, 2002.

55) Steiger B. Survey Results: Doctors Say Morale is Hurting. Physician Executive 2006: 32 (6); 6-15.

56) McGlynn EA, Asch SM, Adams J. et al. The Quality of Health Care Delivered to Adults in the United States. N Eng J Med 2003: 348 (26); 2635-45.

57) Asch SM, Kerr EA, Keesey J, et al. Who Is At Greatest Risk for Receiving Poor Quality Healthcare? N Engl J Med 2006: 354 (11):1147-56.

58) Evans JP. Health Care in the Age of Genetic Medicine. JAMA 2007: 298 (22); 2670-72.

59) Wennberg JE, Cooper MM, Bubolz TA, Fisher EF, et al. The Dartmouth Atlas of Healthcare 1996. American Hospital Publishing, Inc., Chicago, IL, 1996.

60) Wennberg JE, Fisher ES, Goodman DC, Skinner JS. Tracking the Care of Patients with Severe Chronic Illness. The Dartmouth Atlas of Healthcare, 2008. The Dartmouth Institute for Health Policy and Clinical Practice, 2008.

61) Yarnall KS, Pollak KI, Østbye T, Krause KM, Michener JL. Primary Care: Is There Enough Time for Prevention? Am J Public Health. 2003: 93(4); 635-641.

62) Kagan R. Adversarial Legalism. The American Way of Law. Harvard University Press, 2001, p. 27.

63) Levene P. Risk and the Global Economy. Speech delivered to Los Angeles Town Hall, September 15, 2003.

64) Mohr JC. American Medical Malpractice Litigation in Historical Perspective. JAMA 2000: 283(13); 1731-1737.

65) Hickson GB, Federspiel CF, Pichert JW. Patient Complaints and Malpractice Risk. JAMA 2003: 287(22); 2951-2957.

66) Howard PK. A Case of Medical Justice. The Philadelphia Inquirer, May 16, 2004.

67) Tillinghast-Towers Perrin, U.S. Tort Costs and Cross-Border Perspectives: 2005 update. Towers Perrin, 2006, p. 20.

68) Guardado J. Policy Research Perspectives: Professional Medical Liability Insurance Indemnity and Expense Payments, 1997-2006. American Medical Association. December 2007.

69) Gallagher TH, Studdert D, Levinson W. Disclosing Harmful Medical Errors to Patients. N Eng J Med 2007: 356: 2713-19.

70) France M, Woellert L, Mandel MJ. How to Fix the Tort System. Business Week, 3/14/05: Issue 3924, p. 70-78.

71) Carter T. Tort Reform Texas Style. New Laws and Med-Mal Damage Caps Devistate Plaintiff and Defense Firms Alike. ABA Journal, 07470088, October 2006: 92 (10); 30-36.

72) Kane CK, Emmons DW. Policy Research Perspectives: The Impact of Caps on Damages. How are Markets for Medical Liability Insurance and Medical Services Affected? American Medical Association. December 2005

73) Waters TM, Budetti PP, Claxton G, Lundy JP. Impact of State Tort Reforms on Physician Malpractice Payments. Health Affairs 2007: 26 (2); 500-509.

74) Schwartz, GT. Product Liability and Medical Malpractice in Comparative Context. IN: The Liability Maze, Peter W. Huber and Robert E. Litan, Eds., Brookings Institution Press, New York, (1991) p. 64.

75) Mello MM, Studdert DM, Kachalia AB, Brennan TA. Health Courts and Accountability for Patient Safety. The Milbank Quarterly 2006: 84 (3): 459-92.

76) Howard PK. Strong Medicine. Wall Street Journal, January 6, 2007.

77) Manchester W. The Last Lion. Winston Spencer Churchill, Visions of Glory. Little Brown & Co., 1983.

78) Stevens R. In Sickness and In Wealth. Basic Books, New York, 1989, p. 355.

79) Mathews M. Cost Control for Dummies, The Wall Street Journal, August 15, 2007.

80) Keen J, Light D, Mays N. Public-Private Relations in Health Care. The King's Fund: London, England, 2001, Table 2.6-7.

81) Newhouse JP, Reischauer RD. The Institute of Medicine Committee's Clarion Call for Universal Coverage. Health Affairs 2004, Web Exclusive (W4): 179-183.

82) Black D. et al., Inequalities in Health: Report of a Research Working Group. London: Department of Health and Social Security, 1980.

83) Kolata G. A Surprising Secret to a Long Life: Stay in School. The New York Times, January 3, 2007.

84) Gerena-Morales R. U.S. Needs A New Prescription to Slow Health-Care Spending. Wall Street Journal, March 6, 2006.

85) Feachem RGA, Sekhri NK, White KL. "Getting More for Their Dollar: A Comparison of the NHS with California's Kaiser Permanente," Brit Med J 2002: 324; 135-43.

86) Goodman JC. Health Care in A Free Society. Rebutting the Myths of National Health Insurance. Policy Analysis No. 532, 2005.

87) Porter ME, Teisberg EO. How Physicians Can Change the Future of Health Care. JAMA 2007: 297 (10); 1103-11.

88) Fisher JE. Our Health Care System: Where Are We Going? Bull Am Coll Surg 2000; 85 (3): 25-27, 42.

89) Feldstein M. Balancing the Goals of Health Care Provision and Financing. Health Affairs 2006: 25 (6); 1603-11.

90) Hoff JS. Improving the System for Delivering Subsidies: Cap or Scrap the Exclusion? IN. Empowering Health Care Consumers Through Tax Reform. Grace-Marie Arnett, Ed. The University of Michigan Press, 1999, p. 93.

91) Hoff JS. Ibid.

92) Emanuel EJ, Fuchs VR. Who Really Pays for Health Care? The Myth of "Shared Responsibility". JAMA 2008: 299 (9); 1057-59.

93) Health Care Costs: A Primer. The Kaiser Family Foundation, August 8, 2007.

94) Burtless G. Healthcare Consumption and the Relative Well-Being of the Aged. Presented at 10th Annual Joint Conference of the Retirement Research Consortium "Determinants of Retirement Security" August 7-8, 2008, Washington, D.C.

95) Emanuel EJ. The Cost-Coverage Tradeoff. "It's Health Care Costs, Stupid" JAMA 2008: 299 (8); 947-49.

96) Dorn S. Uninsured and Dying Because of It: Updated the Institute of Medicine Analysis on the Impact of Uninsurance on Mortality. Urban Institute. January 2008, pp. 1-8; Institute of Medicine. Care Without Coverage: Too Little, Too Late. Washington, D.C.: Institute of Medicine; 2002.

97) Mechanic D, Tanner J. Vulnerable People, Groups and Populations: Societal View. Health Affairs 2007: 26 (5): 1220-30.

98) Statement of Leonard E. Burman, Senior Fellow, Urban Institute, Before the United States Senate Committee on Finance. Taking a Checkup on the Nation's Health Care Tax Policy: A Prognosis. March 8, 2006, p. 12.

99) DeNavas-Walt C, Proctor BD, Smith J. U.S. Census Bureau, Current Population Reports, P60-233, Income, Poverty, and Health Insurance Coverage in the United States: 2006. U.S. Government Printing Office, Washington, DC, 2007, p. 20.

100) Goodman JC. Employer-Sponsored, Personal, and Portable Health Insurance, Health Affairs 2006: 25 (6): 1556-66.

101) Franklin D. Roosevelt address at Oglethorpe University, May 22, 1932.

102) Steinbrook R. Health Care Reform in Massachusetts—Expanding Coverage, Escalating Costs. N Engl J Med 2008: 358; 2757-63.

103) Weller CD. Two Front Health Care Solution: The Patient Teams Payment Model. Presented at HHS Conference. The Role of Employers and the Workforce in Transforming Health Care. December 11, 2008, Washington, D.C.

104) Thurow LC. Medicine Versus Economics. N Engl J Med 1985: 313 (10); 611-614.

105) Blackwell RD, Williams TE, et al. Consumer-Driven Health Care, Book Publishing Assoc., 2005, p. 127.

106) Cogan JF, Hubbard RG, Kessler DP. Healthy, Wealthy and Wise. Five Steps to a Better Health Care System. AEI Press, Hoover Institution, 2005.

107) Brook RH. Ware Jr. JE, Rogers WH, Keeler EB, et al. Does Free Care Improve Adults' Health? Results From A Randomized Controlled Trial. N Engl J Med 1983: 309; 1426-34.

108) Lohr KN, Brook RH, Kamberg CJ, et al. Effect of Cost-Sharing on Use of Medically Effective And Less Effective Care. Med Care 1986; 24 (9); S31-38.

109) Newhouse JP. Free-for-All. Lessons from the RAND Health Insurance Experiment. Harvard University Press 1996.

110) Lohr KN, Brook RH, Kamberg CJ, et al. ibid.

111) Tanner M. Individual Mandates for Health Insurance. Slippery Slope to National Health Care. Policy Analysis No. 565, April 5, 2006.

CHAPTER 5: THE BUSINESS OF MEDICINE

1) Rettenmaier AJ, Saving TR. Medicare Reform. Issues and Answers. The Bush School Series in the Economics of Public Policy. The University of Chicago Press. 1999. Chapter 9. Paying for Medicare in the Twenty-first Century. p. 184.

2) Exceptional Returns: The Economic Value of America's Investment in Medical Research. Mark Hatfield, Hugo F. Sonnenschein, and Leon E. Rosenberg for *Funding First,* May 2001, p. 2.

3) Cutler DM, Berndt ER. Medical Care Output and Productivity, Chicago: Univ of Chicago Press, 2001.

4) Lichtenberg FR. The Impact of New Drug Launches on Longevity: Evidence from Longitudinal, Disease-Level Data from 52 Countries, 1982-2001. NBER Working Paper no. 9754, June 2003, p. 21, http://www.nberorg/papers/w9754.

5) Cutler DM, Rosen AB, Vijan S. The Value of Medical Spending in the United States, 1960 – 2000, N Engl J Med 355:920-926, 2006.

6) Manton KG, Gu X. Changes in the Prevalence of Chronic Disability in the United States Black and Non-Black Population Above Age 65 from 1982-1999, Proc Natl Acad Sci, USA 2001; 98: 6354-9.

7) Pham HH, Schrag D, O'Malley AS. Care Patterns in Medicare and Their Implications for Pay-for-Performance. N Engl J Med 2007: 356; 1130-39.

8) Bach PB. How Many Doctors Does It Take To Treat a Patient. Wall Street Journal, June 21, 2007, p. A17.

9) Beasley JW, Hankey TH, Erickson R, et al. How Many Problems Do Family Physicians Manage At Each Encounter? Ann Fam Med. 2004;2(5): 405-410.

10) Boyd CM, Darer J, Boult C, et al. Clinical Practice Guidelines and Quality of Care for Older Patients with Multiple Comorbid Diseases. JAMA. 2005;294(6):716-724.

11) Goodson JD. Unintended Consequences of Resource-Based Relative Value Scale Reimbursement. JAMA 2007; 298 (19): 2308-2310.

12) Bigelow B, Arndt M. The More Things Change, The More They Stay the Same. Health Care Management Review. Winter 2000;25(1):65-72.

13) Selected Economic Writings of William J. Baumol, edited by Bailey EE, New York University Press, 1976.

14) Baumol W. Economic Theory and Operations Analysis. Prentice-Hall, Inc., Englewood Cliffs, NJ, 1977; 501-506.

15) Angell M. The Doctor as A Double Agent. Kennedy Inst Ethics J 1993; 3:279-86.

16) Sowell T. Basic Economics: A Common Sense Guide to the Economy. Basic Books, 2007.

17) Palank J. Hospitals Face Financial Squeeze. Wall Street Journal, May 1, 2008.

18) Economic Report of the President. Washington: Government Printing Office, 2004, p. 192.

19) Kelley E, Hurst J. "Health Care Quality Indicators Project: Initial Indicators Report," OECD Health Working Papers no. 22, March 2006.

20) Ohsfeldt RL, Schneider JE. The Business of Health. The Role of Competition, Markets and Regulation. The AEI Press. Washington, D.C., 2006.

21) Schoen CR, Osborn R, et al. Toward Higher-Performance Health Systems: Adults' Health Care Experiences In Seven Countries. 2007, Health Affairs Web Exclusives (October 31). http://www.healthaffairs.org.

22) Hussey PS, Anderson GF, Osborn R, Feek C, McLaughlin V, Millar J, Epstein A. How Does the Quality of Care Compare in Five Countries. Health Affairs 2004: 23 (3); 89-99.

23) Clifton J, Gingrich N. Are Citizens of the World Satisfied with Their Health? Health Affairs 2007: 26 (5): w545-w551.

24) Kelley E. and Hurst J., Ibid.

25) Drucker P. People and Performance: The Best of Peter Drucker on Management. Harvard Business School Publishing Corp., 2007, p. 24.

26) Collins J. Good to Great and the Social Sectors: A Monograph to Accompany Good to Great, HarperCollins 2005.

27) Hamel G. Management à la Google, Wall Street Journal. April 26, 2006.

28) Dodd D, Favaro K. Managing the Right Tension. Harvard Business Review, December 2006, Vol. 84, pp. 62-75.

29) Grove A. Efficiency in Health Care Industries: A View from the Outside. Rotman Magazine, Winter 2006, 58-61.

30) Dick RS, Steen EB, Detmer DE. The Computer-Based Patient Record. An Essential Technology for Health Care (revised edition). National Academy of Press, Washington, D.C., 1997.

31) Hwang J, Christensen CM. Disruptive Innovation in Healthcare Delivery: A Framework for Business-Model Innovation. Health Affairs 2008: 27 (5); 1329-1335.

32) Cited in Kostelanetz R. Beyond Left and Right: Radical Thoughts for Our Times. William Morrow & Co., New York, 1968.

33) Stead WW, Starmer JM. Practical Frontline Challenges to Moving Beyond the Expert – Based Practice. Presented at the 2007 Annual Meeting of the Institute of Medicine. The National Academies.

34) Schoen C, Osborn R, Huynh PT, Doty M, Peugh J, Zapert K. On the Front Lines of Care: Primary Care Doctors' Office Systems, Experiences, and Views in Seven Countries. Health Affairs 2006: 25; w555-71.

35) Wilson JF. Lessons for Health Care Could Be Found Abroad. Ann of Int Med 2007:146 (6); 473-76.

36) Mandl KD, Kohane IS. Tectonic Shifts in the Health Information Economy. N Engl J Med 358:1732-37, 2008.

37) Survey Finds Americans Want Electronic Personal Health Information To Improve Own Health Care. November 2006. Lake Research Partners and American Viewpoint. Connecting for Health, Markle Foundation News Release, http://www.markle.org/downloadable_assets/research_doc_120706.pdf.

38) Bergeson SC, Dean JD. A Systems Approach to Patient—Centered Care, JAMA, Dec 20, 2006, 296:2848-51.

39) Gearon CJ. Perspectives on the Future of Personal Health Records, prepared for California HealthCare Foundation, ihealthreports, June 2007.

40) Kaiser Permanente Puts Personal Health Record Front and Center, Kaiser press release, November 6, 2007.

41) Blackwell RD, Williams TE, et al. Consumer-Driven Health Care, Book Publishing Assoc., 2005, p. 64.

42) Vital Signs Health Law Monthly; IRS issues guidance on hospital physician EHR relationships; a publication of the Health Practice Group of Dorsey and Whitney, LLP, June 2007.

43) Stead WW, Patel NR, Starmer JM. Closing the Loop in Practice to Assure the Desired Performance. Trans Am Clin Climatol Assoc 2008: Vol.119; 185-195.

44) Stead WW, Starmer JM. Ibid, 2007.

45) Smith M, Feied C. 10 Rules of Data Learned from Building a Clinical Information System: Violating Conventional Wisdom. Presentation at National Institutes of Health Biomedical Computing Interest Group, 8 November 2007.

46) Blackstone EH. Generating Knowledge from Information Data and Analysis. IN: Kouchoukos NT, Blackstone EH, Doty DB, Hanley FL, Karp RB. Kirklin/Barratt-Boyes Cardiac Surgery, 3rd ed, Philadelphia: Churchill Livingstone, 2003.

47) Hammer D, Franklin D. Beyond Bolt-Ons: Breakthroughs in Revenue Cycle Information Systems. Healthcare Financial Management 2008: February; 53-59.

48) Carr NG. Does it Matter? Information Technology and the Corrosion of Competitive Advantage. Harvard Business School Press, 2004.

49) Carr NG. The Big Switch. W.W. Norton, 2008.

50) Moody's Analyzes Typical Behaviors of Defaulted Not-For-Profit Hospitals. The Advisory Board, Finance Watch, January 2008.

51) Herzlinger RE. Why Innovation in Health Care is So Hard, Harvard Business Review: 2006; 84(5); 58-66.

52) Enthoven AC, Tollen LA. Toward a 21st Century Health System: The Contributions and Promise of Prepaid Group Practice. San Francisco, Calif., Jossey-Bass, 2004.

53) Enthoven AC, Tollen LA. Competition in Healthcare: It Takes Systems to Pursue Quality and Efficiency. Health Affairs Web Exclusive, September 7, 2005: w5-420-432.

54) Porter ME, Teisberg EO. Redefining Health Care, Creating Value-Based Competition on Results, Harvard Business School Press, 2006.

55) Thorpe KE, Howard DH. The Rise in Spending Among Medicare Beneficiaries: The Role of Chronic Disease Prevalence and Changes in Treatment Intensity, Health Affairs 25 (2006): w378-w388 (published online 22 August 2006; 10.1377/hlthaff.25w378).

56) Supreme Court Justice Sandra Day O'Connor, speech to the National Coalition for Cancer Survivorship, November 3, 1994.

57) Wennberg JE, et al. The Dartmouth Atlas of Health Care 2006: The Care of Patients with Severe Chronic Illness. An Online Report on the Medicare Program by the Dartmouth Atlas Project. The Dartmouth Institute for Health Policy and Clinical Practice, 2006, p. 33

58) Wennberg JE, et al. The Dartmouth Atlas of Health Care 2008: Tracking the Care of Patients with Severe Chronic Illness. The Dartmouth Institute for Health Policy and Clinical Practice, 2008

59) Cortese D, Smoldt R. Taking Steps Towards Integration. Health Affairs 2007: 26 (1); w68-w71.

60) Brown G. State and Market: Towards a Public Interest Test. Speech delivered by the Chancellor of the Exchequer, Gordon Brown, to the Social Market Foundation at the Cass Business School, February 3, 2003.

61) Bender MW, Van Kuiken SJ. IT Remedies for US Health Care: An Interview with WellPoint's Leonard Schaeffer. The McKinsey Quarterly. January 16, 2006.

62) Friedman M. "How to Cure Health Care," The Public Interest 142 (Winter 2001): 8-9, http://www.thepublicinterest.com/archives/2001winter/article1.html.

63) Monheit AC. Persistence in Health Expenditures in the Short Run: Prevalence and Consequences. Medical Care 2003: 41 (7) (Suppl III); III-56.

64) Rosenthal MB. Nonpayment for Performance? Medicare's New Reimbursement Rule. Perspective. N Engl J Med 2007, 357;16.

65) Graves N, McGowan JE. Nosocomial Infection, The Deficit Reduction Act and Incentives for Hospitals. JAMA 2008: 300; 1577-79.

66) Reinhardt U. The Pricing of U.S. Hospital Services: Chaos Behind a Veil of Secrecy. Health Affairs 25, (1) (2006): 57-69.

67) Chang JT, et al., Patients' Global Ratings of Their Health Care Are Not Associated with the Technical Quality of Their Care. Annals of Internal Medicine, Vol. 144, No. 9, May 2006, pp. 665-672.

CHAPTER 6: STRATEGIC PLANNING

1) Viscount Horatio Nelson correspondence with Lady Emma Hamilton and others, Ms Eng 196.5 (84), 31 July 1801. Houghton Library, Harvard University.

2) Lord John Browne, former chief executive officer of BP, speech delivered at Stanford University (2001).

3) Allison M, Kaye J. Strategic Planning For Nonprofit Organizations. A Practical Guide And Workbook. 2nd edition. John Wiley & Sons, Inc., Hoboken, New Jersey, 2005.

4) Oster SM. Modern Competitive Analysis. 2nd edition, Oxford University Press, 1994.

5) Beinhocker ED, Kaplan S. Tired of Strategic Planning? McKinsey & Co., 2002, Special Edition: Risk and Resilience.

6) Barry S. Sternlicht. Cited in Wademan D. The Best Advice I Ever Got. Harvard Business Review 2005: 83 (1); 35-44.

7) Lovallo DP, Mendonca LT. Strategy's Strategist. An Interview with Richard Rumelt. The McKinsey Quarterly 2007: 4; 56-67..

8) Nattermann PM. Best Practice ≠ Best Strategy. The McKinsey Quarterly May 2000: 2; 22-31.

9) Drucker P. Management: Tasks, Responsibilities, Practices, Rev. Ed. 1973, NY, Harper Perennial 1993.

10) Ballmer S. Can Win. Can Win 2001 Conference, Toronto, May 2, 2001.

11) Herb Kelleher. Letter to employees of Southwest Airlines Co., 1990. Cited in Stalk G. and Lachenauer R. Hardball: Five Killer Strategies for Trouncing the Competition. Harvard Business Review, Vol. 82, No. 4, April 2004.

12) Attributed to Clarence Darrow (not Charles Darwin).

13) Muller S. Universities in the Twenty-First Century. Berghahn: Providence, Rhode Island, 1996.

14) Mintzberg H. Crafting Strategy. Harvard Business Review 1987: 65; 66-75.

15) Henderson B. The Logic of Business Strategy, HarperBusiness, NY (new ed), 1986.

16) Barney JB, Clark DN. Resource-Based Theory: Creating and Sustaining Competitive Advantage. Oxford University Press, 2007.

17) Hagstrom R. The Warren Buffett Way. John Wiley & Sons, Inc., Hoboken, New Jersey, 2005.

18) Menniger WJ. Hope and Morale: Critical Elements In Organizational Function presented at the American Psychiatric Association Administrative Psychiatry Lecture, May 6, 1922.

19) Porter ME. Competitive Advantage: Creating and Sustaining Superior Performance. Free Press, New York, 1985, p. 12.

20) Modified from Harrington RJ, Tjan AK. Transforming Strategy One Customer at a Time. Harvard Business Review 2008: 86 (3); 62-72.

21) Drucker PF. Ibid. p. 128.

22) Alfred P. Sloan. Cited in Chatterjee S, Corts K, Ghemawat P, Pisano G, Porter ME, Rivkin JW. Competitive Strategy. Business Fundamentals from Harvard Business School Publishing. HBS No. 1520, 1997.

23) Arrow KJ. I Know a Hawk From A Handsaw. Cited in M. Szenberg, Eminent Economists. Their Life Philosophies. Cambridge University Press, NY, 1993, p. 47.

24) Carroll PB, Mui C. 7 Ways to Fail Big. Harvard Business Review 2008; 86 (9); 82-91.

25) Kim WC, Mauborgne R. Strategy, Value Innovation, and The Knowledge Economy. MIT Sloan Management Review 1999: 40 (3); 41-54.

26) Kay J. Foundations of Corporate Success. How Business Strategies Add Value. Oxford University Press, 1993.

27) Fagerberg J, Mowery DC, Nelson RR. The Oxford Handbook of Innovation. Oxford University Press, 2005.

28) Jeff Bezos. The Institutional Yes. Interview by Julie Kirby and Thomas A. Stewart. Harvard Business Review 2007: 85 (10); 74-82.

29) Kay J. Ibid.

30) Stalk Jr. G. and Haut TM. Competing Against Time. The Free Press, McMillan, Inc., 1990.

31) Kay J. Ibid.

32) Roxburgh C. Hidden Flaws in Strategy. The McKinsey Quarterly, 2: 2003.

33) Townsend D. Engaging the Board of Directors on Strategy. Strategy & Leadership, Vol. 35 Issue 5, 2007, pp. 24-28.

34) Stalk G. Five Future Strategies You Need Right Now. Harvard Business School Press, 2008.

35) de Geus A. Planning as Learning. Harvard Business Review 1988: 66 (2); 70-74.

36) Hand L. The Contribution of an Independent Judiciary to Civilization. Cited in The Spirit of Liberty 155, 155-65 (I. Dilliard ed), 1953.

37) Stalk G. Time – The Next Source of Competitive Advantage. Harvard Business Review 1988; 66 (4): 41-51.

38) Palter RN, Srinivasan D. Habits of the Busiest Acquirers. The McKinsey Quarterly, 2006; 4: 18-27.

39) Lewis JD. Partnerships in Profit: Structuring And Managing Strategic Alliances. The Free Press, New York, 1990.

40) Zuckerman HS, Kluzny AD. Alliances in Health Care: What We Know, What We Think We Know, and What We Should Know. Health Care Management Rev 1995: 20 (1); 54-64.

41) Hamel G. Leading the Revolution. How to Thrive in Turbulent Times By Making Innovation a Way of Life. Harvard Business School Press, Boston, MA, 2002, p. 41.

42) Porter ME. Competitive Strategy. Techniques for Analyzing Industries and Competitors. The Free Press, NY, 1980, p. 98.

43) Stadler C. The Four Principals of Enduring Success. Harvard Business Review 2007: 85 (7/8); 62-72.

44) Fraser CH, Strickland WL. When Organization Isn't Enough. The McKinsey Quarterly 2006; 1; 9-11.

45) General Douglas MacArthur, to the Joint Chiefs of Staff, August 1950.

CHAPTER 7: OPERATIONAL MANAGEMENT

1) Drucker P. Management: Tasks, Responsibilities, Practices, Rev. ed. 1973; Repr., NY: Harper Perennial, 1993.

2) Koch R. The 80 / 20 Principle: The Secret to Success by Achieving More With Less. CurrencyBook/Doubleday&Co.,Inc.,1999.

3) Ford H, Crowther S. My Life and Work. Doubleday, Page & Company. 1922.

4) Drucker PF. The Frontiers of Management: Where Tomorrows Decisions Are Being Shaped Today. HarperCollins, 1987.

5) Smith HA. Cited in Postman N. Now…This! (edited from Amusing Ourselves To Death, 1985). Penguin Books, NY. p. 99.

6) Drucker P. The Practice of Management, Harper and Brothers, New York, 1954, p. 11.

7) Simons R, Davila A. How High is Your Return on Management. Harvard Business Review 1998; 76 (1): 70-80.

8) Edmundson AC. The Competitive Imperative of Learning. Harvard Business Review 2008: 86 (7/8); 60-67

9) Collins J. Chapter 4. Confront the Brutal Facts (Yet Never Lose Faith). Good to Great. Why Some Companies Make the Leap…And Others Don't. Harper Business, New York, 2001, p. 72.

10) Gardner JW. The Role of the Leader. Health Care Forum Journal May-June, 1990, 31-34.

11) Dyer D. Interview with TRW's Frederick C. Crawford. Harvard Business Review 1991: 69(6); 114-126).

12) Selected Speeches of Frederick Coolidge Crawford. Edited by Christopher Johnson. Published privately, Cleveland, Ohio 1992, pp. 130-31.

13) Towers Perrin. Winning Strategies for Global Workplace. Executive Report, 2006.

14) Hamel G. The Future of Management. Harvard Business School Press, 2007, p. 57.

15) Kanter RM. Power Failure in Management Circuits. Harvard Business Review, July-August Harvard Business School Publishing 1979.

16) West African proverb. Part XII. Wisdom. IN: Peck MS. Abounding Grace. An Anthology of Wisdom. Ariel Books, Andrews McMeel Publishing, 1996, p. 258.

17) Heffernan M. Ten Habits of Incompetent Managers. Fast Company, October 2007.

18) Puranam P, Srikanth K. Seven Myths About Outsourcing. Wall Street Journal, July 16-17, 2007, p. R6.

19) Liker J. The Toyota Way. McGraw-Hill, 2003.

20) George J. Stigler of the University of Chicago after leaving a committee meeting. Cited in Sowell T. Knowledge and Decisions. Basic Books, NY, 1980, p. 24.

21) Top Spot in Sight, Toyotas' Not Slacking. Businessweek.com, Dec 13, 2006.

22) Watanabe K, Stuart TA, Raman AP. Lessons from Toyota's Long Drive. Harvard Business Review, 2007: 85(7/8); 74-83.

23) Takeuchi H, Osono E, Chimizu N. The Contradictions That Drive Toyota's Success. Harvard Business Review, 2008: 86(6): 96-104.

24) Schwarzkopf N. Cited in Reichheld F. Satisfaction. The False Path to Employee Loyalty. Harvard Business School Press, 2001, p. 166.

25) Olson MS, Van Bever D, Verry S. When Growth Stalls. Harvard Business Review 2008: 86(3); 50-61.

26) Slater R. Jack Welch & the GE Way. McGraw Hill, 1999, p. 117.

27) Roberts R, Frutos PW, Ciavarella GG, et al. Distribution of Variable Versus Fixed Costs of Hospital Care. JAMA 1999; 281: 644-49.

28) Linking Supply Costs and Revenue: The Time Has Come. Healthcare Financial Management 58 (5) (Special Section); 1-7, 2004.

29) Advisory Board, Inc. SpendCompass. http://www.advisory.com/members/default.asp?program=39&collectionid=1466

30) Seth Greenwald, D. Phil., personal communication.

31) Exploring RFID's Potential Value in Health Care. The Advisory Board, 2006.

32) Kaplan RS, Norton DP. The Balanced Scorecard Measures That Drive Performance. Harvard Business Review 1992: 70: 71-79).

33) Avoiding Financial Flashpoints, Lessons on Foreseeing (and Preventing) Dramatic Decline. The Advisory Healthcare Board. Washington, D.C., 2000.

34) Ferris T. The Whole Shebang. A State-of-the-Universe Report. Touchstone, New York, NY 1997, p. 94.

35) Senge PM. The Fifth Discipline. The Art and Practice of the Learning Organization. Doubleday Currency, 1990.

36) The Advisory Board Company. Facility Innovation Brief, Innovations Center. Hospital of the Future. Lessons for Inpatient Facility Planning and Strategy, 2007:

37) Naik G. To Reduce Errors, Hospitals Prescribe Innovative Designs. Wall Street Journal, May 8, 2006.

38) Mussbaum B. The Power of Design. BusinessWeek, May 17, 2004, p. 86.

39) Berry LL, Bendapudi N. Clueing in Customers. Harvard Business Review 2003: 81(2); February 2003. 100 106.

40) Reiling JG. Safe by Design: Designing Safety in Healthcare Facilities, Processes and Culture. Oakbrook, Ill., Joint Commission Resources, 2007.

41) Landro L. New Standards for Hospitals Call for Patients to Get Private Rooms. Wall Street Journal, March 22, 2006, p. A1.

42) Drucker PF. Management and the World's Work. Harvard Business Review 1988: Sept-Oct; 65-76.

CHAPTER 8: THE LEADERSHIP TEAM

1) Drucker P. There's More Than One Kind of Team. Wall Street Journal, February 11, 1992.

2) Wise H, Beckhard R, Rubin I, Kyte AL. Making Health Teams Work. Ballinger Publishing Co., Cambridge, MA, 1974.

3) Drucker PF. Managing the Non-Profit Organization. Principles and Practices. HarpersCollins, New York, 1990.

4) IN: Drucker P. The Essential Drucker. The Best Sixty Years of Peter Drucker's Essential Writings on Management. Collins, New York, 2003, p. 254.

5) Goodwin DK. Team of Rivals. The Political Genius of Abraham Lincoln. Simon & Schuster, New York, NY, 2005.

6) Stowe HB. Men of Our times; or Leading Patriots of the Day. University of Michigan, 1868 p. 110.

7) Drucker PF. Managing Oneself. Harvard Business Review 1999: 77 (2); 65-74.

8) Amabile TM. How to Kill Creativity. Harvard Business Review 1998: 76 (5): 76-87.

9) Crile G. George Crile: An Autobiography. Philadelphia: J.B. Lippincott Co., 1947. p. 344.

10) de Tocqueville A. Democracy in America: Translated by George Lawrence; Edited by J.P. Mayer, Harper Perennial Modern Classics, 2000, p. 629.

11) Bergdahl M. The Ten Rules of Sam Walton: Success Secrets for Remarkable Results. John Wiley & Sons, Inc., June 2006.

12) Herb E, Leslie K, Price C. Teamwork at the Top. The McKinsey Quarterly 2001: 2; 32-43.

13) Estafanous FG. Personal communication.

14) Katzenbach JR, Smith DK. The Wisdom of Teams: Creating the High Performance Organization. Harper-Collins, 1993, pp. 14-15.

15) Imai M. Kaizen: The Key to Japanese Competitive Success. New York: Random House, 1986.

16) Ross Perot, quoted in BusinessWeek, 6 October 1986.

17) Sowell T. Random Thoughts. Townhall.com February 25, 2004.

18) Needleman J, Buerhaus PI, Stewart M, Zelevinsky K, Mattke S. Nurse Staffing In Hospitals: Is There a Business Case for Quality? Health Affairs 2006; Vol. 25 (1); 204-21.

19) Steinbrook R. Nursing in the Crossfire. N Engl J Med 2002: 346; 1757-66.

20) Aiken L. 7 Myths About the Nursing Shortage, Health Affairs Blog, November 2006.

21) Salmon ME. Richard and Hilda Rosenthal Lecture 2007, Institute of Medicine of the National Academies, National Academy Press, Washington, D.C.

22) Pulley J. What Nurses Want. GHIT Notebook, March 13, 2008; Creating Technology Solutions for the Delivery of Patient Care. Robert Wood Johnson Foundation, March 2008.

23) Hendrich A, Chow MP, Skierczynski BA., Lu Z. A 36-Hospital Time and Motion Study: How Do Medical – Surgical Nurses Spend Their Time? The Permanente Journal 12:25-34. Summer 2008.

24) Pay-for-Performance Drives Importance of Healthy Finance-Nursing Relationship. The Advisory Board, Finance Watch, January 2008.

25) Tucker AL, Edmonson AC. Why Hospitals Don't Learn from Failures: Organizational and Psychological Dynamics that Inhibit System Change. California Management Review 2003: 45 (2): 55-72.

26) Ward D, Berkowitz B. Arching the Flood: How to Bridge the Gap Between Nursing Schools and Hospitals. Health Affairs 2002: 21 (5); 42-52.

27) Adair J. Effective Team Building. Pan McMillan, London 1986.

28) Wilde O. A Woman of No Importance. 1893.

29) Barker J. Agincourt. Little Brown & Co., NY, 2006, p. 51.

30) Cited by Robert Sobel, Past and Imperfect: History According to the Movies. Electronic News, Vol. 42, Issue 2124, p. 52. IN: Koch CG. The Science of Success. John Wiley & Sons, Inc., Hoboken, New Jersey, 2007.

31) Skarsten MO. George Drouillard of the Lewis and Clark Expedition and Fur Traders. 1807- The Arthur H. Clark Co., Glendale, CA, 1964.

32) U.S. Government Accountability Office, Medicare Physician Services. Washington, D.C.: U.S. Government Accountability Office, July 2006.

33) Osler W. A Way of life. IN: Franklin WF, ed., "A Way of Life" and Selected Writings of Sir William Osler. New York: Dover Publications, 1958.

34) Sides H. The Ghost Soldiers: The Forgotten Epic Story of World War II's Most Dramatic Mission. Knopf Publishing Group, May 2002.

35) Sharon A, Chanoff D. Warrior: An Autobiography. Simon & Schuster, 2001.

36) Adair J. Ibid.

37) Johann von Goethe IN: Maurois, A. The Art of Living. Harper & Brothers, 1940, p. 208.

38) Levitt, T. Marketing Myopia. Harvard Business Review. July-August 1960, pp. 45-56.

39) Dilenschneider, RL. Power and Influence. Mastering the Art of Persuasion. Prentice Hall Press, 1990.

40) As Intuitive Surgical, Inc. President Gary Guthart was buying tires, he saw and recorded businessman Karl Eller's philosophy which was posted on a wall in the store.

41) Kemmons Wilson Founder and Chairman Holiday Inn. Speech presented to Hillsdale College, September 1966.

42) McConnell JM, Director of National Intelligence. Address to George Washington University Columbian College of Arts and Sciences graduation, May 17, 2008.

43) Thurber J. The Scotty Who Knew Too Much, *The New Yorker*, February 18, 1939.

44) Thomke S. Enlightened Experimentation. The New Imperative for Innovation. Harvard Business Review 2001: 79 (2);67-75.

45) Burns LR, Cacciamani J, Clement J and Aquino W. The Fall of the House of AHERF: The Allegheny Bankruptcy. Health Affairs. January/February 2000. Volume 19. Number 1.

46) Surowiecki J. The Wisdom of Crowds. Doubleday, NY, 2004, p. xix.

47) Hammond JS, Kenney RL, Raiffa H. The Hidden Traps in Decision Making. Harvard Business Review. September-October 1998, pp. 47-58.

48) Kanter RM. Power Failure in Management Circuits. Harvard Business Review 1979: 57(4); 65-75).

49) Buffett W. Letter from the Chairman. Berkshire Hathaway Annual Report, 1984.

50) Jim Bennett, retired Director, McKinsey and Co. Personnel Communication.

51) Shapiro M. Personnel Communication.

52) Katzenbach JR, Smith DK. Ibid.

CHAPTER 9: INNOVATION

1) Fagerberg J, Mowery DC, Nelson RR. The Oxford Handbook of Innovation. Oxford University Press 2005.

2) Rogers EM. Diffusion of Innovations. 4th ed. New York: The Free Press, 1995.

3) Kline SJ, Rosenberg N. (1986), An Overview of Innovation, in R. Landau and N. Rosenberg (eds.), The Positive Sum Strategy: Harnessing Technology for Economic Growth, Washington, DC: National Academy Press, 275-305.

4) Adair J. Effective Innovation, Pan Books 1996.

5) Smith K. Measuring Innovation. The Oxford Handbook of Innovation. Oxford University Press, 2005, pp. 148-177.

6) Barsh J, Capozzi MM, Davidson J. Leadership and Innovation. The McKinsey Quarterly 2008: Issue 1; 36-47.

7) Porter M, Stern S. National Innovative Capacity. In The World Economic Forum Global Competitiveness Report, 2002.

8) Kandybin A, Kihn M. Raising Your Return on Innovation Investment. Resilience Report, Strategy + Business e-news, 5/11/04.

9) Foster R, Kaplan S. Creative Destruction. Doubleday Publishing 2003.

10) Christensen CM. The Innovator's Dilemma. Boston: Harvard School Press, 1997.

11) Smith MD. Disruptive Innovation: Can Health Care Learn from Other Industries? A Conversation with Clayton M. Christensen. Health Affairs. November 21, 2006-May 1, 2007. Web Exclusives.

12) Foster R, Kaplan S. Ibid.

13) Hesselbein F. Hesselbein on Leadership, Jossey-Bass California, 2002, p.101.

14) Center for Information Technology Leadership. The Value of Provider-to-Provider Telehealth Technologies. Partners Healthcare System, Inc., 2007.

15) Herzlinger RE. Why Innovation in Health Care is So Hard. Harvard Business Review, May 2006: 84 (5); 58-66.

16) Christensen CM, Overdorf M. Meeting the Challenge of Disruptive Change. Harvard Business Review: 2000: 78 (2); 66-76).

17) Berwick DM, Calkins DR, McCannon CJ, Hackbarth AD. The 100,000 Lives Campaign. Setting a Goal and a Deadline for Improving Healthcare Quality. JAMA 2006: 295; 324-27.

18) Remoussenard C. Innovation, Making Change. It Isn't Easy to Disturb the Status Quo. Wall Street Journal, June 16, 2007, p. R6.

19) Drucker PF. Innovation and Entrepreneurship. Harper Business, 1985.

20) Davidson A, Leavy B. Interview with Innovation Guru Geoffrey Moore: Seeking Solutions to Intractable Problems. Strategy & Leadership. Vol. 35 No. 5, 2007, p.4.

21) Tapscott D, Williams AD. Wikinomics: How Mass Collaboration Changes Everything. Penguin Group USA 2006.

22) Manyika JM, Roberts RP, Sprague KL. Eight Business Technology Trends to Watch. McKinsey Quarterly 2007: December, pp. 1-10.

23) Mitka M. New Innovation Web Site Helps Spread Ideas Through the Health Care Community. JAMA, May 28, 2008-Vol 299, No. 20 p. 2377.

24) Lafley AG, Charan R. The Game Changer: How You Can Drive Revenue and Profit Growth with Innovation. Crown Business, 2008.

25) Berkun S. The Myths of Innovation. O'Reilly Media, Inc. 2007. p. 88.

26) Lessons from Innovation's Frontlines: An Interview with IDEO's CEO, Tim Brown. McKinsey Quarterly, November 2008.

27) Hurson T. Think Better (Your Company's Future Depends on It...and So Does Yours). McGraw Hills, New York, 2007.

28) Foster R, Kaplan S. Ibid.

29) Mourkogiannis N: Purpose and Innovation. How to Optimize Corporate R & D Efforts. Strategy + Business e-news, 10/26/06.

30) Rogers EM. Diffusion of Innovation, 4th ed, The Free Press 1995.

31) Confucius, Analects, 7:1

32) Carr N. How to Be a Smart Innovator. Wall Street Journal, September 11, 2006, p. R7.

33) Jobs S. The Next Insanely Great Thing. Wired, February 1996: Issue 4.02.

34) Carlson CR and Wilmot WW. Innovation: The Five Disciplines For Creating What Customers Want. Crown Publishing, 2006.

35) Friedman TL. The World is Flat. A Brief History of the 21st Century. New York: Farrar, Straus and Giroux, 2005.

36) Arndt M. 3M's Seven Pillars of Innovation. BusinessWeek, May 10, 2006.

37) Nonaka I, Takeuchi H. The Knowledge-Creating Company. How Japanese Companies Create the Dynamic Innovation. Oxford University Press, 1995.

38) Thomas Alva Edison. Cited in McCormick B, At Work with Thomas Edison: 10 Business Lessons from America's Greatest Innovator. Eliot House Productions 2001, p. 15.

39) Eccles T. Succeeding with Change: Implementing Action-Driven Strategies. McGraw-Hill Companies April 1994.

40) Chesbrough H. Open Innovation: The New Imperative for Creating and Profiting from Technology. Boston: Harvard Business School Press, 2003.

41) Walton S. Sam Walton: Made In America. Bantam, New York, 1993.

42) Carlson CR, Wilmot WW. Ibid.

43) Butler NM. "These United States," Looking Forward: What Will the American People Do About It? New York, London: Charles Scribner's Sons, 1932, p. 17.

44) Drucker PF. Ibid.

45) Novak M. The Hemisphere of Liberty: A Philosophy of the Americas. American Enterprise Institute, 1992, p. 104.

46) Morgenthaler DT. A Quiet Crisis. The Plain Dealer, March 23, 2006.

47) Pisano GP. Science Business: The Promise, The Reality, And the Future of Biotech. Harvard Business School Press. 2006.

48) Mullins B, Crow J. Technology Transfer: A Roadmap. College and University Auditor, Feb. 1999.

49) Henry Ford. Ford News. March 15, 1926.

50) Klinger D: Angelou Economics. The Promise of Academic Tech Transfer in Economic Development, November 2006; www.Angelouseconomics.com/ techtransfer.html.

51) Chesbrough H, Vanhaverbeke W, West J. Open Innovation. Researching the New Paradigm. Oxford University Press, 2006.

52) Chesbrough H. Open Business Models: How to Thrive in the New Innovation Landscape. Boston: Harvard Business School Press, 2006.

53) Michael Novak. Cited in Choate P. Hot Property. Alfred A. Knopf, NY, 2005, p. 224.

54) Burns LR. The Business of Health Care Innovation. Cambridge University Press, 2005.

55) Fagerberg J, Mowery DC, Nelson RR. The Oxford Handbook of Innovation. Oxford University Press, 2006. (http://www.iaspworld.org/ information/definitions.php).

56) Pisano GP. Ibid.

57) Azoulay P, Michigan R, Sampat B. The Anatomy of Medical School Patenting. N Engl J Med 2007: 357: 20; 2049-56.

58) Kassirer JP. On the Take: How Medicine's Complicity with Big Business Can Endanger Your Health. Oxford University Press, New York, 2005, p. 50.

59) American Association of Medical Colleges Task Force on Financial Conflicts of Interest in Clinical Research. Protecting Subjects, Preserving Trust, Promoting Progress: Policy And Guidelines For The Oversight Of Individual Financial Interests In Human Subjects Research. 2001 www.aamc.org/coitf.

60) Rothman DJ. Academic Medical Centers and Financial Conflicts of Interest. JAMA 2008: 299; 695-97.

61) Moses III H, Braunwald E, Martin JB,Thier SO. Collaborating with Industry—Choices for the Academic Medical Center, N Engl J Med, 2002: 347:1371-75

62) Kassirer JP. Ibid. pp. 212-13.

63) Devol R, Bedroussian A, et al. Mind to Market: A Global Analysis of University Bio-Technology Transfer and Commercialization; Milken Institute, Sept 2006.

64) Graff G, Heiman A, Zilberman D, et al. Universities Technology Transfer and Industrial R & D in Economic and Social Issues in Agricultural Biotechnology, Evenson RE, ed, Yale Univ, July 2002.

65) Pisano GP. Ibid.

66) Bercovitz J, Feldmann M. Entrepreneurial Universities and Technology Transfer: A Conceptual Framework for Understanding Knowledge-Based Economic Development, Journal of Technology Transfer, 31:175-188, 2006.

67) Hamel G. Leading the Revolution. Harvard Business Press, 2002.

68) Kanter RM. Innovation: The Classic Traps. Harvard Business Review, Vol. 84 (11) November 2006, p. 72-83.

69) Teisberg EO, Porter ME, Brown GB. Making Competition in Health Care Work. Harvard Business Review 1994: July-August; 131-41.

CHAPTER 10: HEALTHCARE DELIVERY

1) Coble YD. AMA Presidential Installation Speech. Passion, Perseverance and Professionalism: A Prescription for Renewing Medicine for the 21st Century. 2002 AMA Annual Meeting. June 19, 2002.

2) Morita A. (Sony co-founder) Quoted in International Management, April 1988.

3) Reingold E. Interview with Peter Drucker. Facing the "Totally New and Dynamic." Time, January 22, 1990.

4) Sirower ML. Chapter 1: Introduction the Acquisition Game. The Synergy Trap. How Companies Lose the Acquisition Game. The Free Press, New York, 1997, p. 6.

5) Ellwood PM. Shattuck Lecture. Outcome Management. N Engl J Med 1988: 318; 1549-56.

6) Chatterjee S, Corts KS, Ghemawat P, Pisano G, Porter ME, Rivkin JW. Business Fundamentals: Competitive Strategy. Harvard Business School Publishing, HBS #1520, 2002, p. 104.

7) Starfield B, Shi L, Macinko J. Contribution of Primary Care to Health Systems and Health. Milbank Quarterly 2005: 83(3); 457-502.

8) Baicker K, Chandra A. Medicare Spending, the Physician Workforce, and Beneficiaries' Quality of Care. Health Affairs 23 (2004): w184-w197 (published online 7 April 2004; 10.1377/hlthaff.w4184).

9) Sepulveda MJ, Bodenheimer T, Grundy P. Primary Care: Can It Solve Employers' Health Care Dilemma? Health Affairs 2008: 27 (1); 151-158.

10) Langley M. Tearing Down the Walls, The Free Press, 2004, p. 114.

11) Herzlinger R. Who Killed Healthcare? McGraw Hill 2007, p. 137.

12) Attributed to Tony Blair. Cited in Micklethwait J, Wooldridge A. The Right Nation. Conservative Power in America. The Penguin Press, New York, 2004, p. 389.

13) Berenson RA, Ginsburg PB, May JH: Hospital-Physician Relations: Cooperation, Competition, or Separation? Health Affairs 2007: 26(1);w31-w43.

14) Chiefs Head Coach Herm Edwards Press Conference. January 9, 2006. . http://www.kcchiefs.com/news/2006/01/09/chiefs_head_coach_herm_edwards_press_conference/

15) Berenson RA, Ginsburg PB, May JH. Ibid.

16) Baker B. The Hospitalists. Washington Post, September 11, 2007.

17) Goodman DC, Grumbach K. Does Having More Physicians Lead to Better Health System Performance? JAMA 2008: 299 (3); 335-337.

18) Goodman DC, Grumbach K. Ibid.

19) Cooper RA, Getzen TE, Laud P. Economic Expansion is a Major Determinant of Physician Supply and Utilization. Health Serv Res 2003: 38(2); 675-696.

20) Shaw SR. Network Advantage: Scale Economies and Cost Savings. Health Care Advisory Board, Washington, D.C., 1994.

21) First Consulting Group, Healthcare Industry News Summary, February 2007, Research.

22) Center for Studying Health System Change. Research Brief. Development of State Level Health Information Exchange Initiatives, Final Report. September 1, 2006. www.ahima.org/fore.

23) Cited in Robeznieks A. P4P Programs Quadruple; Physicians, Regulators Still Question Use of Plan. Modern Healthcare, 9/3/07; 37(35); 10.

24) FYA – For Your Advantage, Volume 6, Issue 9, May 7, 2007, Patients Give Hospitals Higher Score, p.4.

25) Reichheld F. The Loyalty Affect. The Hidden Force Behind Growth Profits and Lasting Value. Harvard Business School Press, 1996.

26) Grote KD, Newman JRS, Sutaria SS. A Better Hospital Experience. The McKinsey Quarterly, November 30, 2007.

27) Francis T. How to Size Up Your Hospital. Wall Street Journal, July 10, 2007.

28) The Advisory Board Marketing and Planning Leadership Council 2007 Drivers of Consumer Choice.

29) Russell TR. I Need an Operation...Now What? The Patients Guide to a Safe and Successful Outcome. American College of Surgeons. Thompson Healthcare, 2008.

30) Dans PE. Passengers and Patients: Some Ruminations About Quality of Care. Pharos, Summer 1988; 2-7.

31) Studer Q. Hardwiring Excellence: Purpose, Worthwhile Work, Making a Difference, Fire Starting Publishing, Gulf Breeze, FL, 2003 by The Studer Group, LLC.

32) Studer Q. Ibid.

33) Waterman RH. Frontiers of Excellence. Nicholas Brealey Publishing Ltd., London, 1994.

34) Kenagy JW. How Your Hospital Can Deliver an Exceptional Patient Experience. FYA, Vol. 7 (4): 1, February 19, 2008; Lee F. If Disney Ran Your Hospital. Second River Healthcare, 2004.

35) LaPorte TR. High Reliability Organizations: Unlikely, Demanding and at Risk. Journal of Contingencies and Crisis Management 1996: 4 (2); 60-71.

36) To Err is Human: Building a Safer Health System. Institute of Medicine, November 1999.

37) Reason J. Managing the Risks of Organizational Accidents. Ashgate Publishing Co., 1997

38) Keckley P. Roundtable, Healthcare Quality: The Dynamic System. HealthLeaders, October 2006. Daily Healthcare News at www.healthleadersmedia.com.

39) CMS, "HCAHPS: Patient Perspectives on Care," http://www.cms.hhs.gov/HospitalQualityInits /30_HospitalHCAHPS.asp and http://www.cms.hhs.gov/HospitalQualityInits/downloads/ HospitalSurvey2.pdf, accessed August 21, 2007; Marketing and Planning Leadership Council interviews.

40) Donabedian A. Quality Assessment and Assurance: Unity of Purpose, Diversity of Means. Inquiry 1988: 25(1); 173-192.

41) Kahn MW. Etiquette-Based Medicine. N Engl J Med 2008: 358 (19); 1988-89.

42) Reichheld FF. Learning from Customer Defections. Harvard Business Review. March-April 1996.

43) Groopman J. How Doctors Think. Houghton Mifflin Company, 2007.

44) Reichheld FF. The Loyalty Effect, Ibid.

45) United States Office of Consumer Affairs. Consumer Complaint Handling In America: An Update Study. Completed in 1986 and released during National Consumers Week, 1986, Washington, Technical Assistance Research Programs Institute (TARP), for the United States of Consumer Affairs, 1986.

46) Hertzer NR. Presidential Address. Carotid Endarterectomy – A Crisis in Confidence. J Vasc Surg 1988; 7(5): 611-19.

47) Ingelfinger F. Arrogance. N Engl J Med 1980; 303: 1507-1511.

48) Feinstein A. Clinical Judgment. Williams and Wilkins, Baltimore, 1967

49) Landro L. The Informed Patient: Teaching Doctors How to Interview. The Wall Street Journal, September 21, 2005.

50) Lord Beaverbrook. Quoted in Johnson P. A Rich Man's Best Friend is Health. Forbes 2005: 176 (7); 39.

51) Jamieson KH. Eloquence in an Electronic Age. The Transformation of Political Speechmaking. Oxford University Press, New York, 1988.

52) Horowitz CR, Suchman AL, Branch, Jr. WT, Frankel RM. What Do Doctors Find Meaningful About Their Work? Ann Intern Med 2003: 138 (9); 772-775.

53) Groopman J. Ibid.

54) Steinbeck J. East of Eden. Penguin Press, 2002, Chapter 34, p. 411, 1952.

55) Crile Jr. G. Cancer in Common Sense. Viking Press 1955. p. 104.

I N D E X

FLOYD D. LOOP, M.D.

Floyd D. Loop grew up in Indiana, was educated at Purdue University and received his M.D. from The George Washington University. He began surgical residency there, served in the Air Force as a surgeon and returned to The George Washington University to complete general surgery training. After a further postgraduate fellowship in cardiothoracic surgery at the Cleveland Clinic, he joined the Department of Thoracic and Cardiovascular Surgery and became chairman of the department in 1975, a post he held until 1989 when he was appointed chief executive of the Cleveland Clinic Foundation. He served as CEO and chairman of the Board of Governors for 15 years, until October 2004.

He and his colleagues gained an international reputation in cardiac surgery. Dr. Loop's surgical team was responsible for today's widespread use of arterial conduits in coronary artery surgery, innovations in valve repair and many technical improvements for reoperations.

At the Clinic, cardiologists and surgeons together developed one of the first patient registries, which was the source for advancing clinical research in coronary atherosclerosis. Despite long days in surgery, Dr. Loop has been a prolific author and deeply respected leader whose style has inspired great loyalty to theCleveland Clinic.

During his 15-year tenure as chief executive, Dr. Loop selected a new administrative team, which reorganized the Clinic and added greatly to the academic enterprise. A new health delivery system was created by acquiring eight hospitals, building 14 outpatient clinics and starting a medical school for physician-investigators. In Florida, new clinics and hospitals were built in Ft. Lauderdale and Naples. The revenues grew from $645 million in 1989 to $3.6 billion in 2004. The Cleveland Clinic is consistently recognized as one of the top 10 hospitals in the United States and honored as one of the best managed medical centers. Beginning in 1990, each year has brought about a new record for patient activity and overall academic performance.

Dr. Loop has served on editorial boards of numerous periodicals and was editor of *Seminars in Thoracic and Cardiovascular Surgery*. He has been a guest lecturer at many cardiology and surgical meetings internationally, and has demonstrated surgical techniques in many countries. Among the awards and honors accorded him, Dr. Loop received the American College of Cardiology Cummings Humanitarian Award in 1975, the American Heart Association Citation for International Service in 1980, and the Order of Merit, the highest civilian award given in Brazil, in 1982. He chaired the Residency Review Committee for Thoracic and Cardiovascular Surgery in 1993, was president of the American Association for Thoracic Surgery in 1997, and was a director of the American Board of Thoracic Surgery, 1993-1999. From 1999-2002, Dr. Loop served on the Medicare Payment Advisory Commission (MedPAC). He has received Honorary Doctor of Science degrees from Cleveland State University, St. Louis University and Purdue University.

Currently Dr. Loop serves on public and private corporate boards and has interests in medical product development.

He and his wife, Dr. Bernadine Healy, a renowned physician, former director of the National Institutes of Health and now health editor and columnist at *U.S. News and World Report*, live outside Cleveland, Ohio. Always more comfortable in the greenhouse than in social settings, Dr. Loop spends hours growing beautiful orchids, gardening, working in his apple orchard and playing with their dogs, Lewis and Clark.

My friend has written a great book on leadership and you will better understand the complicated field of medicine. This book perfectly unites two of Dr. Loop's greatest areas of expertise.

— Bill Belichick, Head Coach, New England Patriots

Dr. Loop has written a great leadership book that will also teach you a little about healthcare. Brimming with complex ideas conveyed in a plain-spoken style, *Leadership and Medicine* blends lessons from the author's distinguished career with insights on the future of healthcare in America. The leaders who will reshape this most vital industry would be well advised to heed his words.

— Jeb Bush, Former Governor of Florida (1998-2007)

Dr. Loop demonstrates an unparalleled understanding of leadership, the hospital industry and the broader healthcare challenges that we face. A wide and deep perspective that explains his success in running one of America's preeminent health institutions.

— Regina Herzlinger, Nancy R. McPherson Professor of Business
Administration Chair, Harvard Business School

This wonderful book has captured the critical elements of leadership in a professional enterprise. He distinguishes the differences between leadership, management and professional activity in a way that is useful for all of us who lead. It is a great read for all who lead professionals, especially those in medicine.

— Edward A. Kangas, Former Global Chairman and CEO of Deloitte

Wise, learned and perceptive, Dr. Loop has created a field manual for those men and women who have chosen leadership positions, especially those on the front lines of the heroic and imperfect effort to give care to the sick and injured. *Leadership and Medicine* is a source of inspiration, particularly useful in the midst of those moments when the burdens and loneliness of being in charge threaten to defeat the will of those who have made this choice.

— J. Robert Kerrey, President, The New School
Former U.S. Senator (Nebraska) (1989-2001)

Leadership and Medicine is a great collection of lessons originated by Dr. Loop and filled with many philosophical thoughts by thought-leaders throughout history. Although targeted toward leadership in medicine, the many lessons in this book apply to all walks of life and institutions. This is a "must-read" for anyone in a leadership role in today's society, anyone aspiring to a leadership role or anyone simply interested in understanding the tenets of good leadership. This book could easily become the foundation for a graduate-level MBA course in leadership.

— Dane Miller, Ph.D.
Founder and Board Member of Biomet, Inc.

This book provides invaluable insight regarding how one of the world's preeminent heart surgeons translated his passion for medicine into a transformational approach to leadership. Over 15 years, Dr. Loop's keen intellect and commitment to excellence lifted the Cleveland Clinic to unprecedented progress in innovative treatments, economic stability and system expansion. His account of this time is as fascinating as it is instructive, and should be read by anyone interested in healthcare or management.

— Barbara R. Snyder, President, Case Western Reserve University

Dr. Loop has provided a comprehensive view of what it takes to effectively lead in today's dynamic healthcare environment. Certainly, the Cleveland Clinic stands as a shining testament to what can be achieved. This book provides an inside look as to how to make this happen and serves as a wonderful guide for emerging healthcare leaders.

— Frank Williams
Chairman, The Advisory Board Company

HOW TO ORDER ADDITIONAL COPIES OF

Leadership and Medicine

Orders may be placed:

Online at:

www.firestarterpublishing.com

www.studergroup.com

By phone at: 866-354-3473

By mail at: Fire Starter Publishing

913 Gulf Breeze Parkway, Suite 6

Gulf Breeze, FL 32561

(Bulk discounts are available.)

Leadership and Medicine
is also available online at www.amazon.com.